Materials for Total Joint Arthroplasty

Biotribology of Potential Bearings

Materials for Total Joint Arthroplasty

Biotribology of Potential Bearings

Robert Sonntag
Jan Philippe Kretzer
Heidelberg University Hospital, Germany

ICP
Imperial College Press

Published by

Imperial College Press
57 Shelton Street
Covent Garden
London WC2H 9HE

Distributed by

World Scientific Publishing Co. Pte. Ltd.
5 Toh Tuck Link, Singapore 596224
USA office: 27 Warren Street, Suite 401-402, Hackensack, NJ 07601
UK office: 57 Shelton Street, Covent Garden, London WC2H 9HE

Library of Congress Cataloging-in-Publication Data
Materials for total joint arthroplasty : biotribology of potential bearings / [edited] by
Robert Sonntag & Jan Philippe Kretzer.
p. ; cm.
Includes bibliographical references.
ISBN 978-1-78326-716-3 (alk. paper)
I. Sonntag, Robert, editor. II. Kretzer, Jan Philippe, editor.
[DNLM: 1. Joint Prosthesis. 2. Arthroplasty, Replacement--instrumentation.
3. Biocompatible Materials. WE 312]
RD686
617.5'810592--dc23
2015021098

British Library Cataloguing-in-Publication Data
A catalogue record for this book is available from the British Library.

In-house Editors: Mary Simpson/Dipasri Sardar

Typeset by Stallion Press
Email: enquiries@stallionpress.com

Printed in Singapore by Mainland Press Pte Ltd.

Preface

Total joint replacement has a 125-year history, beginning when Themistocles Gluck replaced a degenerated joint with an ivory prosthesis in 1890. At that time, biotribological issues had not been of particular interest, since the implant stability limited clinical use for a long period. Once the issue of stable prosthesis fixation was solved with the introduction of PMMA for cemented fixation and titanium surface treatments for cementless fixation, the focus has returned to the most central aspect of joint function: The articulation. In addition to being confronted with increasingly demanding patients, who tend to be younger and more active, surgeons now are confronted with more choices for bearing materials than ever before. Furthermore, the continuous advances in science and clinical study design allow us to better evaluate clinical outcomes and consequently set new standards in quality assurance. However, the available literature on both experimental and clinical studies is not uniformly distributed for all bearing materials under consideration. Due to the discrepancies in the amount of research on the various materials, in addition to the dates they were introduced to the market, some newer approaches and implant materials may only have been evaluated in an *in vitro* as opposed to clinical setting, while others may still lack mid- or long-term clinical results. Hence, the surgeon is confronted with making a choice on which bearing material to use based upon available clinical studies while weighing future perspectives based upon experimental data.

This comprehensive book aims to investigate the different materials and implants to allow for a better understanding of which material to choose in a particular clinical setting. The various material characteristics, current laboratory and clinical studies, and the future implant potential are discussed in order to inform and to enable an orthopaedic surgeon, bioengineer or the interested reader to evaluate the available treatment options. We hope you enjoy it!

Heidelberg, Germany Robert Sonntag and J. Philippe Kretzer

Contents

Chapter 1

Bio-Tribological Demands

Robert Sonntag, Joern Reinders and J. Philippe Kretzer

Laboratory of Biomechanics and Implant Research, Clinic for Orthopedics and Trauma Surgery, Center for Orthopedics, Trauma Surgery and Spinal Cord Injury, Heidelberg University Hospital, Heidelberg, Germany

1. Description of the Bio-Technical System

From an engineer's point of view, an artificial joint represents a technical system with well-defined components under individual boundary conditions that are difficult to predict. History has shown that materials which were demonstrated to have considerable potential as biomaterials for joint reconstruction under *in vitro* conditions, failed *in vivo* after a short period due to a bad mechanical or biological outcome. Examples of this are polytetrafluoroethylene (PTFE, or 'teflon') and zirconia ceramics (Charnley, 1961, 1963; Derbyshire *et al.*, 1994; Dowson, 2001; Haraguchi *et al.*, 2001; Hernigou and Bahrami, 2003). Bio-engineers and surgeons often must wait for years to discover if a new material or implant design will have a proven clinical outcome.

Materials are used for joint prostheses according to their function. For example, a distinction can be drawn between materials made for components used to achieve the best possible long-term fixation within the bone stock and those that are made for reconstruction of the deceased joint articulation function. The latter are included in the present book. This chapter explains the choice of materials used today and what the bio-tribological demands for a new bearing material are.

2. Factors Influencing Longevity of Joint Replacements

Surgical intervention to replace a deceased natural joint with an artificial one has proven to be very successful (Learmonth *et al.*, 2007), even though early as well as long-term failures are reported by national joint registries and numerous clinical studies (Park *et al.*, 2005; Swedish Hip Arthroplasty Register, 2010; Willert *et al.*, 1990) (Figure 1-1). The main reason for long-term failure is aseptic loosening of the fixating components, which is associated with a biological reaction that wears debris, resulting in osteolysis. Special attention is therefore paid to the tribological performance of articulating components so as to minimise the biological potential of the bulk materials and wear products. Registry data from Sweden (Figure 1-1) reveals

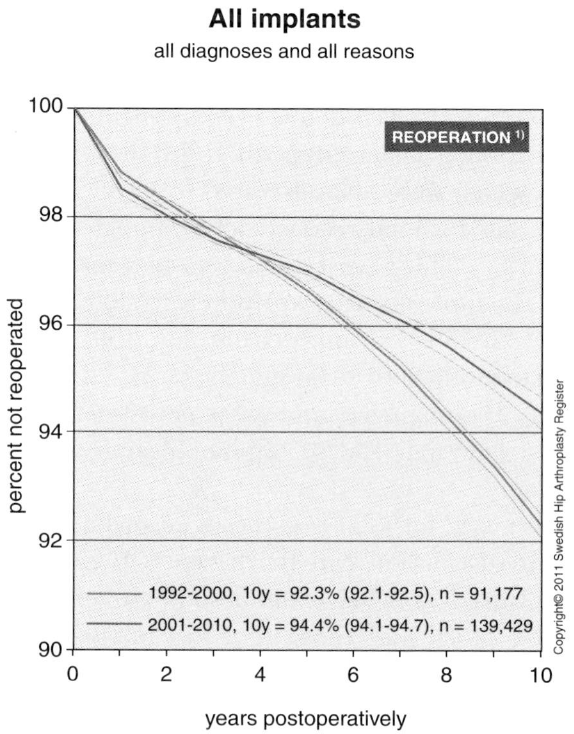

Figure 1-1. Hip implant survival rates from Swedish registry data (Swedish Hip Arthroplasty Register, 2010).

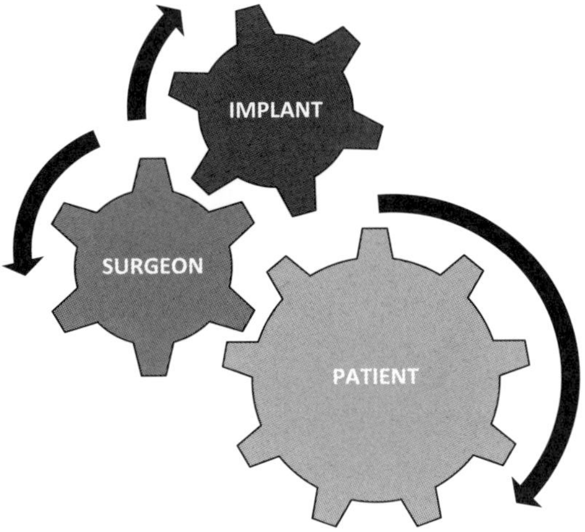

Figure 1-2. Factors influencing the long-term outcome of an implant system.

a clearly increased survival rate for modern implant systems compared to total hip replacements that were implanted more than 20 years ago.

The main factors that influence a joint's short- and long-term performance are the actual implant, which is the product of investigation at the manufacturer, the orthopaedic surgeon, who significantly influences the boundary conditions under which the implant is working and, often underestimated, the patient who receives the artificial joint and defines the loading conditions and kinematics by his/her individual lifestyle (Figure 1-2).

2.1. *Implant*

The tribological components of an implant for joint reconstruction (e.g. head and insert of a THA) are defined by their material and technical design. Nowadays, the components are generally made of metals, ceramics and polymers and are advanced products designed by highly experienced engineers. They are developed under boundary conditions that are provided by standardisation organisations such as the International Organization for Standardization (ISO) or ASTM International, for example, surface specifications (Table 1-1)

Table 1-1. Topological specifications for articulating surfaces given by the ISO 7206-2 and ISO 7207-2.

	ISO 7206-2: Hip	ISO 7207-2: Knee
	Implants for surgery — partial and total hip joint prostheses — Part 2: Articulating surfaces made of metallic, ceramic and plastic materials	Implants for surgery — components for a partial and total knee joint prostheses — Part 2: Articulating surfaces made of metal, ceramic and plastic materials
Surface finish (total joint replacement)	Metal: $R_{a,max} = 0.05\,\mu m$ Ceramics: $R_{a,max} = 0.02\,\mu m$ Plastics: $R_{a,max} = 2\,\mu m$	Metal: $R_{a,max} = 0.1\,\mu m$ Ceramics: $R_{a,max} = 0.1\,\mu m$ Plastics: $R_{a,max} = 2\,\mu m$
Radial sphericity (total joint replacement)	Femoral component: Max. $10\,\mu m$ Acetabular component: Max. $100\,\mu m$	— —

or pre-clinical tribological testing (Chapter 3). The general aim of these standards is to guarantee a high and comparable product quality under the control of independent testing laboratories and Notified Bodies.

Regarding their function during articulation, today's materials are evaluated according to their wear resistance, mechanical strength and biocompatibility of the bulk material and wear products, but also economic factors. Most of today's articulation materials follow the principle of hard and smooth surfaces that wear off at a very low rate (Figure 1-3). However, besides low wearing properties, implant materials are also evaluated according to their aging resistance in an oxidative environment *in vivo* and during sterilisation processes (Kurtz *et al.*, 2003; Muratoglu *et al.*, 2003).

The contact conditions within the bearing are determined by the contact area and pressure that are a function of the material, the design and the loading conditions. The synovial fluid plays a major role in the lubrication of the bio-tribological system. This is,

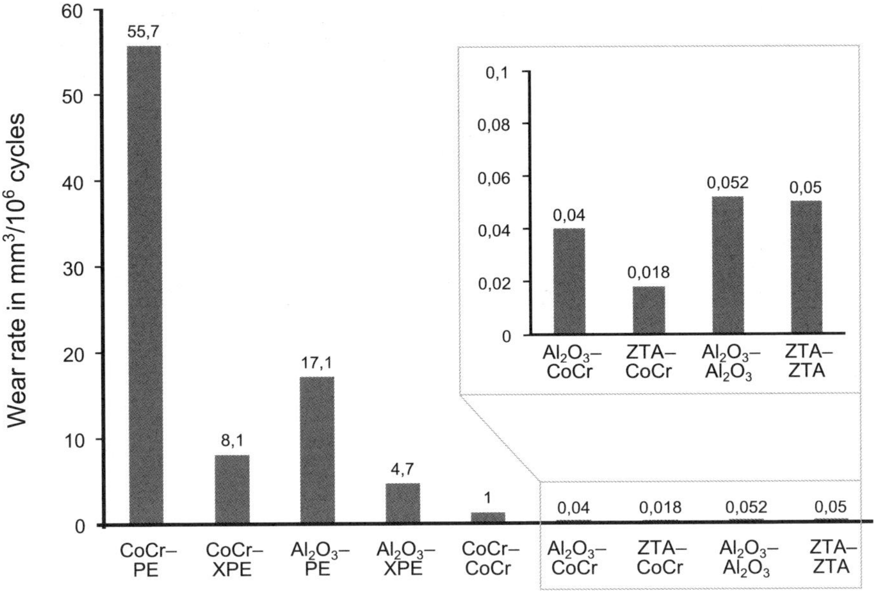

Figure 1-3. Volumetric wear rates after *in vitro* testing of conventional hip bearings (Sonntag *et al.*, 2012).

however, dependent on the material combinations: While hard-on-hard bearings ideally build up a separating fluid film between the articulating surfaces by (elasto-)hydrodynamic effects, bearings using polyethylene as an articulating partner are meant to be completely or partly in physical contact during articulation (boundary or mixed lubrication conditions) (Jin *et al.*, 2006; Sonntag *et al.*, 2013). Based on the height of these fluid films, frictional forces and moments are generated. From a technical point of view, the physiological periprosthetic environment presents a challenging condition for bio-medical engineers, as the implant is working under a corrosive environment and dynamic loading conditions. High punctual stresses may act on the surface of a bearing, for instance under adverse alignment of the articulating components, such as edge loading or impingement of the femoral neck to the cup rim in total hip arthroplasty (Habermann *et al.*, 2006; Park *et al.*, 2006) (Figure 1-4). Under these conditions, lubrication of the joint may be limited.

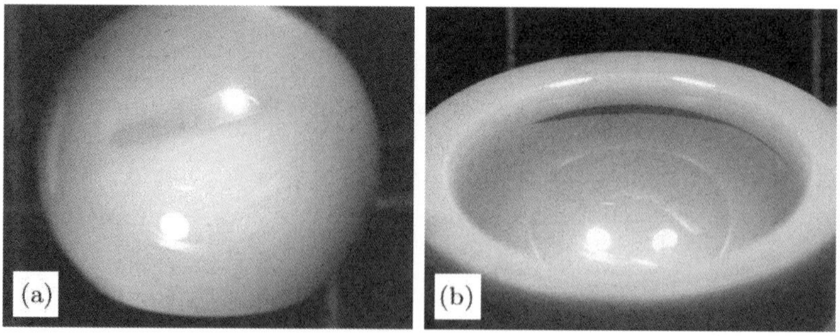

Figure 1-4. Typical stripe wear after edge-loading of an alumina–alumina bearing after eight months *in vivo* (Walter *et al.*, 2004).

2.2. *Surgeon*

The surgeon plays a significant role in the clinical outcome as malalignment, for example, may lead to an early implant failure. It is the surgeon's expert opinion in the first instance that determines whether the patient should receive an artificial joint or not and, if an artificial joint is given, the choice of the appropriate implant system. These decisions, together with the operating theatre team's experience and skills, define the clinical starting conditions that are crucial for the quality of implantation and create the framework for the longevity of the implant.

In several studies, it has been shown that a malalignment, for example of the acetabular cup/insert in total hip arthroplasty, can result in catastrophic wear or mechanical failure that may subsequently lead to early revision (Fisher, 2011; Waewsawangwong and Goodman, 2012). In 1978, Lewinnek *et al.* defined a so-called 'safe zone' based on clinical observations. Within an acetabular cup inclination between 30° and 50° of abduction and 5–25° in anteversion, the implant showed less risk of dislocation due to impingement between stem and cup (Lewinnek *et al.*, 1978). In that context, recent clinical data give a more distinct correlation between cup inclination, metal ion level and the formation of pseudotumours after metal-on-metal hip resurfacing with a recommended maximum inclination angle of 55° (De Haan *et al.*, 2008; Grammatopoulos *et al.*, 2010). These findings have further promoted pre-clinical adverse testing protocols to mimic critical situations that may occur in the patient's daily use and are particularly crucial for these hard-on-hard bearings (Fabry *et al.*, 2013).

In addition, the volume of implantations per surgeon is a critical factor that is purported to influence the outcome of the artificial joint, as low-volume surgeons are associated with an increased risk of early revision (Losina *et al.*, 2004; Manley *et al.*, 2008). These facts have opened up the discussion in the orthopaedic community about a minimum number of implantations per year for a surgeon.

2.3. *Patient*

The endoprosthetic patient addresses the orthopaedic specialist because of pain, decreased function and quality of life. In general, the surgical intervention using a joint replacement enables the patient to recover and resume a quality of life regarded as 'normal'. From this point on, it is the patient's responsibility to take care of the new joint. Gait analysis and studies on instrumented artificial joint components have shed some light on the bio-mechanics of artificial joints during daily activities (Bergmann *et al.*, 2001; Damm *et al.*, 2010; D'Lima *et al.*, 2006; Kutzner *et al.*, 2010). The most important aspects are:

- Relevant loading conditions act during most daily activities such as normal walking (approximately 300% of the body weight) and vary between other activities (Bergmann *et al.*, 2001; Kutzner *et al.*, 2010) (Figure 1-5).
- The highest loads have been measured under conditions that have not been previewed before (spontaneous stumbling with up to 900% of the body weight) and, more importantly, that were not possible to reproduce under controlled conditions (Bergmann *et al.*, 2004).

These findings need to be addressed to verify the implant's performance in pre-clinical testing (Fabry *et al.*, 2013) and will be part of future adaptations of the testing standards developed by the ISO and ASTM International organisations.

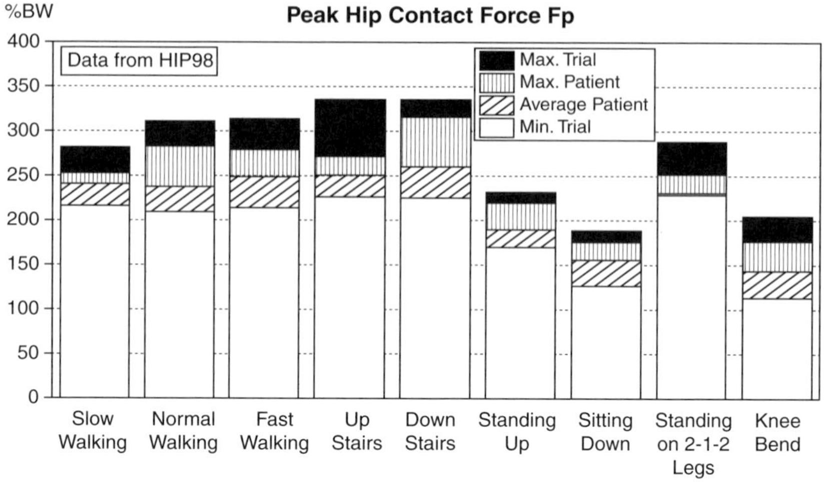

Figure 1-5. Contact forces during daily activities measured *in vivo* using instrumented total hip replacements (Bergmann *et al.*, 2001).

A meta-analysis by Prokopetz *et al.* (2012) revealed some factors that affect patient outcome by increasing the risk of a revision surgery after total hip replacement. These include male and younger patients. The register data confirm this as well (Australian National Joint Replacement Registry, 2013) (Figure 1-6). Furthermore, greater comorbidity and a diagnosis for avascular necrosis as compared to osteoarthritis have been shown to be risk factors for an early revision.

3. Approaches for New Bearings

New approaches for bearing materials may be classified according to the scheme of Sonntag *et al.* (2012) (Figure 1-7).

The approaches can be summarised as follows:

- New bulk material, for example ceramics:
  One or both articulation components are made of a new material that wears off at a very low rate and presents a minimal risk of a biological reaction on the bulk material as well as the wear products.

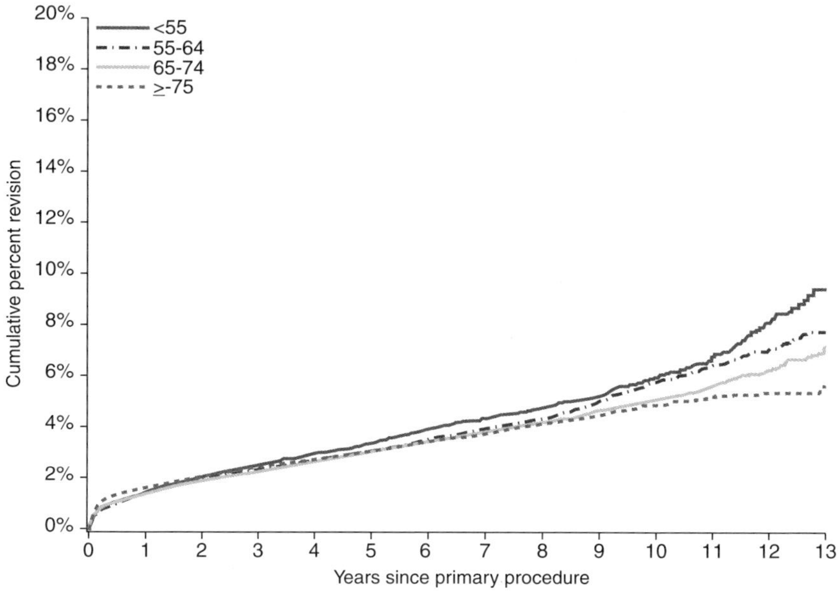

Figure 1-6. Cumulative percent revision of primary total hip replacement by patient age (Australian National Joint Replacement Registry, 2014).

- Cushion bearings, in order to replicate the physiological situation: Soft bearing materials that attempt to mimic the natural joint, which is covered by a smooth cartilage. They are intended to work under better lubrication conditions than the established hard materials used for artificial articulation.
- Surface coatings, for example implants for patients suffering allergies: Surface properties are adapted (e.g. metal ion release) without changing the properties of the underlying substrate material. Adhesion of the coating on the substrate under high punctual loads is a limiting factor and needs to be addressed during development by the manufacturer.
- Surface modification, such as controlled oxidisation processes: Compared to coatings, no material is added to the substrate but the bulk material is chemically modified by diffusion into the outer layers of the substrate.

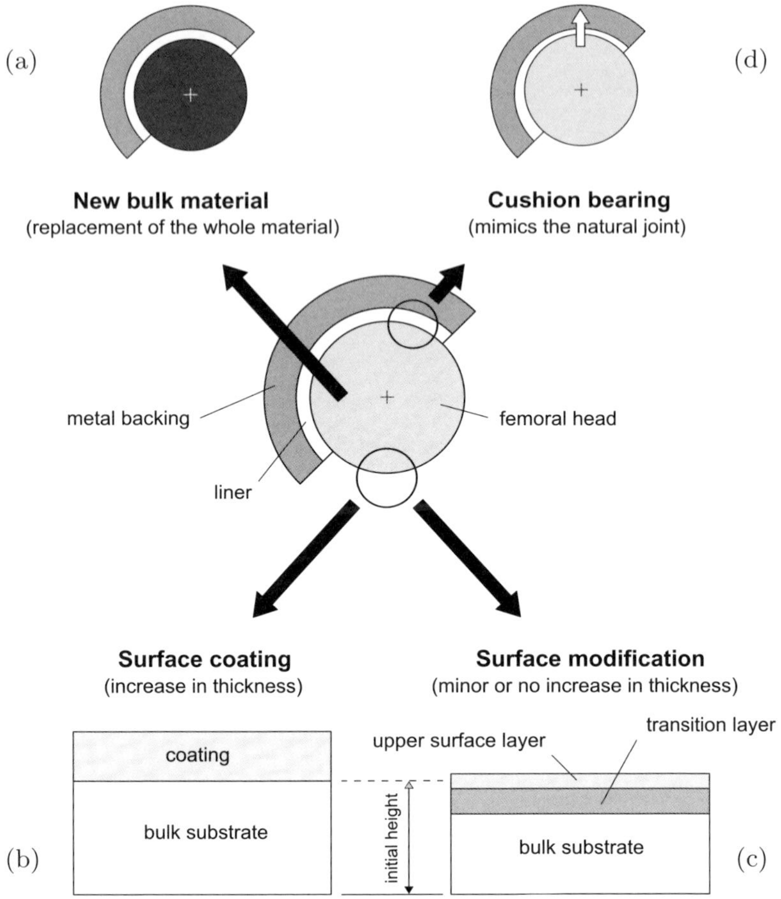

Figure 1-7. Classification of new bearing materials: (a) — new bulk material; (b) — surface coatings; (c) — surface modification; (d) — soft cushion bearings (Sonntag *et al.*, 2012).

Based on these theoretical approaches, new bearing materials have been developed. Some are still under consideration in the laboratory, while others have already been introduced in the clinic. The aim of this book is to give a detailed overview on the material science aspects as well as the *in vitro* and *in vivo* performances of these new bearings so that a more rigorous evaluation of them can take place.

References

Australian National Joint Replacement Registry (2014). *Annual Report*, AOA, Adelaide.

Bergmann, G., Deuretzbacher, G., Heller, M., Graichen, F., Rohlmann, A., Strauss, J. *et al.* (2001). Hip contact forces and gait patterns from routine activities, *J Biomech*, **34**(7), 859–871.

Bergmann, G., Graichen, F. and Rohlmann, A. (2004). Hip joint contact forces during stumbling, *Langenbecks Arch Surg*, **389**(1), 53–59.

Charnley, J. (1961). Arthroplasty of the hip: A new operation, *Lancet*, **277**(7187), 1129–1132.

Charnley, J. (1963). Tissue reactions to polytetrafluororethylene, *Lancet*, **282**(7322), 1379.

D'Lima, D.D., Patil, S., Steklov, N., Slamin, J.E. and Colwell Jr., C.W. (2006). Tibial forces measured *in vivo* after total knee arthroplasty, *J Arthroplasty*, **21**(2), 255–262.

Damm, P., Graichen, F., Rohlmann, A., Bender, A. and Bergmann, G. (2010). Total hip joint prosthesis for *in vivo* measurement of forces and moments, *Med Eng Phys*, **32**(1), 95–100.

De Haan, R., Pattyn, C., Gill, H.S., Murray, D.W., Campbell, P.A. and De Smet, K. (2008). Correlation between inclination of the acetabular component and metal ion levels in metal-on-metal hip resurfacing replacement, *J Bone Joint Surg Br*, **90-B**(10), 1291–1297.

Derbyshire, B., Fisher, J., Dowson, D., Hardaker, C. and Brummitt, K. (1994). Comparative study of the wear of UHMWPE with zirconia ceramic and stainless steel femoral heads in artificial hip joints, *Med Eng Phys*, **16**(3), 229–236.

Dowson, D. (2001). New joints for the millennium: Wear control in total replacement hip joints, *Proc Inst Mech Eng H*, **215**(4), 335–358.

Fabry, C., Herrmann, S., Kaehler, M., Klinkenberg, E.D., Woernle, C. and Bader, R. (2013). Generation of physiological parameter sets for hip joint motions and loads during daily life activities for application in wear simulators of the artificial hip joint, *Med Eng Phys*, **35**(1), 131–139.

Fisher, J. (2011). Bioengineering reasons for the failure of metal-on-metal hip prostheses: An engineer's perspective, *J Bone Joint Surg Br*, **93-B**(8), 1001–1004.

Grammatopoulos, G., Pandit, H., Glyn-Jones, S., McLardy-Smith, P., Gundle, R., Whitwell, D. *et al.* (2010). Optimal acetabular orientation for hip resurfacing, *J Bone Joint Surg Br*, **92**(8), 1072–1078.

Habermann, B., Ewald, W., Rauschmann, M., Zichner, L. and Kurth, A.A. (2006). Fracture of ceramic heads in total hip replacement, *Arch Orthop Trauma Surg*, **126**(7), 464–470.

Haraguchi, K., Sugano, N., Nishii, T., Miki, H., Oka, K. and Yoshikawa, H. (2001). Phase transformation of a zirconia ceramic head after total hip arthroplasty, *J Bone Joint Surg Br*, **83**(7), 996–1000.

Hernigou, P. and Bahrami, T. (2003). Zirconia and alumina ceramics in comparison with stainless-steel heads. Polyethylene wear after a minimum ten-year follow-up, *J Bone Joint Surg Br*, **85**(4), 504–509.

Jin, Z.M., Stone, M., Ingham, E. and Fisher, J. (2006). Biotribology, *Curr Orthopaed*, **20**(1), 32–40.

Kurtz, S.M., Hozack, W., Marcolongo, M., Turner, J., Rimnac, C. and Edidin, A. (2003). Degradation of mechanical properties of UHMWPE acetabular liners following long-term implantation, *J Arthroplasty*, **18**(7 Suppl 1), 68–78.

Kutzner, I., Heinlein, B., Graichen, F., Bender, A., Rohlmann, A., Halder, A. *et al.* (2010). Loading of the knee joint during activities of daily living measured *in vivo* in five subjects, *J Biomech*, **43**(11), 2164–2173.

Learmonth, I.D., Young, C. and Rorabeck, C. (2007). The operation of the century: Total hip replacement, *Lancet*, **370**(9597), 1508–1519.

Lewinnek, G.E., Lewis, J.L., Tarr, R., Compere, C.L. and Zimmerman, J.R. (1978). Dislocations after total hip-replacement arthroplasties, *J Bone Joint Surg Am*, **60**(2), 217–220.

Losina, E., Barrett, J., Mahomed, N.N., Baron, J.A. and Katz, J.N. (2004). Early failures of total hip replacement: Effect of surgeon volume, *Arthritis Rheum*, **50**(4), 1338–1343.

Manley, M., Ong, K., Lau, E. and Kurtz, S.M. (2008). Effect of volume on total hip arthroplasty revision rates in the United States Medicare population, *J Bone Joint Surg Am*, **90**(11), 2446–2451.

Muratoglu, O.K., Merrill, E.W., Bragdon, C.R., O'Connor, D., Hoeffel, D., Burroughs, B. *et al.* (2003). Effect of radiation, heat, and aging on *in vitro* wear resistance of polyethylene, *Clin Orthop Relat R*, (417), 253–262.

Park, Y.S., Hwang, S.K., Choy, W.S., Kim, Y.S. and Moon, Y.W. (2006). Ceramic failure after total hip arthroplasty with an alumina-on-alumina bearing, *J Bone Joint Surg Am*, **88**(4), 780–787.

Park, Y.S., Moon, Y.W., Lim, S.J., Yang, J.M., Ahn, G. and Choi, Y.L. (2005). Early osteolysis following second-generation metal-on-metal hip replacement, *J Bone Joint Surg Am*, **87**(7), 1515–1521.

Prokopetz, J.J., Losina, E., Bliss, R.L., Wright, J., Baron, J.A. and Katz, J.N. (2012). Risk factors for revision of primary total hip arthroplasty: A systematic review, *BMC Musculoskelet Disord*, **13**, 251.

Sonntag, R., Reinders, J. and Kretzer, J.P. (2012). What's next? Alternative materials for articulation in total joint replacement, *Acta Biomaterialia*, **8**(7), 2434–2441.

Sonntag, R., Reinders, J., Rieger, J.S., Heitzmann, D.W.W. and Kretzer, J.P. (2013). Hard-on-hard lubrication in the artificial hip under dynamic loading conditions, *PLoS ONE*, **8**(8), e71622.

Swedish Hip Arthroplasty Register (2010). *Annual Report.*

Waewsawangwong, W. and Goodman, S.B. (2012). Unexpected failure of highly cross-linked polyethylene acetabular liner, *J Arthroplasty*, **27**(2), 323.e1–323.e4.

Walter, W.L., Insley, G.M., Walter, W.K. and Tuke, M.A. (2004). Edge loading in third generation alumina ceramic-on-ceramic bearings: Stripe wear, *J Arthroplasty*, **19**(4), 402–413.

Willert, H.G., Bertram, H. and Buchhorn, G.H. (1990). Osteolysis in alloarthroplasty of the hip: The role of ultra-high molecular weight polyethylene wear particles, *Clin Orthop Relat R*, **258**, 95–107.

Chapter 2

Evolutionary History of Arthroplasty

Robert Sonntag[a], Nicholas A. Beckmann[a,b], Joern Reinders[a] and J. Philippe Kretzer[a]

[a]*Laboratory of Biomechanics and Implant Research, Clinic for Orthopedics and Trauma Surgery, Center for Orthopedics, Trauma Surgery and Spinal Cord Injury, Heidelberg University Hospital, Heidelberg, Germany*

[b]*Clinic for Orthopedics and Trauma Surgery, Center for Orthopedics, Trauma Surgery and Spinal Cord Injury, Heidelberg University Hospital, Heidelberg, Germany*

1. Early Treatment of Joint Diseases

Until the mid 19th century, the accepted treatment for degenerative joint disease or traumatic joint injury was arthrodesis of the joint or amputation of the affected limb, necessitated by the lack of anesthesia and sterile technique and the level of surgical knowledge and expertise at that time. Amputation of the limb was practiced widely in Europe and North America, particularly after traumatic injury (Hernigou, 2013).

At that time the separate components of the joint were not considered individually, and the joint was considered to be one unit in its entirety. However, there were early attempts to maintain some function and mobility of the joint. One step in this direction was the utilization of excision arthroplasty (Figure 2-1), where the goal was

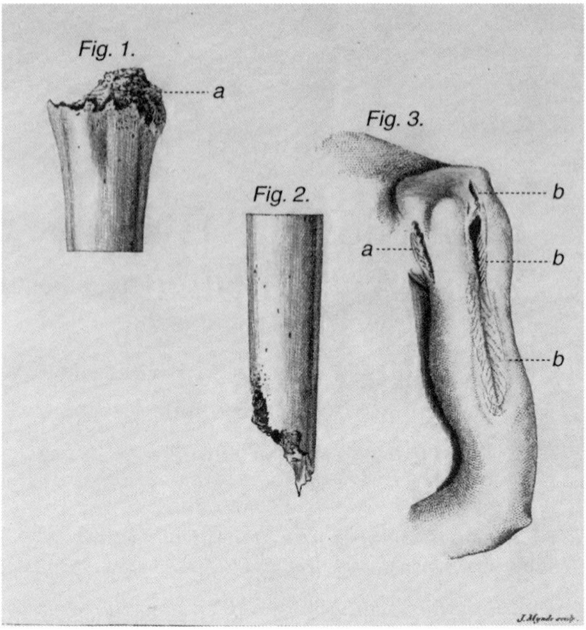

Figure 2-1. Resected humerus head (Reproduction was made from a volume held in the Boston Medical Library in the Francis A. Countway Library of Medicine) (White, 1770).

to preserve joint mobility by removing only the degenerated portions of the bones of the effected joint and thereby form a pseudo-joint with the remaining bone stumps. (White, 1770).

In 1826, the American surgeon John Rhea Barton (1794–1871) in Philadelphia successfully performed a femoral osteotomy of the hip to retain joint motion and subsequently became recognized as the pioneer of this procedure. After 20 days post-operatively, Barton began gentle motion of the operated limb in order to prevent the development of ankylosis and to promote the fibrous attachment of the severed bone and form a pseudarthrosis. The patient was reported to be able to walk with the assistance of crutches for six years after the surgery (Hernigou, 2013).

At the time, it was known that early mobilization of the joint post-operatively was a necessity in order to reduce the likelihood of ankylosis occurring between the cut surfaces of the bones (femoral head and acetabulum in cases of hip surgery). It was also known that there was a considerable loss of muscle strength as a result of the necessary sectioning of muscle tissue during the surgical procedure. Despite these disadvantages, arthroplasty of the hip according to the Whitman technique (resecting of the femoral head, placement of the femoral neck into the acetabulum and transplantation of the greater trochanter inferiorly on the femoral shaft, a process named after the noted orthopedic surgeon Royal Whitman (1857–1946)) remained the standard of care for degenerative joint disease in many places, including France, until the middle of the 20th century (Lowendorf, 1932). Long term results were poor, with ankylosis occurring in many cases (Judet and Judet, 1950). Modifications of the procedure were attempted with variable success since it was necessary to sacrifice either mobility or stability of the joint in order to achieve remission of pain (Gomez and Morcuende, 2005).

1.1. *Interposition Arthroplasty*

The poor results of excision arthroplasty and osteotomy procedures that resulted from the frequent long-term development of joint ankylosis led to the introduction of interposition arthroplasty. This involves the separation of the articulating surfaces by various intermediate materials, after the resecting of the degenerated joint surfaces. August S. Verneuil (1823–1895) in France performed soft tissue hip interpositions in 1860, but it was Leopold Ollier (1830–1900), also working in France, who popularized the concept of interpositional arthroplasty utilizing adipose tissue in uninfected joints. However, the interposed tissue was not anchored to the bone, and these procedures failed (Gomez and Morcuende, 2005). The materials used for interposition were many and varied, and included wood (John Carnochan, 1817–1871), muscle and pig bladder (Gomez and Morcuende, 2005; Hernigou, 2013). Pig bladder was found to be effective in withstanding pressure, and by 1918 was popularized for interposition arthroplasty by William S. Baer (1872–1931) at the Johns Hopkins Hospital. In Britain, Sir Robert Jones (1855–1933) used a strip of gold foil over reconstructed femoral heads with limited positive results (Gomez and Morcuende, 2005). Vitezlav Chlumsky

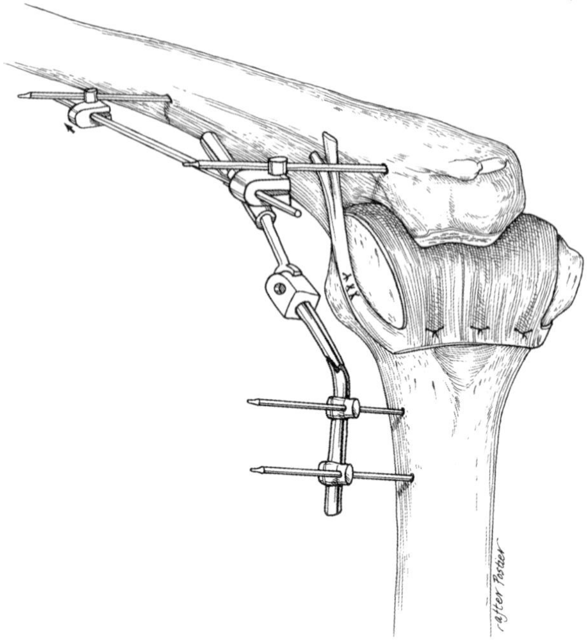

Figure 2-2. Interposition arthroplasty of the elbow (Cheung *et al.*, 2008).

(1867–1943) in Germany experimented with many materials including metals, rubber, glass, wax, and celluloid (Hernigou, 2013).

The results were generally poor, and the materials used were called into question. Pain and instability of the joint were continuing concerns, particularly in the lower limb weight bearing joints. Positive results were only achieved in joints exposed to lesser loads, such as in the shoulder and elbow (Figure 2-2). Even today, this procedure of interposition arthroplasty continues to be performed in young, active patients with degenerative joint conditions of the elbow, such as inflammatory or post-traumatic arthritis, which are considered appropriate indications for the procedure (Papatheodorou *et al.*, 2013). This procedure allows these patients to participate in activities such as weight lifting at an earlier post-operative stage compared to patients who have received total elbow arthroplasty.

1.2. *First Joint Replacements in the Late 19th Century*

Several surgeons, including the Russian Nikolai Iwanowitsch Pirogow (1810–1881) in 1830, had already considered the possibility of artificial joints replacing resected ones to fill the created void, but it was the German surgeon Themistocles Gluck (1853–1942) who became the pioneer in the development and implementation of joint implants (Hernigou, 2013). His interest was piqued during his work as a wartime surgeon between the years 1877 and 1885, when he successfully repaired a fractured femur by using two steel plates secured to the bone by screws, and also repaired a mandibular defect (resulting from the excision of a tumor) with steel plate and screws (Hernigou, 2013). Gluck also pursued the replacement of entire joints that were resected as a result of disease, with artificial joints that he designed and implanted. He successfully utilized extensive animal trials before embarking on joint replacements in patients. In 1890, at the 10th International Surgical Congress in Berlin, Gluck presented the novel idea of utilizing the void that had been created after resection of the diseased joint for the insertion of an artificial joint. This contradicted the prevailing philosophy of the orthopedic community at the time and was not well received (Brand *et al.*, 2011). In addition to hip joint implants, Gluck devised implants for the wrist, elbow, shoulder, ankle, and knee. Early implants were made of ivory and fixed inside the marrow cavity with bone cement made from copper amalgam, plaster of Paris and stony putty (Brand *et al.*, 2011).

The procedures were successful initially, with satisfactory post-surgical mobility, but failed long term due to infection that was related to his choice of patients, who had suffered preoperatively with joint tuberculosis, and also to the use of ivory that proved to have insufficient stability. Gluck's work on joint replacement was dismissed during his lifetime, but his many accomplishments were eventually recognized and by the end of his life he had been listed on the honor roll of the German Surgical Society. Among other achievements, he pioneered the concept of biocompatibility: tolerance of foreign materials by the body, including those used in hip joint replacements. The technical drawings of his hinged knee joint made of ivory (Figure 2-3) became popular all over the world and

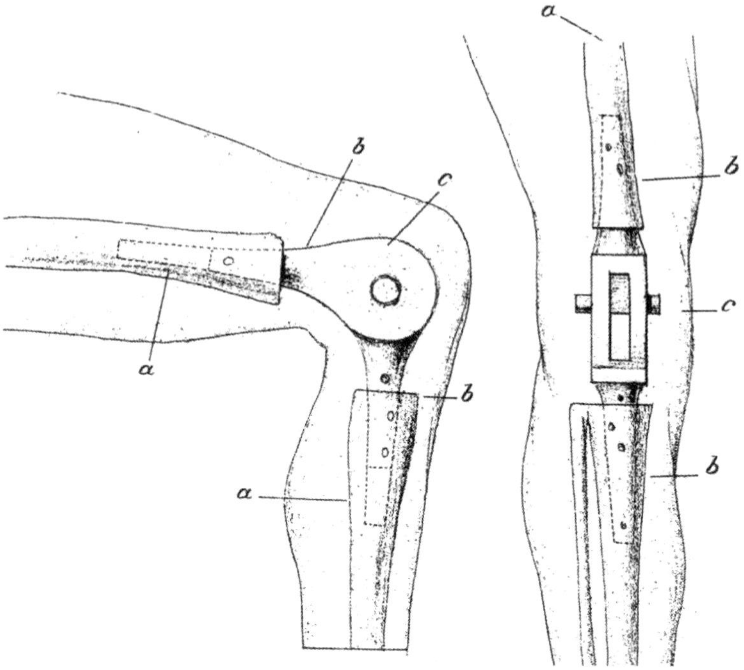

Figure 2-3. Sketch of a hinged knee implant by Themistocles Gluck, 1890 (Gluck, 2011).

had some similarity to the constraint total knee prosthesis introduced decades later (Brand *et al.*, 2011; Hernigou, 2013).

Other procedures done around the turn of the 20th century included hip cheilotomy, which involved the resection of overhanging bone osteophytes from the head of the femur and the rim of the acetabulum in cases of localized osteoarthritis of the hip. This procedure was promoted by John Benjamin Murphy (1857–1916) of Chicago (Hernigou, 2013).

In 1927, the British surgeon Ernest William Hey Groves (1872–1944) described a procedure where the degenerated femoral head was replaced by an ivory nail (Figure 2-4), with dubious results (Ratliff, 1983).

Pierre Delbet (1861–1925) in France used a rubber femoral prosthesis in 1919 to replace half of the hip joint (Gomez and Morcuende, 2005).

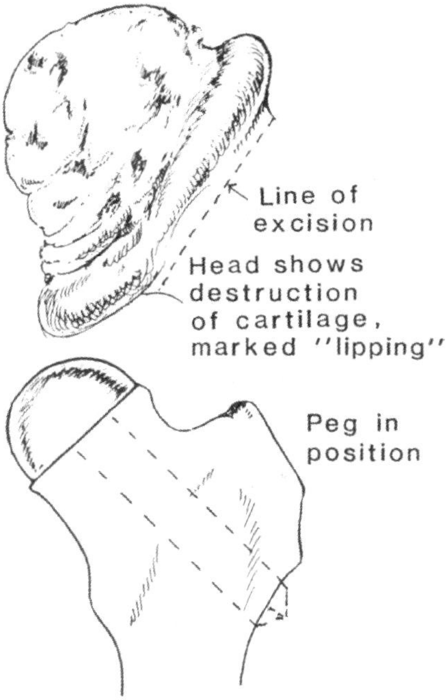

Figure 2-4. Illustration of an early hip arthroplasty by Hey Groved, 1933 (Ratliff, 1983) (Copyright The Royal College of Surgeons of England. Reproduced with permission).

In parallel, Erich Lexer (1867–1937) in Germany pioneered tissue transplantation and transplanted partial bones of fresh cadavers or amputees into the femoral head and neck of patients. The results of these and other transplantation surgeries he performed on the knee were unsatisfactory because of misalignments, joint instability, and infection (Lexer, 1914).

2. Early Milestones

2.1. *Mold Hemiarthroplasty: Another Step Forward*

At the beginning of the 20th century, after the failure of both the excision arthroplasty and the first total joint arthroplasty, the focus of the surgical community returned to interposition arthroplasty for the treatment of degenerative hip disease. In 1923, the

Norwegian-born American surgeon Marius Nygaard Smith-Petersen (1886–1953) introduced the mold arthroplasty. This development followed an observation he had made during removal of a piece of glass from a patient during an unrelated procedure. Smith-Petersen noted that a smooth synovial-like membrane had developed around the glass, and deduced that the presence of the glass had stimulated the development of this tissue and could similarly stimulate the development of cartilage and synovial tissue. Smith-Petersen believed that a mold of similar glassy material placed between the surgically reshaped surfaces of the femur and acetabulum would stimulate the natural growth of new reparative joint tissue that would provide smooth articular surfaces. This observation led to the development of a mold shaped as a hollow hemisphere of glass that could fit over the shaped femoral head of the hip joint, and he thought that with gentle motion against the natural acetabular cartilage and modified weight bearing, it would lead to the regeneration of cartilage on each side of the mold. In 1932, Smith-Petersen began to implant these glass molds utilizing an anterior surgical approach that he devised and that still bears his name to this day. The device was designed to fit over the femoral head between it and the acetabulum and it was intended that after the successful development of a new covering of smooth surface tissue, the mold would be removed during the second stage of a two-step procedure (Smith-Petersen, 1939). However, he was reluctant to perform the second step of the procedure in patients who were showing positive signs. The glass proved biocompatible but could not withstand the stress of weight bearing and broke, and his method was abandoned. However, when the pieces were removed, Smith-Peterson found that the bones were covered with a glistening membrane and this encouraged him to search for a more suitable material for the molds (Smith-Petersen, 1948). Various materials were tried unsuccessfully, including celluloid that provoked a foreign body reaction, and later viscaloid, borosilicate glass, and bakelite. At the suggestion of his dentist, he tried Vitallium (a cobalt chromium molybdenum alloy) and employed the research findings of Charles S. Venable (1827–1900) regarding the necessary properties of metal alloys that make them suitable for use in arthroplasty (Venable

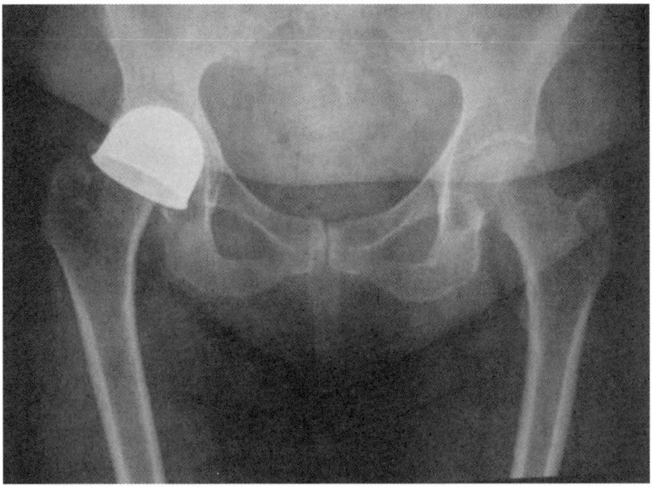

Figure 2-5. Smith-Petersen cup after 62 years *in vivo* (Landham *et al.*, 2006).

et al., 1937). Venable had experimented for many years in testing the effects of various metals on bone, and concluded that Vitallium was superior to all others. Vitallium was originally developed in the submarine industry for military purposes, and is a highly corrosion-resistant ion-free material that was also used successfully in patients for dental implants (Hernigou *et al.*, 2014). Smith-Petersen implanted the first vitallium mold in 1938 followed by an additional 500 molds over the following decade, with good clinical results (Figure 2-5) (Berntsen and Bertelsen, 1952; Smith-Petersen, 1948). This Vitallium cup and further modifications of the cup, including those by his associate Otto Aufranc (1909–1990), which were also placed as interposed devices that articulated against the natural cartilage of the acetabulum, provided the first routinely predictable and moderately satisfactory clinical results. Several publications have reported well-functioning Smith-Petersen cups after 45–62 years placement *in vivo* (Baker *et al.*, 2011; Mahalingam and Reidy, 1996; Santanapipatkul and Udomkiat, 2012). However, the unilateral replacement of the degenerated tissue by Smith-Petersen cups led to increased stress on the adjacent natural acetabular cup, resulting in continued pain and osteophyte formation, osteolysis, necrosis, and fractures of the acetabulum in some cases (Wiles, 1958).

2.2. *The Hip Hemiarthroplasty*

Other surgeons, including Harold Bohlmann (1893–1979) in the United States, introduced a hemiprosthesis that replaced the entire femoral head and the covering cartilage. Incorporating the work of Venable, he implanted the first femoral prosthesis made of Vitallium. The prosthesis had a short stem and was fixed at the cortical external femoral neck by a nail (Hernigou *et al.*, 2014). Other materials such as acrylic and various metals were also used between the years 1939 and 1950.

In 1946, the French surgeons and brothers Jean Judet (1905–1995) and Robert Judet (1901–1980) introduced a mold hemiprosthesis utilizing acrylic (polymethylmethacrylate, or PMMA) that was thought to be biologically inert. These surgeons removed the femoral head and replaced it with the synthetic acrylic one that was designed to fit the femoral bearing surface of the underlying bone, and had a short stem that extended through the neck of the femur and penetrated the lateral cortex of the femur (Figure 2-6) (Judet and Judet, 1950). The stem was reinforced by a steel core that was covered by the acrylic resin. Without the steel core, the stem had fractured in 12 cases.

The operation garnered a lot of attention at the time since it was relatively easy to perform and produced impressive early results. However, despite the positive short-term results, the longer-term outcome was less favorable, with recurrence of pain, massive wear of the head of the prosthesis, and an increasing incidence of implant fracture (Figure 2-7) (Wiles, 2003). Consequently, the Judet prosthesis was losing favor by the early 1950s (Pridie, 1955; Scales and Zarek, 1954). However, as with the Smith-Petersen design, there are occasional cases of long-term survival of the prosthesis of 42–51 years (Kovac *et al.*, 2004; Schreurs *et al.*, 2001; Tatari *et al.*, 2001).

In addition to the shortcomings of the Judet prosthesis noted above, short-stem prostheses in general were found to be limited biomechanically and were subject to high shear stresses that resulted in early loosening, failure, and recurrent pain in a large number of patients (Wiles, 2003). They were gradually replaced by next generation designs which had stems that were anchored in the femoral

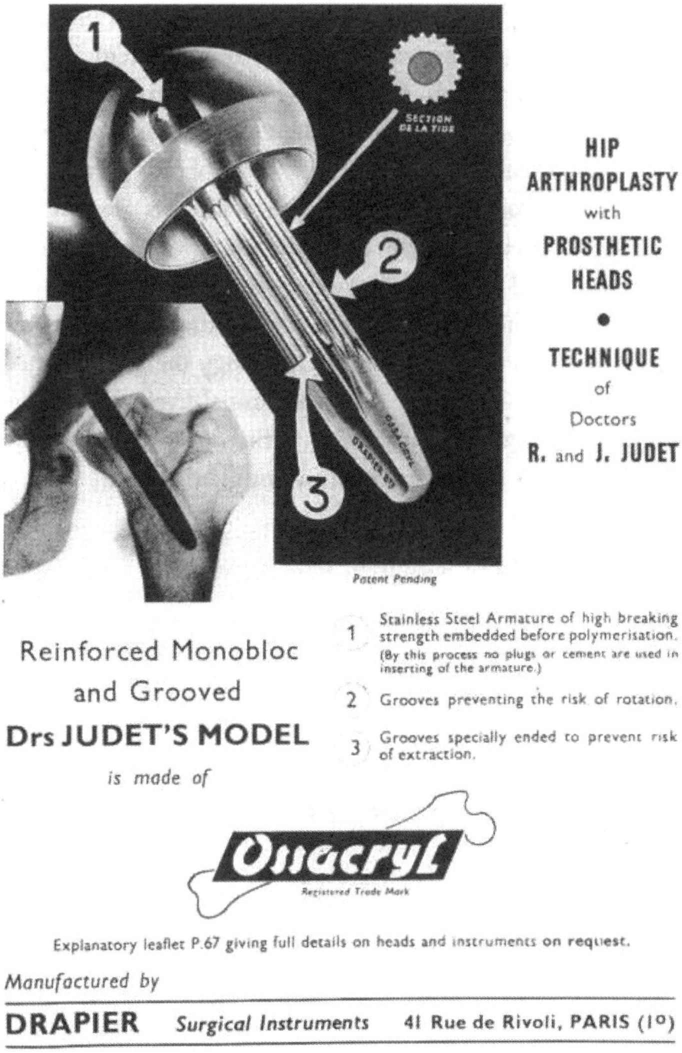

Figure 2-6. Advertisement of the Judet prostheses in 1950 in the *Journal of Bone and Joint Surgery* (Tennent and Eastwood, 1998).

shaft in order to improve the shear stress capabilities by transferring the weight bearing forces to the femur through the intramedullary stem. In the United States in 1943, Austin T. Moore (1899–1963) collaborated with Harold Böhlmann to devise a long-stem prosthesis. Both surgeons had some prior experience with a modified form of a

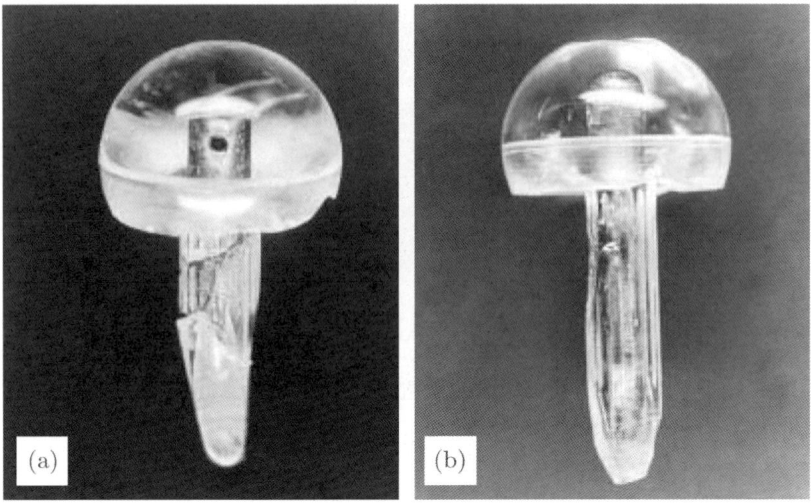

Figure 2-7. Judet prostheses revised after 42 years *in vivo*: (a) broken rod; (b) worn head and partly broken rod (Tatari *et al.*, 2001).

long-stem prosthesis that they had devised for treatment of a patient with a bone tumor. In 1940, the tumor was excised and replaced by a Vitallium prosthesis that was 12 inches long and was designed to replace the head and upper portion of the femur, articulate against the natural cartilage of the acetabulum, and had incorporated loops of metal for the attachment of muscles. The patient died within three years of other causes, and autopsy revealed the Vitallium implant to be free of any corrosion (Hernigou *et al.*, 2014; Moore and Böhlman, 1943). Moore and Böhlmann refined their design and proposed a revolutionary method of fixing the implant by driving a long metal stem into the medullary cavity of the femur (Figure 2-8(a)). In 1952 they produced a model with a fenestrated stem that allowed bone ingrowth. The Vitallium implant also featured a window in the prosthetic tail that allowed bone ingrowth and a hole at the upper part of the collar to facilitate extraction, if necessary (Hernigou *et al.*, 2014).

These were the first hip arthroplasty products that became widely distributed. They eventually became the product of choice and continue to be used for the replacement of the femoral head and neck,

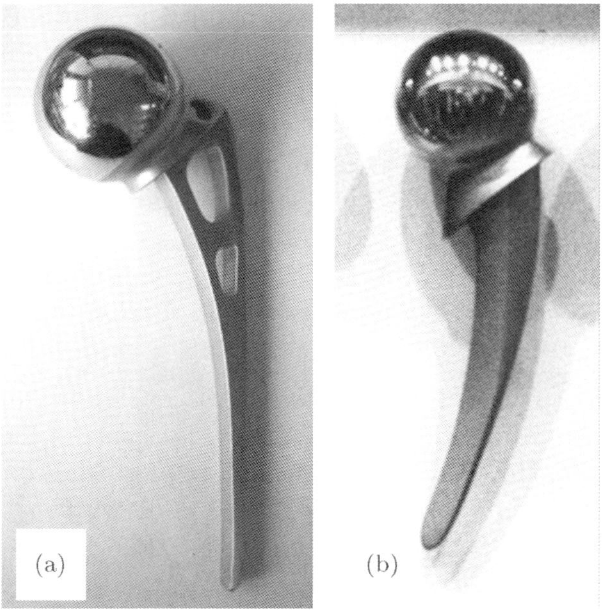

Figure 2-8. Hemiprostheses by Moore/Böhlmann (a) and Thompson (b) (Hernigou *et al.*, 2014).

especially following femoral neck fractures in the elderly (Gomez and Morcuende, 2005; Hernigou *et al.*, 2014). The concept of the intramedullary stem has been universally adopted and has transformed the outlook for femoral neck fractures. Prior to this, fracture of the femoral neck was a frequent cause of death in older patients. With this development, patients were able to ambulate a few days after the operation (Hernigou *et al.*, 2014).

In 1950, Frederick Roeck Thompson (1907–1983) developed a cemented Vitallium prosthesis that featured a flared collar below the head and had a vertical intramedullary stem (Figure 2-8(b)). The cement used by Thompson was polymethylmethacrylate (PMMA), which is still in use today. Prior to its use in orthopedics, early applications of the cement were in industry. It was first used in orthopedics by Judet and Judet, then later by Edward Haboush (1904–1973) and Kenneth McKee (1905–1991) for fixation of the devices that they developed (Gomez and Morcuende, 2005). Like the Austin Moore prosthesis, the Thompson prosthesis is still used extensively today in some countries to treat femoral neck fractures (Hernigou *et al.*, 2014).

Despite many successes with these prostheses, there remained some disadvantages that included instances of arthritic destruction of the acetabular socket and loosening of the implant with resultant pain (Anderson *et al.*, 1964).

2.3. *Replacement of Both Articulation Partners: First Generation Metal-On-Metal*

In 1958, the British surgeon Philip Wiles (1899–1966) published his account of replacing both articulating components of the hip, which he first attempted in 1938 by utilizing a pre-formed acetabulum and femoral head, both made of stainless steel and with surfaces ground to fit accurately. The acetabulum was prevented from rotating by a couple of screws and the femoral head was secured by a bolt passing through the neck of the femur (Wiles, 1958). In all but one of the patients the necessary follow-up to the surgery was unfortunately rendered impossible thanks to the destruction of patient records during World War II, but one patient was able to be followed for 13 years and was found to have very limited hip motion. Her metal-on-metal total joint replacement remained in place (Figure 2-9(a)), although the acetabular screws were disintegrating and the bolt had broken away from the head of the femur without any pain.

Wiles later designed a second generation model, also of stainless steel, that was designed to transfer the stress from the cancellous bone of the femoral head to the dense cortical bone of the shaft by a screwed plate (Figure 2-9(b)). The acetabulum was designed with a flange around the rim with the goal of reducing scar tissue; rotation was prevented by three pins projecting from the rim. The femoral component was designed to fit closely to the bone with a stem that could slide outward if bone was resorbed. Only eight patients were operated on and the results were poor: Only two of the eight had a tolerably satisfactory result (Wiles, 2003).

Further developments were interrupted by World War II. However, in Norwich (UK) from 1951, Kenneth McKee (1909–1991),

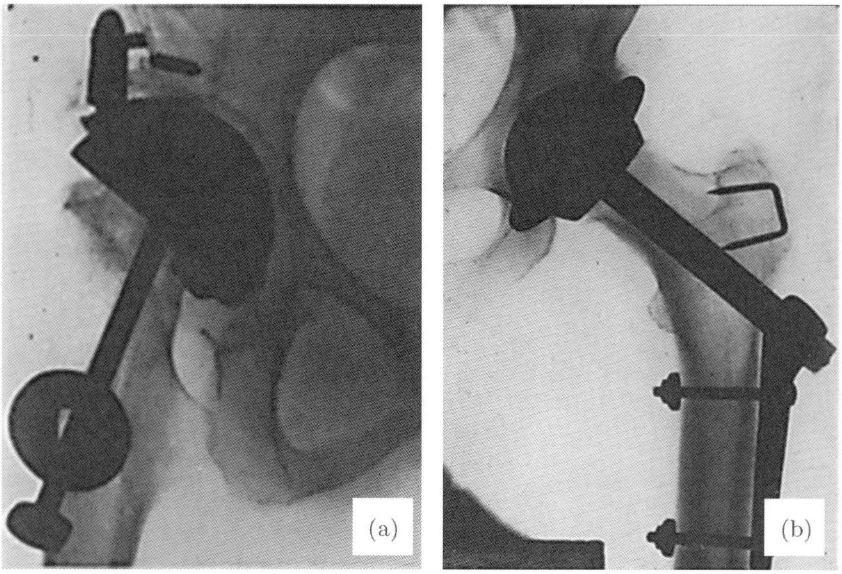

Figure 2-9. Wiles prostheses: (a) implanted in 1938 after 13 years *in vivo*; and, (b) second generation design (Wiles, 2003).

who had trained with Wiles, together with John Watson Farrar (1926–1999) used a ball-and-socket joint with limited success. Of three such appliances, two were of stainless steel and became corroded and loose. Vitallium cobalt-chromium alloy was subsequently used with a modified Thompson prosthesis with a smaller femoral head that articulated with a three claw cup that screwed into the acetabulum (Figure 2-10) (McKee and Watson-Farrar, 1966). The success of the procedure was determined by the integrity of the joint. Loosening of the components occurred in some patients and led to recurrent pain on weight bearing (August *et al.*, 1986). There were a number of additional attempts to completely replace degenerated joints. There were some successes but the major problem in all cases remained the same: The loosening of the implant over time. It was the re-introduction of PMMA as a fixing bone cement by Charnley in 1960 that reduced the problem of implant loosening and allowed for the further development of hip prostheses, including a second

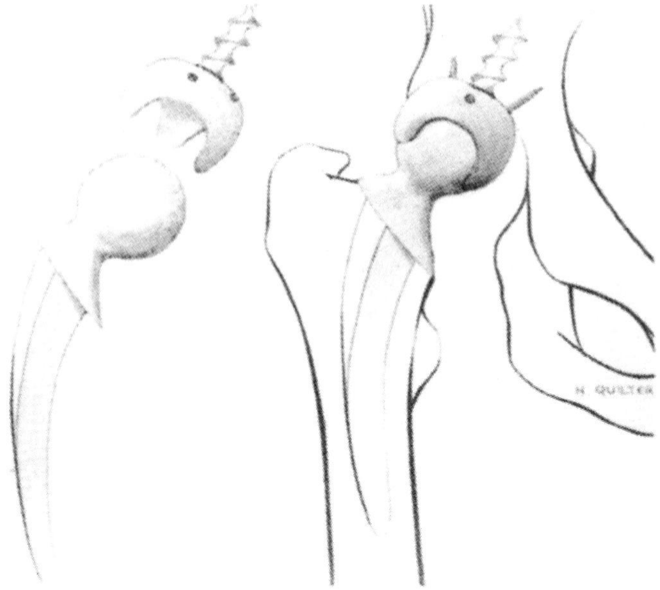

Figure 2-10. First generation McKee–Farrar prosthesis (Amstutz and Grigoris, 1996).

generation McKee–Farrar model (Figure 2-11(a)) (Gomez and Morcuende, 2005). The acetabular cup was modified in this model, and had a round form with small pegs on the acetabular aspect and was cemented deeper into the acetabulum. This allowed for the use of a standard Thompson prosthesis with a large femoral head, leading to reduced weight bearing stress per unit area of the acetabulum and therefore reduced acetabular destruction and improved long-term results. Vitallium with a lower coefficient of friction than most other metals was used for both components (August *et al.*, 1986; Brown *et al.*, 2002).

Despite the use of PMMA cement, acetabular loosening in particular continued to be a problem in some cases. The acrylic cement (PMMA) used was also associated with a slightly increased risk of infection and was thought to have occasionally precipitated an intensive hypotensive reaction at the time of insertion (Ring, 1968). Consequently, in Britain, Peter Ring (1922) devised a cementless metal-on-metal prosthesis consisting of a deeply seated acetabular cup with

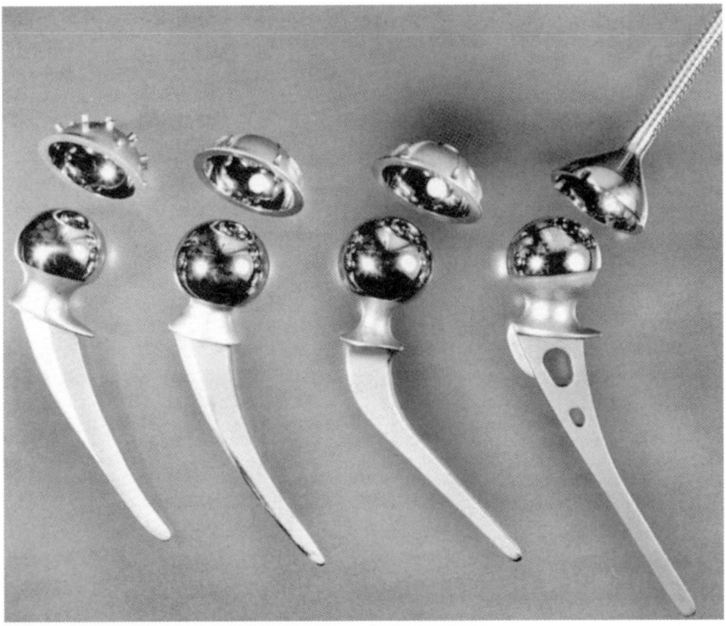

Figure 2-11. Examples of early metal-on-metal total hip replacements. Left: Second generation McKee-Farrar; Right: Ring prostheses (McKellop *et al.*, 1996).

a long threaded metal stem placed in line with the weight bearing plane of the pelvis (Figure 2-11(b)). The femoral component was a modified Moore–Böhlmann prosthesis. These devices began to be used in 1964 (Ring, 1968), with the results achieved comparable to those found with the McKee–Farrar prosthesis (Bryant *et al.*, 1991).

Following excision arthroplasty, interposition arthroplasty, and hemiarthroplasty, total joint arthroplasty was successfully introduced all over the world in the 1950s, and became a more reliable intervention for the average orthopedic surgeon. However, studies showed that despite promising and successful results in the short term, a resounding success in the long term remained elusive. This was attributed to the manufacturing limitations of the times, particularly the inadequacy of the materials utilized in terms of their ability to withstand the high stress loads placed on the devices by the body during weight bearing. The McKee–Farrar and other first generation prostheses failed at a high rate long term because of component (acetabular and femoral) loosening as a result of impingement of the femoral component on the acetabular rim, and there were instances of fracturing of the femoral stem, and also of tissue reaction to the metal used. These issues were partially corrected by improving manufacturing quality and the utilization of second generation devices with more favorable head:neck ratios (Fabi *et al.*, 2012; Long, 2005). However, tissue reaction to the metals used remains an issue in some cases, and cases of metallosis have been reported since the 1970s. The release of metal ions has been found to cause local tissue necrosis and resultant pain, bone loss, and fracture, and more rarely can affect distant organ systems (Cohen, 2012).

3. Focus on Friction: Charnley and the Utilization of Polyethylene

Sir John Charnley (1911–1982) in Britain was very active in investigational research directed at understanding the friction and lubrication of animal and artificial joints (Charnley, 1959, 1960). Charnley and his associates recognized that the inadequacies of the prosthetic devices were a result of the materials used and the resulting frictional forces that occurred in the artificial joints. He recognized that the increased frictional resistance was the cause of the squeaking on movement in the Judet prosthesis. Charnley developed the concept of low friction arthroplasty (Charnley, 1961) and as a result deduced the necessity of reducing frictional resistance at the articular surface of the implant. He achieved this by reducing the size of the femoral head component, and introduced a 22.2 mm diameter Vitallium femoral head to minimize femoral torque, while recognizing the increased risk of dislocation with a small diameter femoral head (Figure 2-12) (Gomez and Morcuende, 2005).

In 1956, Charnley began using self-lubricating polytetrafluoroethylene (PTFE) in the hip joint, initially as synthetic articular cartilage lining the acetabulum and also covering the femoral head as a hollow cup. Unexpectedly, the post-operative results obtained defied lab expectations and early failure as a result of severe wear was

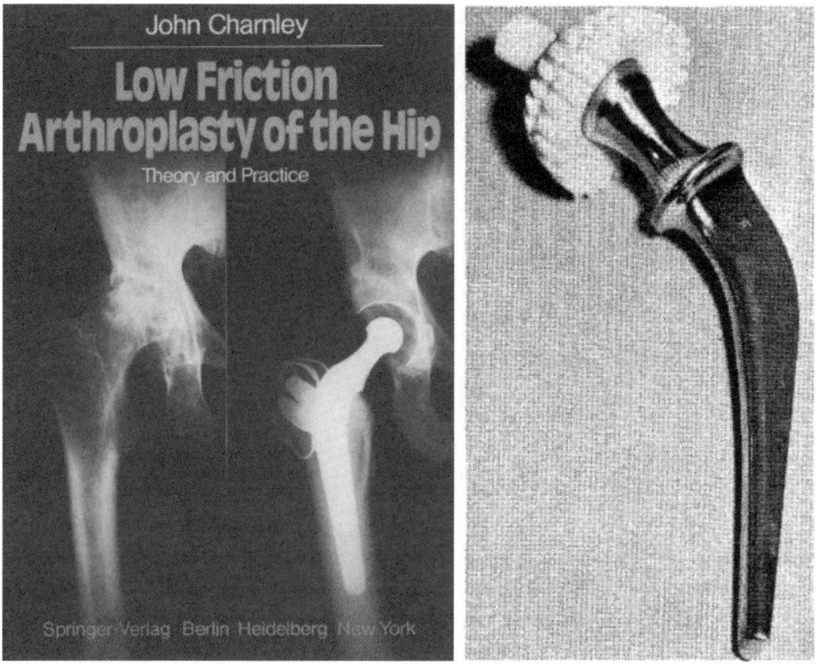

Figure 2-12. Charnley prostheses according to the concept of Low Friction Arthroplasty (Charnley, 1961).

observed. Charnley then used thick PTFE acetabular inserts articulating with a small femoral head, which also resulted in excessive wear and an intense foreign body reaction to the debris produced by the wear, after implantation in 300 patients. Despite discouragement from Charnley, one of his technical assistants mechanically tested ultra-high molecular weight polyethylene (UHMWPE) and found it to have much improved wear resistance by a factor of 1,000 compared to PTFE and only slightly increased friction. In addition, the biological reaction to UHMWPE was far less than to PTFE, as demonstrated by a self-experiment when Charnley introduced samples of both substances subcutaneously into his thigh (Charnley, 1963). The PTFE site developed marked nodularity after nine months whereas the UHMWPE site had almost no reaction and was almost nonpalpable (Gomez and Morcuende, 2005). Although Charnley had pioneered the use of PTFE years before, these findings convinced him to abandon its use and substitute it with UHMWPE, and in 1962 he implanted the first UHMWPE hip socket. Use of this material has allowed more extensive employment of joint reconstructions by artificial hip joints and has remained the state-of-the-art model for decades (Gomez and Morcuende, 2005). Charnley can also be credited with advancing the concept of tribological effect as it applies in orthopedics, and the significance of friction wear and lubrication of implant materials for their longevity and function, and particularly the body's reaction to the particulate debris produced as a result of implant wear (Knahr, 2013).

4. Ceramics as a Bearing Material

Ceramic implants were introduced in hip arthroplasties in the early 1970s by Piere Boutin (1924–1989) and were subsequently used as femoral heads, monolithic sockets and liners for acetabular cups (Figure 2-13) (Boutin, 1972).

Also around this time, reports began to surface about the previously unknown risks of adverse biological responses to polyethylene and its wear products and to the wear products of metals (Willert and Semlitsch, 1977). Charnley therefore advocated restriction of the use of metal-on-polyethylene joint replacements in elderly patients. Boutin advocated, as an alternative, the use of ceramic components made of aluminum oxide (Al_2O_3) as a bearing surface material for the femoral head and acetabular cup (ceramic-on-ceramic). He had already carried out tribological studies and reported on 200 clinical cases and *in vivo* animal studies. Based on his findings, he suggested ceramic-on-ceramic joints as an appropriate alternative to metal-on-polyethylene bearings, especially for younger patients (Boutin *et al.*, 1988). Other experimental studies at that time (Fritsch and Gleitz, 1996; Hannouche *et al.*, 2005; Willmann, 2000) confirmed the superior mechanical and tribological properties of ceramics; they are very hard, scratch resistant, show increased wettability with liquids, and have excellent biocompatibility. In early ceramic-on-ceramic designs by Sedel and Mittelmeier, the femoral head was fitted using a tapered

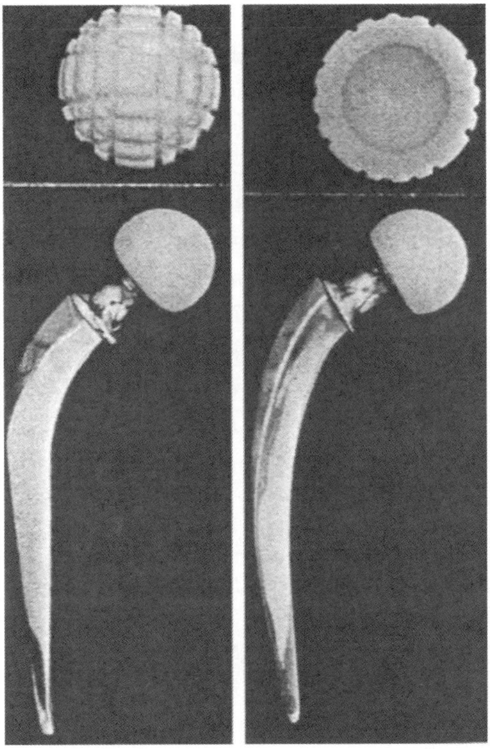

(a) (b)

Figure 2-13. Boutin ceramic hip bearings (Reproduced from Boutin P (2014). Total arthroplasty of the hip by fritted alumina prosthesis. Experimental study and 1st clinical applications. *Orthop Traumatol Surg Res*, **100**(1), 15–21. Copyright © 2014 Elsevier Masson SAS. All rights reserved).

interlock to the metallic stem, while the monolithic acetabular component was fixed to the pelvis without cement by the use of tapered screw threads or spikes on the back surface of the acetabular component (Mittelmeier, 1984; Sedel *et al.*, 1990).

Primarily because of the significantly reduced wear, ceramic-on-ceramic joints were felt to be a good alternative for younger patients (Mittelmeier and Heisel, 1992). However, due to the brittleness of ceramics an increased fracture rate of the ceramic-on-ceramic bearings in the long term was encountered in the early designs (Fritsch and Gleitz, 1996; Michaud and Rashad, 1995).

Simultaneously in Europe and Japan, ceramic heads were combined with polyethylene acetabular liners (ceramic-on-polyethylene) (Semlitsch *et al.*, 1977; Sugano *et al.*, 1995). Semlitsch *et al.* showed in tribological studies that with ceramic-on-polyethylene bearings, polyethylene wear could be reduced by a factor of 20 when compared to metal-on-polyethylene bearings. In addition, the ceramic-on-polyethylene bearings had shown a significant reduction in the ceramic head fracture rate when compared to the ceramic-on-ceramic bearings (Heisel and Schmitt, 1987).

There were still isolated cases of catastrophic failure of alumina femoral heads reported in ceramic-on-polyethylene bearings (Michaud and Rashad, 1995). For this reason zirconia femoral heads were introduced. They exhibit superior mechanical strength in comparison to alumina and when properly manufactured should reduce the risk of catastrophic failures. Zirconia is a complex, metastable material that exists in different phases (Cales, 2000). Depending on different environmental conditions (temperature, humidity, mechanical stress) it can undergo a phase transformation resulting in volume loss. Because of this, metastable zirconia is typically stabilized by the use of additives (e.g. yttria, magnesium). However, in the 2000s an unexpectedly high number of fractures were reported and were blamed on a change in the manufacturing process (Clarke *et al.*, 2003). This resulted in the withdrawal of yttria-stabilized zirconia-based ceramics from orthopedic application (Bal *et al.*, 2007) and ceramics thus fell out of favor as a major joint replacement material. However, the majority of zirconia femoral heads implanted at that time appear to be working well still. Since then, further improvements have been made using different stabilizing agents such as magnesium and alumina–zirconia composites. Additional improvement was achieved by the use of crosslinked polyethylene liners, which led to a further reduction in both the fracture and wear rates (Jameson *et al.*, 2013; Lang *et al.*, 2008).

Studies with a follow up period of 17 years by Legenstein *et al.* (2006) and Yoon *et al.* (2008), and at 18 years by Urban *et al.* (2001) showed a fracture rate in their collectives approaching 0% using alumina components that are not currently regarded as state-of-the-art.

Using the newer designs and materials it is speculated that further improvement of long-term results can likely be expected. Recent indications are that these ceramic-on-polyethylene bearings are again becoming used with increased frequency in Europe and are again considered clinically relevant, particularly in younger patients.

References

Amstutz, H.C. and Grigoris, P. (1996). Metal on metal bearings in hip arthroplasty, *Clin Orthop Relat Res*, **329**, S11–S34.

Anderson, L.D., Hamsa Jr., W.R. and Waring, T.L. (1964). Femoral head prostheses. A review of three hundred and fifty-six operations and their results, *J Bone Joint Surg Am*, **46**, 1049–1065.

August, A.C., Aldam, C.H. and Pynsent, P.B. (1986). The McKee-Farrar hip arthroplasty: A long-term study, *J Bone Joint Surg Br*, **68**(4), 520–527.

Baker, J.F., Vioreanu, M.H. and Khan, H.A. (2011). Smith-Petersen Vitallium mould arthroplasty: A 62-year follow-up, *J Bone Joint Surg Br*, **93**, 1285–1286.

Bal, B.S., Garino, J., Ries, M. and Rahaman, M.N. (2007). A review of ceramic bearing materials in total joint arthroplasty, *Hip Int*, **17**(1), 21–30.

Berntsen, A. and Bertelsen, A. (1952). Preliminary experience with Smith-Petersen's hip cup arthroplasty, *Acta Orthop Scand*, **22**(2), 147–152.

Boutin, P. (1972). Arthroplastie totale de la hanche par prothese en alumine frittee. Etude experimentale et premieres applications cliniques, *Rev Chir Orthop*, **58**, 229–246.

Boutin, P. (2014). Total arthroplasty of the hip by fritted alumina prosthesis. Experimental study and 1st clinical applications, *Orthop Traumatol Surg Res*, **100**(1), 15–21.

Boutin, P., Christel, P., Dorlot, J.M., Meunier, A., de Roquancourt, A., Blanquaert, D. *et al.* (1988). The use of dense alumina–alumina ceramic combination in total hip replacement, *J Biomed Mater Res*, **22**(12), 1203–1232.

Brand, R., Mont, M. and Manring, M. (2011). Biographical Sketch: Themistocles Gluck (1853–1942), *Clin Orthop Relat R*, **469**, 1525–1527.

Brown, S.R., Davies, W.A., DeHeer, D.H. and Swanson, A.B. (2002). Long-term survival of McKee-Farrar total hip prostheses, *Clin Orthop Relat R*, **402**, 157–163.

Bryant, M.J., Mollan, R.A.B. and Nixon, J.R. (1991). Survivorship analysis of the ring hip arthroplasty, *J Arthroplasty*, **6**, S5–S10.

Cales, B. (2000). Zirconia as a sliding material: Histologic, laboratory, and clinical data, *Clin Orthop Relat R*, **379**, 94–112.

Charnley, J. (1959). The lubrication of animal joints, *Inst Mech Eng: Symp Biomech*, **17**, 12–19.

Charnley, J. (1960). The lubrication of animal joints in relation to surgical reconstruction by arthroplasty, *Ann Rheum Dis*, **19**(1), 10–19.

Charnley, J. (1961). Arthroplasty of the hip: A new operation, *Lancet*, **277**(7187), 1129–1132.

Charnley, J. (1963). Tissue reactions to polytetrafluororethylene, *Lancet*, **282**(7322), 1379.

Cheung, E.V., Adams, R. and Morrey, B.F. (2008). Primary osteoarthritis of the elbow: Current treatment options, *J Am Acad Orthop Surg*, **16**(2), 77–87.

Clarke, I.C., Manaka, M., Green, D.D., Williams, P., Pezzotti, G., Kim, Y.H. *et al.* (2003). Current status of zirconia used in total hip implants, *J Bone Joint Surg Am*, **85**(Suppl 4), 73–84.

Cohen, D. (2012). How safe are metal-on-metal hip implants?, *Brit Med J*, **344**, e1410.

Fabi, D., Levine, B., Paprosky, W., Della Valle, C., Sporer, S., Klein, G. *et al.* (2012). Metal-on-metal total hip arthroplasty: Causes and high incidence of early failure, *Orthopedics*, **35**(7), e1009–e1016.

Fritsch, E.W.M.D. and Gleitz, M.M.D. (1996). Ceramic femoral head fractures in total hip arthroplasty, *Clin Orthop Relat R*, **328**, 129–136.

Gluck, T. (2011). Report on the positive results obtained by the modern surgical experiment regarding the suture and replacement of defects of superior tissue, as well as the utilization of re-absorbable and living tamponade in surgery. 1891, *Clin Orthop Relat R*, **469**(6), 1528–1535.

Gomez, P.F. and Morcuende, J.A. (2005a). Early attempts at hip arthroplasty — 1700s to 1950s, *Iowa Orthop J*, **25**, 25–29.

Gomez, P.F. and Morcuende, J.A. (2005b). A historical and economic perspective on Sir John Charnley, Chas F. Thackray Limited, and the early arthoplasty industry, *Iowa Orthop J*, **25**, 30–37.

Hannouche, D., Hamadouche, M., Nizard, R., Bizot, P., Meunier, A. and Sedel, L. (2005). Ceramics in total hip replacement, *Clin Orthop Relat R*, **430**, 62–71.

Heisel, J. and Schmitt, E. (1987). Implant fractures in ceramic hip endoprostheses, *Z Orthop Grenzgeb*, **125**(5), 480–490.

Hernigou, P. (2013). Earliest times before hip arthroplasty: From John Rhea Barton to Themistocles Glück, *Int Orthop*, **37**(11), 2313–2318.

Hernigou, P., Quiennec, S. and Guissou, I. (2014). Hip hemiarthroplasty: From Venable and Bohlman to Moore and Thompson, *Int Orthop*, **38**(3), 655–661.

Jameson, S.S., Mason, J.M., Baker, P.N., Jettoo, P., Deehan, D.J. and Reed, M.R. (2013). Factors influencing revision risk following 15 740 single-brand hybrid hip arthroplasties: A cohort study from a National Joint Registry, *J Arthroplasty*, **28**(7), 1152–1159.

Judet, J. and Judet, R. (1950). The use of an artificial femoral head for arthroplasty of the hip joint, *J Bone Joint Surg Br*, **32**(2), 166–173.

Knahr, K. (2013). Tribology and total hip arthroplasty implants, *Orthopedics*, **36**(11), 854–855.

Kovac, S., Pisot, V., Trebse, R. and Rotter, A. (2004). Fifty-one-year survival of a Judet polymethylmethacrylate hip prosthesis, *J Arthroplasty*, **19**(5), 664–667.

Landham, P.R., Abbas, N. and Jähnich, H. (2006). The oldest surviving arthroplasty?, *J R Soc Med*, **99**(12), 640.

Lang, J.E., Whiddon, D.R., Smith, E.L. and Salyapongse, A.K. (2008). Use of ceramics in total hip replacement, *J Surg Orthop Adv*, **17**(1), 51–57.

Legenstein, R., Huber, W., Ungersboeck, A. and Boesch, P. (2006). Long-term clinical and radiographic outcome of the PPF system in ceramic-on-polyethylene hip bearings, *Hip Int*, **16**(2), 75–80.

Lexer, E. (1914). Free transplantation, *Ann Surg*, **60**(2), 166–194.

Long, W.T. (2005). The clinical performance of metal-on-metal as an articulation surface in total hip replacement, *Iowa Orthop J*, **25**, 10–16.

Lowendorf, C.S. (1932). Whitman reconstruction operation on the hip joint: An analysis of late results, *Arch Surg*, **25**(5), 863–869.

Mahalingam, K. and Reidy, D. (1996). Smith-Petersen Vitallium mould arthroplasty: A 45-year follow-up, *J Bone Joint Surg Br*, **78**(3), 496–497.

McKee, G.K. and Watson-Farrar, J. (1966). Replacement of arthritic hips by the McKee–Farrar prosthesis, *J Bone Joint Surg Br*, **48**(2), 245–259.

McKellop, H., Park, S.H., Chiesa, R., Doorn, P., Lu, B., Normand, P. *et al.* (1996). *In vivo* wear of 3 types of metal on metal hip prostheses during 2 decades of use, *Clin Orthop Relat R*, **329**, 128–140.

Michaud, R.J. and Rashad, S.Y. (1995). Spontaneous fracture of the ceramic ball in a ceramic-polyethylene total hip arthroplasty, *J Arthroplasty*, **10**(6), 863–867.

Mittelmeier, H. (1984). Hip joint replacement in young patients, *Z Orthop Unfallchir*, **122**(01), 20–26.

Mittelmeier, H. and Heisel, J. (1992). Sixteen-years' experience with ceramic hip prostheses, *Clin Orthop Rel R*, **282**, 64–72.

Moore, A.T. and Böhlman, H.R. (1943). Metal hip joint. A case report, *J Bone Joint Surg Am*, **25**(3), 688–692.

Papatheodorou, L.K., Baratz, M.E. and Sotereanos, D.G. (2013). Elbow arthritis: Current concepts, *J Hand Surg-Am*, **38**(3), 605–613.

Pridie, K.H. (1955). The problem of the broken Judet prosthesis, *J Bone Joint Surg Br*, **37**(2), 224–227.

Ratliff, A.H. (1983). Ernest William Hey Groves and his contributions to orthopaedic surgery, *Ann Roy Coll Surg*, **65**(3), 203–206.

Ring, P.A. (1968). Complete replacement arthroplasty of the hip by the ring prosthesis, *J Bone Joint Surg Br*, **50**(4), 720–731.

Santanapipatkul, P. and Udomkiat, P. (2012). Smith–Petersen mould arthroplasty: A 48-year follow-up, *Siriraj Med J*, **64**(4), 127–128.

Scales, J.T. and Zarek, J.M. (1954). Biomechanical problems of the original Judet prosthesis, *Brit Med J*, **1**(4869), 1007–1013.

Schreurs, B.W., Kats, J., Buma, P. and Gardeniers, J.W. (2001). Histology of the bone-implant interface 45 years after bilateral implantation of a Judet acrylic hip prosthesis: A case report, *Acta Orthop Belg*, **67**(4), 403–406.

Sedel, L., Kerboull, L., Christel, P., Meunier, A. and Witvoet, J. (1990). Alumina-on-alumina hip replacement. Results and survivorship in young patients, *J Bone Joint Surg Br*, **72**(4), 658–663.

Semlitsch, M., Lehmann, M., Weber, H., Doerre, E. and Willert, H.G. (1977). New prospects for a prolonged functional life-span of artificial hip joints by using the material combination polyethylene/aluminium oxide ceramic/metal, *J Biomed Mater Res*, **11**(4), 537–552.

Smith-Petersen, M.N. (1939). Arthroplasty of the hip: A new method, *J Bone Joint Surg Am*, **21**(2), 269–288.

Smith-Petersen, M.N. (1948). Evolution of mould arthroplasty of the hip joint, *J Bone Joint Surg Br*, **30**(1), 59–75.

Sugano, N., Nishii, T., Nakata, K., Masuhara, K. and Takaoka, K. (1995). Polyethylene sockets and alumina ceramic heads in cemented total hip arthroplasty. A ten-year study, *J Bone Joint Surg Br*, **77**(4), 548–556.

Tatari, H., Alici, E. and Havitcioglu, H. (2001). Forty-two year survival with bilateral Judet hip prostheses, *Arch Orthop Traum Su*, **121**(1–2), 112–113.

Tennent, T.D. and Eastwood, D.M. (1998). Survival of the Judet hip prosthesis, *J Roy Soc Med*, **91**(7), 385–386.

Urban, J.A., Garvin, K.L., Boese, C.K., Bryson, L., Pedersen, D.R., Callaghan, J.J. *et al.* (2001). Ceramic-on-polyethylene bearing surfaces in total hip arthroplasty. Seventeen to twenty-one-year results, *J Bone Joint Surg Am*, **83**(11), 1688–1694.

Venable, C.S., Stuck, W.G. and Beach, A. (1937). The effects on bone of the presence of metals; based upon electrolysis: An experimental study, *Ann Surg*, **105**(6), 917–938.

White, C. (1770). *Cases in Surgery, With Remarks*, W. Johnston, London.

Wiles, P. (1958). The surgery of the osteoarthritic hip, *Brit J Surg*, **45**(193), 488–497.

Wiles, P. (2003). The Classic: The Surgery of the osteo-arthritic hip, *Clin Orthop Rel R*, **417**, 3–16.

Willert, H.G. and Semlitsch, M. (1977). Reactions of the articular capsule to wear products of artificial joint prostheses, *J Biomed Mater Res*, **11**(2), 157–164.

Willmann, G.M.S.P. (2000). Ceramic femoral head retrieval data, *Clin Orthop Rel R*, **379**, 22–28.

Chapter 3

In Vitro and *In Vivo* Wear Evaluation

J. Philippe Kretzer[a], Jörn Reinders[a], Ulrike Müller[a], Christian Schröder[b], Carmen Zietz[c], Christian Gibney[a] and Robert Sonntag[a]

[a]*Laboratory of Biomechanics and Implant Research, Clinic for Orthopedics and Trauma Surgery, Center for Orthopedics, Trauma Surgery and Spinal Cord Injury, Heidelberg University Hospital, Heidelberg, Germany*

[b]*Department of Orthopaedic Surgery, Physical Medicine and Rehabilitation Campus Großhadern Ludwig-Maximilians-University Munich, Germany*

[c]*Biomechanics and Implant Technology Research Laboratory, Department of Orthopaedics, University Medical Center Rostock, Rostock, Germany*

Ever since the implementation of artificial joints for young and active patients began to increase, the demand for long-term durability of these implants has also been on the rise. Wear debris (e.g. particles and ions), which is generated through the articulation of the sliding surfaces of these implants, is then released into the surrounding tissue (Hallab and Jacobs, 2009; Purdue *et al.*, 2007; Revell, 2008). The consequences experienced by the patient depend upon the quantity, size, form, and chemical composition of the wear debris from the artificial joint (Fisher *et al.*, 2004; Gallo *et al.*, 2010; Libouban *et al.*, 2009; Purdue *et al.*, 2007; Wooley *et al.*, 2002). Negative consequences from the infiltration of wear debris into the periprosthetic tissue include particle-induced osteolysis and, as more recently observed, metal ion-induced cytotoxic and tissue-corroding processes (Glyn-Jones *et al.*, 2009; Langton *et al.*, 2010).

Frictional forces that result from the articulation of the artificial joints are immediately transferred to the implanted prosthetic components (Bishop *et al.*, 2008). With increasing friction in the joint comes a higher stress on implant–bone interfaces or on modular connections.

New implantation concepts, designs, and materials have become higher priorities in the tribologic studies in arthroplasty. Pre-clinical wear studies have been conducted to determine the mass or volume of the wear products, with respect to the quantity, size, and morphology of wear particles *in vitro*. However, these experiments are often limited as the clinical demands are influenced by an excessive amount of parameters. The clinical evaluation normally targets specific parameters, such as the functionality or longevity of the joint replacements, and as such the quantification of wear is thereby dependent on the joint replacement. Therefore, the success or otherwise of a new material or design will only be established following a final and comprehensive assessment after several years.

In addition to planned clinical trials, which usually only take a limited number of cases into account and are often only performed at specialized centers, nationwide surveys from the implant registries can provide the basis of the probability of joint replacement revisions in the long-term. However, no substantial conclusions about the materials' wear behaviors can be drawn from the registries; rather, it simply describes the plethora of causes which can lead to the joint replacement revision.

1. *In Vitro* Wear Evaluation

Generally, experimental studies in tribology are divided into friction and wear experiments. Friction studies aim to ascertain the sources of the frictional forces while wear studies serve to generate relevant quantities of wear products in order to evaluate their quantity and morphology and to test their biological reactivity (Section 3.1 has been adopted from (Kretzer *et al.*, 2012) with kind permission of Springer Science+Business Media).

1.1. *Simulation*

Screening tests offer different assessment options compared to complex simulator studies. Joint simulators are intended to reflect joint-specific movements and loading while the screening tests only consider the area of contact (i.e. the point at which the surfaces articulate). In doing so, it has been established that environmental conditions such as temperature and the ambient fluid (synovial fluid) are based on physiological constraints. Proteins in the synovial fluid, for example, have an effect on the lubricating performance of the joint partners (Scholes and Unsworth, 2006). Therefore, as a replacement for the synovial fluid, bovine serum, which is adjusted to a protein content of 20–30 g/L and tempered at 37°C, is often used.

1.1.1. *Screening tests*

The development of new articulating materials is often evaluated at earlier stages under simplified *in vitro* conditions. The purpose of these screening tests is a fast, cost-effective, and reproducible test of the intrinsic material and system properties as an alternative to the extensive wear simulator tests.

Simple test specimens and varying testing concepts are used: (A) a pin articulates along a curved path on a plate (pin-on-plate, Figure 3-1); or, (B) a pin articulates on a rotating plate (pin-on-disk) or is rotated on a surface plate (ring-on-disk).

From this, a distinction can be made between unidirectional motion (e.g. linear movement) and multidirectional motion (any trajectory). With the help of such screening test units, which are used widely in industry and research, a large number of samples can be simultaneously analyzed and statistically evaluated. These results should be viewed with consideration of movement patterns, specimen geometries, and loading behavior, and without the need to reflect the constraints of clinically expected conditions.

1.1.2. *Hip wear simulator*

In order to simulate the loads and movements of the hip joint, two simulator concepts are primarily employed: (a) multi-axial hip

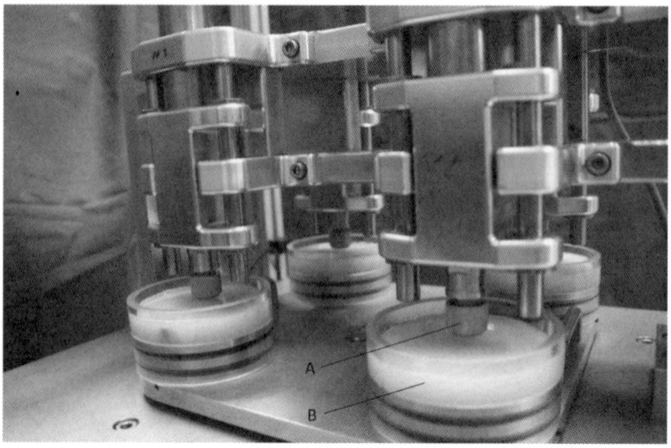

Figure 3-1. An example of a 'pin on plate' testing device with four stations. The pin is held in a fixture (A) and articulates with the plate in the test medium (B) (reproduced with kind permission of Springer Science+Business Media) (Kretzer *et al.*, 2012).

simulators (in accordance with ISO 14242-1), by which various degrees of freedom can be simulated (e.g. running, walking up stairs); and, (b) orbital (bi-axial rocking) simulators (in accordance with ISO 14242-3) where the motion sequence is defined by the orientation of the implant fixture. These differences should be considered while interpreting the results of the wear tests.

Laboratory trials limitedly reflect *in vivo* conditions. In accordance with ISO 14242-1, all degrees of freedom of the hip joint (flexion, abduction, rotation, and axial loading) will therefore be achieved, but only the kinematics and loading for the condition of level walking are simulated at a frequency of 1 Hz (Figure 3-2). In reality, multiple activity patterns may act on the hip joint that can lead to conditions that are not considered in ISO 14242-1. McKellop classified the clinically relevant wear forms into four wear modes (Mode 1–4, Figure 3-3) (Kretzer, 2010; Kretzer *et al.*, 2012; McKellop, 2007).

Only mode 1, which describes the wear caused by the primary articulation of the sliding components, is covered by the ISO 14242-1 standard. On the other hand, wear modes 2–4 illustrate the phenomena of an increased proportion of clinical failure

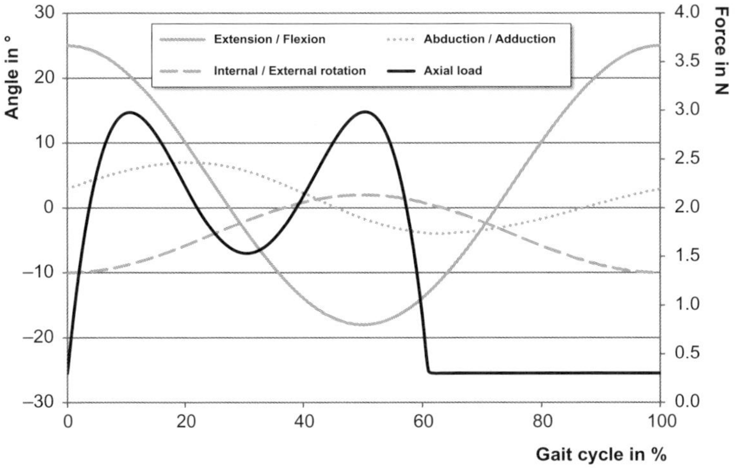

Figure 3-2. Boundary conditions for the level walking according to ISO 14242-1. Gait of the hip joint (reproduced with kind permission of Springer Science+Business Media) (Kretzer *et al.*, 2012).

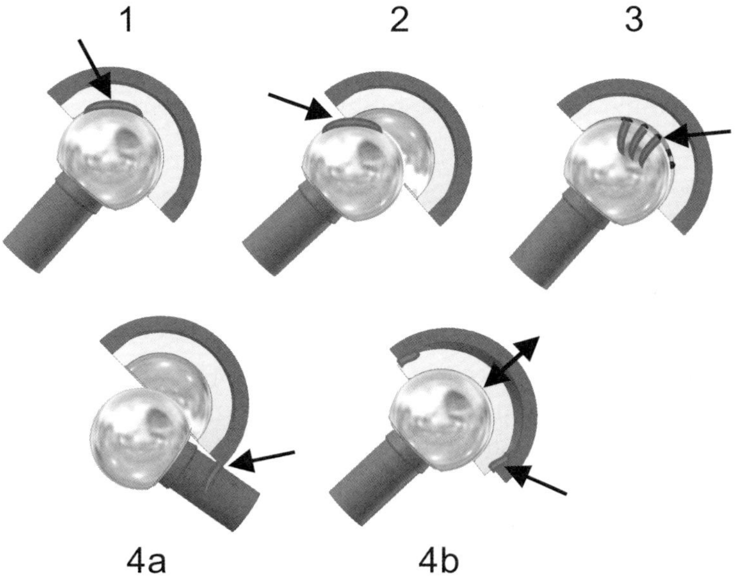

Figure 3-3. Wear modes in context of the hip joint. Wear can take place through various interfaces; ideally, only those surfaces intended for articulation are in contact (mode 1). However, clinically, the articulation may also occur on unintended surfaces (reproduced with kind permission of Springer Science+Business Media and ISTE Ltd.) (Kretzer *et al.*, 2012; Kretzer, 2010).

cases particularly found in hard-on-hard bearings (metal-on-metal or ceramic-on-ceramic) due to design and application problems, such as high cup inclination (De Haan *et al.*, 2008) or smaller clearances between the head and acetabular component (Heisel *et al.*, 2009; Underwood *et al.*, 2011). In wear mode 2, one sliding surface articulates with another component that is not supposed to be an articulating surface. This occurs, for example, in subluxation, when the femoral head slides over the acetabular rim (edge loading) resulting in a characteristic, half moon-shaped wear pattern (stripe wear) (Walter *et al.*, 2004).

Mode 3 describes the influence of third-body particles (e.g. cement particles that penetrate the joint space), which can lead to increased wear, even with polyethylene bearing couples (Bragdon *et al.*, 2003). In mode 4, two surfaces articulate with each other that are not intended to do so, such as the neck at the outer rim of the socket (impingement) or micro motions along the posterior surface (back side wear) (Malik *et al.*, 2007).

The implementation of these clinically relevant wear modes in existing simulator concepts is a crucial issue in current research (such as the dynamic integration of subluxation effects in motion pattern of the hip joint).

1.1.3. *Knee wear simulator*

The knee joint involves complicated kinematics. In addition to extension and flexion, the joint shows a complex rolling and sliding movement in the sagittal plane in conjunction with rotation in the transverse plane. The extent of these coarse movements are determined by the active muscle forces and limited by passive structures like the cruciate and collateral ligaments.

Knee wear simulators are used in order to replicate these movements (Figure 3-4). There are two standardized test methods: Force-controlled (ISO 14243-1) and displacement-controlled (ISO 14243-3) simulation. In the displacement-controlled simulation, the extent of the anterior–posterior (AP) translation, as well as the internal and external rotation (IE) are given. The knee design (e.g. conformity), ligament laxity, and changes to the components due to abrasion are

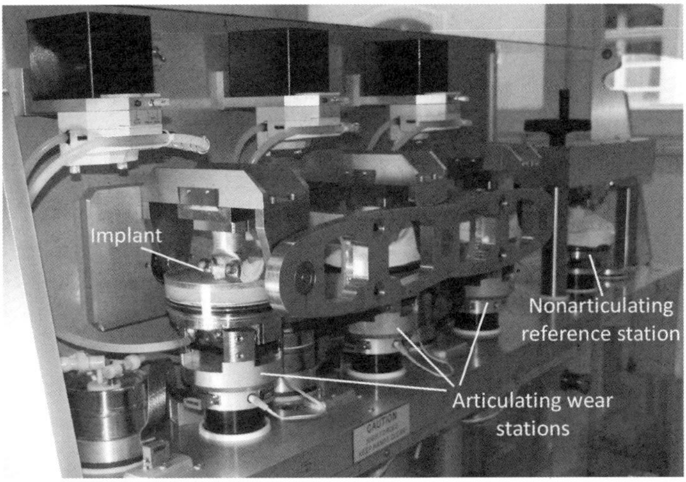

Figure 3-4. Example of a knee wear simulator.

not taken into account in this simulation mode as motions are independent of these parameters. Contrarily, in the force-controlled simulation, neither displacements nor angles are predefined; rather, the forces and moments drive these motions (AP and IE) with the exception of flexion angle. The kinematic range is determined by the active forces, implant design, and motion inhibition of soft tissue structures. Up until now, the soft tissue structures are most easily simulated through mechanical springs. Newer concepts simulate the ligament and soft tissue structures based on non-linear virtual ligament models in contrast to the linear behavior of mechanical springs. This allows for the definition of individual ligament parameters, which have been shown to influence the wear behavior (Kretzer *et al.*, 2010a).

The kinematics of the knee joint influence wear to a large extent, which means that increased AP translation and IE rotation leads to increased polyethylene wear (McEwen *et al.*, 2005). However, not only the magnitude of the unidirectional movements is important. The combination of both movements lead to multidirectional movement and, consequently, cross-shear. The reduction of cross-shearing is an approach to wear reduction. Thus, the mobile-bearing knee designs follow the approach via two articulating surfaces (femoral and tibial) in order to achieve a decoupling of multidirectional motions and consequentially, wear reduction. Furthermore, the contact pressures should be reduced through increased conformity, whereby the wear is believed to be further reduced. Both clinical and experimental studies showed controversial results regarding the effectiveness of these approaches (Barbour *et al.*, 1997; Grupp *et al.*, 2009; Manson *et al.*, 2010; McEwen *et al.*, 2005). Low-congruent, fixed-bearing knee designs have also shown lower wear as compared to high-conforming or mobile bearing designs (Galvin *et al.*, 2009; Kretzer *et al.*, 2011). It then becomes clear that it is a combination of several mechanisms that influence the wear behavior of artificial knee joints.

Standardized wear tests, however, often lead to different wear behaviors in comparison to retrieval studies (Harman *et al.*, 2009). In keeping with wear studies at the hip, test methods that simulate extreme cases of clinical situations such as incorrect component positioning or third-body wear are of interest in current research (Ezzet *et al.*, 2011).

1.2. *Wear Analytics*

In order to determine and morphologically evaluate wear products, different methods are available that should be chosen based on the research in question. It is important here not to derive information only from the total wear mass (with respect to total wear volume), but also from the size and morphology of the wear products; together these parameters determine the biological potential of the wear products. As part of tribological implant studies, wear measurements are performed primarily at defined intervals (about every 0.5 or 1.0 million steps/cycles). The wear rate is then determined from the accumulated results (wear mass or wear volume in relation to the number of steps/cycles).

1.2.1. *Gravimetry*

In order to determine the gravimetric wear rate of the implant components, the loss of mass from the individual articulating components during the wear process in the simulator is determined (e.g. in accordance with ISO 14242-2). After careful cleaning, the samples are weighed with an analytical balance at least three times. This is necessary as the samples can absorb or give off humidity through their surface. The results gathered are acceptable if the measured differences in mass is less than 0.1 mg. Additionally, polymeric components (e.g. polyethylene) can increase in mass due to liquid absorption during the simulator tests. To minimize this error, all the polymeric components are stored in the test fluid for several weeks before the actual wear test until no measureable gain in mass is detected (conditioning). Furthermore, the wear mass of the articulating components is adjusted with a non-articulating control that is also stored in liquid (load–soak–control). Through this process, the gravimetric wear analysis achieved high accuracy and precision that led to a standard analytical procedure, especially in the wear analysis of polyethylene (Grupp *et al.*, 2010; Kretzer *et al.*, 2011; McEwen *et al.*, 2005; Utzschneider *et al.*, 2009a).

1.2.2. *Geometry*

The approach to geometric wear analysis works to determine the corresponding change in wear volume due to changes in the geometry of the implant. In addition, further information on the wear scar regions and discrepancies in roundness of the implant can be ascertained. The measurement of the implant is normally acquired by means of tactile scanning in a coordinate measuring machine (CMM). Because of the low wear volumes in artificial joints, the CMM measurements must exhibit very high accuracy and precision (within a few microns). As disturbances emerge, particularly in terms of temperature fluctuations, volumetric changes in the measured object become more common. For polymeric materials, creep (deformation) of the material under loading and the liquid intake has a direct effect on the volumetric measurement. Due to these limitations, geometric wear analysis is not often employed for the *in vitro* determination of wear. In contrast, geometric wear analysis has been shown to be the most appropriate method in determining wear on clinically retrieved components (Figure 3-5).

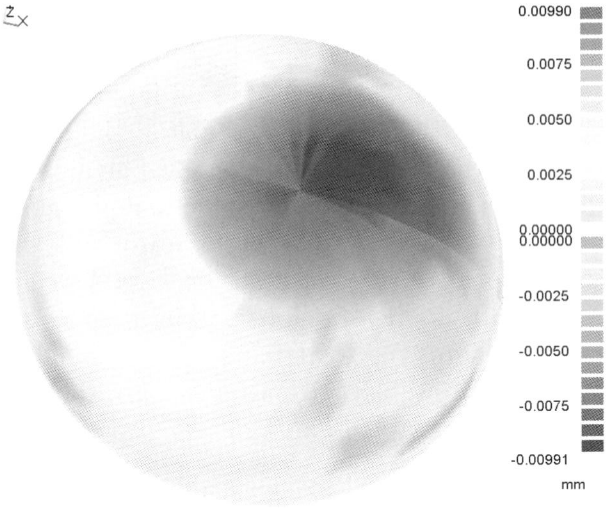

Figure 3-5. Geometric analysis of a worn femoral head by measurements from a coordinate measuring machine.

1.2.3. *Ion analysis*

While the gravimetric or geometric measuring methods determine the changes in geometry or mass of the implant, ion analysis examines the ambient medium for wear products. In order to accomplish this, the ambient medium must first be chemically broken down so that all of the wear particles can be resolved to their atomic constituents. Depending on the material, this can be achieved through the addition of acids at elevated temperatures and pressures (e.g. in a microwave high-pressure autoclave). Finally, the solution is analyzed by atomic absorption spectroscopy or inductively coupled plasma mass spectroscopy. The wear mass or the wear volume is then calculated based on the ion concentration (Kretzer *et al.*, 2010b).

The ion analytic methodology is advantageous as it offers high detection sensitivity and accuracy. This renders it particularly suitable for materials with very low wear and for the detection of individual chemical constituents. Furthermore, ion values that have been collected experimentally can be correlated with clinical ion values from the patient (Heisel *et al.*, 2008). A highly purified environment that is free from contamination is necessary, however. The disadvantages to this are the high methodological effort and the procedural inability for pairings with polyethylene since carbon (which is an essential constituent in polyethylene) is also contained within the surrounding liquid.

1.2.4. *Particle analysis*

Particle characterization is a sophisticated analytical method for determining the morphology and size of wear particles. Joint fluid (from patients), serum (from simulator studies), or tissue samples that have been collected during revision surgery have to be treated chemically or enzymatically. Depending on the implant material, the samples may be subjected to degeneration by highly concentrated hydrochloric acid, sodium hydroxide, or proteinase K in conjunction with a strong solvent such as methanol (Niedzwiecki *et al.*, 2001). All of the organic ingredients go into a solution so that the wear particles remain in their solid states. The degenerated and diluted particle suspension is subsequently filtered off via a fine porous filter (pore size 15–100 nm) and then examined using a scanning electron microscope (SEM) (Figure 3-6). The generated SEM micrographs of

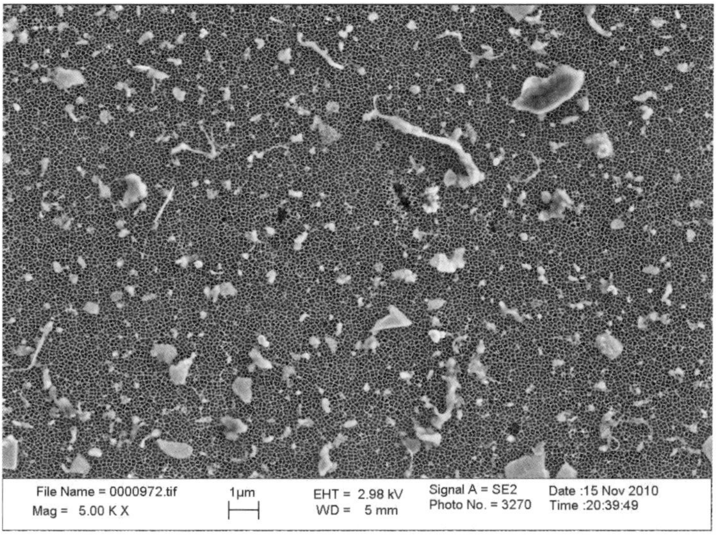

Figure 3-6. Isolated polyethylene wear particles in SEM.

the wear particles are evaluated quantitatively and qualitatively with special particle analysis software. Parameters such as the number and size of the particles as well as the shape of the particles play a role in the evaluation. The shape parameters can be calculated in order to differentiate and distinguish the particles into spherical, fibrilar, rough, or smooth (Sieving *et al.*, 2003; Utzschneider *et al.*, 2009b). Because this methodology lacks three-dimensional imaging capabilities (only length and width can be measured in SEM), no direct conclusions can be made in terms of the particle size and quantity in terms of the gravimetric or volumetric wear rate. However, the particle analysis allows for the estimation of biological damage potential for the examined wear particles, as numerous studies have shown a correlation between particle number, size, morphology, and material along with their biological activity (Catelas *et al.*, 2011; Fang *et al.*, 2003; Utzschneider *et al.*, 2010).

2. *In Vivo* Wear Evaluation

The clinical wear behavior can be determined either radiologically on implanted components within the clinical follow-up or on retrieved components after revision surgery.

2.1. *Radiographic Studies*

Radiographic wear measurements are based generally on the change in position of the implant components due to wear between the components themselves. This is illustrated in Figure 3-7 with the example of the hip joint. Assuming that the femoral head is initially centered with the acetabular shell, an example of migration of the femoral head after 20 years can be seen. This shift can be measured and is expressed as linear penetration.

It is important, however, to consider that radiographic wear measurements can only be taken on polyethylene bearing couples. Because of the X-ray density and the low wear rates of hard-on-hard bearings (e.g. metal-on-metal or ceramic-on-ceramic), off-centering of the femoral head is difficult to detect precisely. With regards to polyethylene bearing couples, it must also be noted that the head

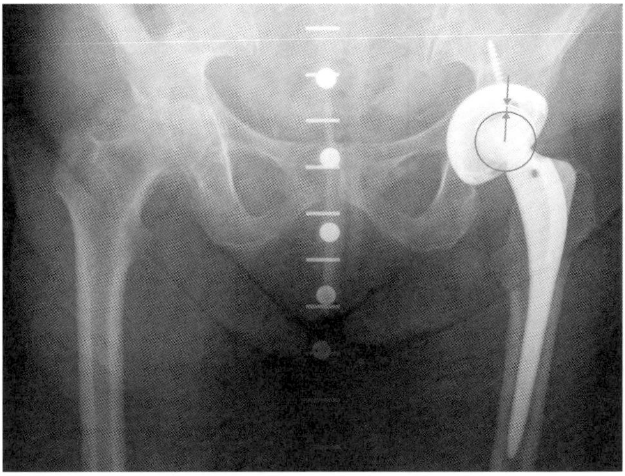

Figure 3-7. X-ray of the pelvis: After 20 years, a migration of the femoral can be seen. The linear displacement can be quantified as head penetration.

penetration is not solely a result of wear, but also is a result of the cold flow (creep) of the material. Therefore, it is most practical to compare numerous X-rays with each other over an extended period of time. While the wear of a material over a number of years is viewed to resemble a linear relationship, cold flow-induced deformation is, instead, initially increased and becomes noticeably reduced over time. Figure 3-8 shows the profile of head penetration as an example; during the first two years, increased penetration occurs, which is mainly due to the cold flow-induced deformation denoted by the dashed line. As the process persists, cold flow plays a minor role and wear becomes the relevant factor in terms of head penetration. Based on the slope of the solid line, the annual linear wear rate can be calculated.

In order to determine the linear and volumetric wear, the head dimensions and direction of the head penetration must be known. For this, numerous methods for the quantification of head penetration have been established which are divided into two-dimensional manual techniques, two-dimensional computer-assisted techniques, and three-dimensional computer-assisted techniques (McCalden *et al.*, 2005). While these methods work well for hip implants and are widely applied (Charnley *et al.*, 1969; Devane *et al.*, 1995a; Devane *et al.*,

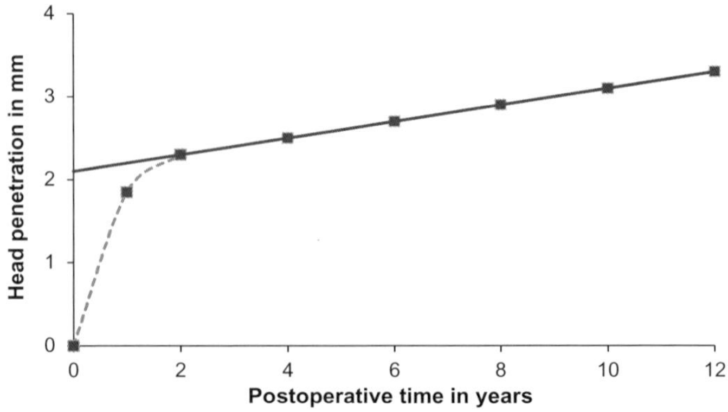

Figure 3-8. An example of a follow-up study of head penetration: It can be seen that in the first two years, there is a stronger influence of penetration due to cold flow-induced deformation (dashed line). During subsequent observations, however, cold flow only plays a minor role in penetration and wear became the dominating factor.

1995b; Hui *et al.*, 2003; Ilchmann *et al.*, 1995; Kang *et al.*, 2003; Livermore *et al.*, 1990; Martell and Berdia, 1997; Pedersen *et al.*, 1998), they are limited in terms of wear measurements in knee replacements. Although the linear wear can be measured (Collier *et al.*, 2003; Engh *et al.*, 2013; Hide *et al.*, 2000), any conclusion on the wear volume remains elusive as the inlay geometry, individual kinematics, and thus the resulting wear area are largely unknown. Nevertheless, a method that has been postulated to circumvent this problem has been described in the literature (Gill *et al.*, 2006).

2.2. *Retrieval Analysis*

In addition to determining the wear of the implanted prostheses, the retrievals must also be investigated for their wear behavior. However, the reasons for revision should be taken into account as the retrievals can come from a clinical situation that does not necessarily correspond to an ideal condition (e.g. misalignment) and, therefore, does not warrant general conclusions.

In order to determine the linear or volumetric wear for the explanted components, the geometric wear analysis (see Section 1.2.2) has been shown to be a common and reliable method. It is especially

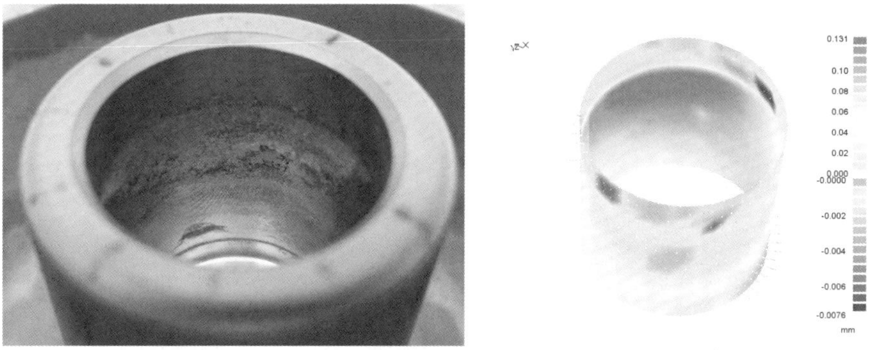

Figure 3-9. Left: Heavily corroded and worn taper connection on an explanted femoral head. Right: A geometric measurement and calculation of wear.

suitable when the components to be analyzed correspond to simple geometric elements (e.g. femoral head/acetabulum liner — spherical, taper — conical), which allows them to be compared to an ideal geometry (Figure 3-9). It should be considered that a change in volume is not just a product of wear; rather, it can also be caused by deformation (see Section 1.2.2).

There are numerous retrieval studies that quantify the linear or volumetric wear for explanted components through geometric wear analysis (Bishop *et al.*, 2013; Hall *et al.*, 1995; Morlock *et al.*, 2008; Raimondi *et al.*, 2000; Sieber *et al.*, 1999).

In addition to the quantification of wear, qualitative and semi-quantitative methods have been established in order to describe the wear or the extent of damage to retrieved components. One often applied method is described by Hood *et al.* in which a reproducible evaluation of the type, prevalence, and the intensity of damage to polyethylene components in knee arthroplasty is achievable (Hood *et al.*, 1983).

The articulation surface of polyethylene inlays is divided into ten regions (see Figure 3-10) and the retro-patellar articulating surfaces in four regions. The surface are examined regarding damage via light microscopy with 10× magnification. Seven types of damage are distinguished: Pitting, embedded debris, scratching, delamination, surface deformation, burnishing, and abrasion. In each region of the

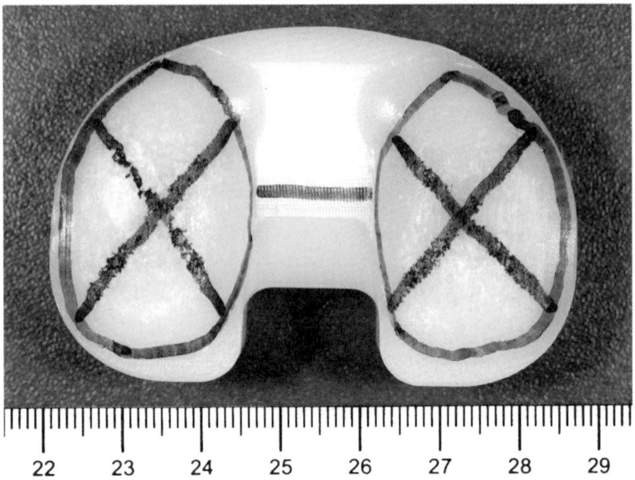

Figure 3-10. Explanted polyethylene inlays with scoring by Hood (Hood *et al.*, 1983).

polyethylene inlay and the retro-patellar articulating surfaces, the prevalence and extent of damage is rated on a scale from 0 to 3 based on the aforementioned criteria. A score of 0 means that no damage was detected in the corresponding zone. The scores 1, 2, and 3 correspond to <10%, 10–50%, and >50% detected wear in the zone under consideration. Through this method, the extent of the damage is evaluated along with the intensity. The total score is calculated by summing the score for each damage type across every examined region. Accordingly, a maximum score of 210 (3 as a maximum score/region × 10 regions × 7 damage types) is possible for the tibia component and a maximum score of 84 (3 as a maximum score/region × 4 regions × 7 damage types) for the retro-patellar replacement.

Furthermore, the extent of oxidation OH the polyethylene can also be used as an assessment criterion for material degradation or aging (Currier *et al.*, 2013; Hara *et al.*, 2008; MacDonald *et al.*, 2011, 2012). This can be achieved through Fourier transform infrared spectroscopy (FTIR). This method is standardized according to ASTM F2102-13. The IR absorption of a sample (20–300 nm thin slices) is measured in a FTIR spectrometer and the resulting spectrum of absorbance is plotted against the wavelength. The oxidation index is usually specified in order to quantify the damage or oxidation of polyethylene by FTIR analysis. The oxidation index is calculated from the ratio of the area under the carbonyl band to the area under the methyl band or, alternatively, to the area under the H_2O or CH_2 bands. Since the oxidation index is not constant over the entire profile, it is usually plotted over the height of the sample.

3. Summary and Conclusion

In total joint replacement, materials and implant design concepts are continuously being developed. Reliable and valid methodologies are required to assess these developments accurately. Since wear is an important evaluation criterion, several methods have been established which initially permit *in vitro* assessments in the context of experiments and then can evaluate their clinical use *in vivo*. Even with failures in the development of arthroplasty, it can be stated unequivocally that the overall performance and durability of implants have become increasingly better to which experimental and clinical wear analysis have contributed significantly.

References

Barbour, P.S., Barton, D.C. and Fisher, J. (1997). The influence of stress conditions on the wear of UHMWPE for total joint replacements, *J Mater Sci-Mater M*, **8**, 603–611.

Bishop, N., Witt, F., Pourzal, R., Fischer, A., Rutschi, M., Michel, M. *et al.* (2013). Wear patterns of taper connections in retrieved large diameter metal-on-metal bearings, *J Orthop Res*, **31**, 1116–1122.

Bishop, N.E., Waldow, F. and Morlock, M.M. (2008). Friction moments of large metal-on-metal hip joint bearings and other modern designs, *Med Eng Phys*, **30**, 1057–1064.

Bragdon, C.R., Jasty, M., Muratoglu, O.K., O'Connor, D.O. and Harris, W.H. (2003). Third-body wear of highly cross-linked polyethylene in a hip simulator, *J Arthroplasty*, **18**, 553–561.

Catelas, I., Wimmer, M.A. and Utzschneider, S. (2011). Polyethylene and metal wear particles: Characteristics and biological effects, *Semin Immunopathol*, **33**, 257–271.

Charnley, J., Kamangar, A. and Longfield, M.D. (1969). The optimum size of prosthetic heads in relation to the wear of plastic sockets in total replacement of the hip, *Med Biol Eng*, **7**, 31–39.

Collier, M.B., Jewett, B.A. and Engh Jr., C.A. (2003). Clinical assessment of tibial polyethylene thickness: Comparison of radiographic measurements with as-implanted and as-retrieved thicknesses, *J Arthroplasty*, **18**, 860–866.

Currier, B.H., van Citters, D.W., Currier, J.H., Carlson, E.M., Tibbo, M.E. and Collier, J.P. (2013). *In vivo* oxidation in retrieved highly crosslinked tibial inserts, *J Biomed Mater Res B Appl Biomater*, **101**, 441–448.

De Haan, R., Pattyn, C., Gill, H.S., Murray, D.W., Campbell, P.A. and de Smet, K. (2008). Correlation between inclination of the acetabular component and metal ion levels in metal-on-metal hip resurfacing replacement, *J Bone Joint Surg Br*, **90**, 1291–1297.

Devane, P.A., Bourne, R.B., Rorabeck, C.H., Hardie, R.M. and Horne, J.G. (1995a). Measurement of polyethylene wear in metal-backed acetabular cups. I. Three-dimensional technique, *Clin Orthop Relat R*, **319**, 303–316.

Devane, P.A., Bourne, R.B., Rorabeck, C.H., MacDonald, S. and Robinson, E.J. (1995b). Measurement of polyethylene wear in metal-backed acetabular cups. II. Clinical application, *Clin Orthop Relat R*, **319**, 317–326.

Engh Jr., C.A., Collier, M.B., Hopper Jr., R.H., Hatten, K.M. and Engh, G.A. (2013). Radiographically measured total knee wear is constant and predicts failure, *J Arthroplasty*, **28**, 1338–1344.

Ezzet, K.A., Hermida, J.C., Steklov, N. and D'Lima, D.D. (2011). Wear of polyethylene against oxidized zirconium femoral components effect of aggressive kinematic conditions and malalignment in total knee arthroplasty, *J Arthroplasty*, **27**(1), 116–121.

Fang, H.W., Hsu, S.M. and Sengers, J.V. (2003). Generation of narrowly distributed ultra-high-molecular-weight polyethylene particles by surface texturing techniques, *J Biomed Mater Res B Appl Biomater*, **67**, 741–749.

Fisher, J., McEwen, H.M., Tipper, J.L., Galvin, A.L., Ingram, J., Kamali, A. *et al.* (2004). Wear, debris, and biologic activity of cross-linked polyethylene in the knee: Benefits and potential concerns, *Clin Orthop Relat R*, **428**, 114–119.

Gallo, J., Slouf, M. and Goodman, S.B. (2010). The relationship of polyethylene wear to particle size, distribution, and number: A possible factor explaining the risk of osteolysis after hip arthroplasty, *J Biomed Mater Res B Appl Biomater*, **94**, 171–177.

Galvin, A.L., Kang, L., Udofia, I., Jennings, L.M., McEwen, H.M., Jin, Z. *et al.* (2009). Effect of conformity and contact stress on wear in fixed-bearing total knee prostheses, *J Biomech*, **42**, 1898–1902.

Gill, H.S., Waite, J.C., Short, A., Kellett, C.F., Price, A.J. and Murray, D.W. (2006). In vivo measurement of volumetric wear of a total knee replacement, *Knee*, **13**, 312–317.

Glyn-Jones, S., Pandit, H., Kwon, Y.M., Doll, H., Gill, H.S. and Murray, D.W. (2009). Risk factors for inflammatory pseudotumour formation following hip resurfacing, *J Bone Joint Surg Br*, **91**, 1566–1574.

Grupp, T.M., Stulberg, D., Kaddick, C., Maas, A., Fritz, B., Schwiesau, J. *et al.* (2009). Fixed bearing knee congruency — influence on contact mechanics, abrasive wear and kinematics, *Int J Artif Organs*, **32**, 213–223.

Grupp, T.M., Utzschneider, S., Schroder, C., Schwiesau, J., Fritz, B., Maas, A. *et al.* (2010). Biotribology of alternative bearing materials for unicompartmental knee arthroplasty, *Acta Biomater*, **6**, 3601–3610.

Hall, R.M., Unsworth, A., Craig, P.S., Hardaker, C., Siney, P. and Wroblewski, B.M. (1995). Measurement of wear in retrieved acetabular sockets, *Proc Inst Mech Eng H*, **209**, 233–242.

Hallab, N.J. and Jacobs, J.J. (2009). Biologic effects of implant debris, *Bull NYU Hosp Jt Dis*, **67**, 182–188.

Hara, K., Kaku, N., Tsumura, H. and Torisu, T. (2008). Analysis of wear and oxidation on retrieved bipolar polyethylene liner, *J Orthop Sci*, **13**, 366–370.

Harman, M.K., Desjardins, J., Benson, L., Banks, S.A., Laberge, M. and Hodge, W.A. (2009). Comparison of polyethylene tibial insert damage from *in vivo* function and *in vitro* wear simulation, *J Orthop Res*, **27**, 540–548.

Heisel, C., Kleinhans, J.A., Menge, M. and Kretzer, J.P. (2009). Ten different hip resurfacing systems: Biomechanical analysis of design and material properties, *Int Orthop*, **33**, 939–943.

Heisel, C., Streich, N., Krachler, M., Jakubowitz, E. and Kretzer, J.P. (2008). Characterization of the running-in period in total hip resurfacing arthroplasty: An *in vivo* and *in vitro* metal ion analysis, *J Bone Joint Surg Am*, **90**(Suppl 3), 125–133.

Hide, I.G., Grainger, A.J., Wallace, I.W., Hui, A. and Campbell, R.S. (2000). A radiological technique for the assessment of wear in prosthetic knee replacements, *Skeletal Radiol*, **29**, 583–586.

Hood, R.W., Wright, T.M. and Burstein, A.H. (1983). Retrieval analysis of total knee prostheses: A method and its application to 48 total condylar prostheses, *J Biomed Mater Res*, **17**, 829–842.

Hui, A.J., McCalden, R.W., Martell, J.M., MacDonald, S.J., Bourne, R.B. and Rorabeck, C.H. (2003). Validation of two and three-dimensional radiographic techniques for measuring polyethylene wear after total hip arthroplasty, *J Bone Joint Surg Am*, **85**, 505–511.

Ilchmann, T., Mjoberg, B. and Wingstrand, H. (1995). Measurement accuracy in acetabular cup wear. Three retrospective methods compared with Roentgen stereophotogrammetry, *J Arthroplasty*, **10**, 636–642.

Kang, J.S., Park, S.R., Ebramzadeh, E. and Dorr, L.D. (2003). Measurement of polyethylene wear in total hip arthroplasty — accuracy versus ease of use, *Yonsei Med J*, **44**, 473–478.

Kretzer, J.P. (2010). Biotribology of total hip replacement: The metal-on-metal articulation, in Davim, J.P. (ed.), *Biotribology*, Wiley, Hoboken.

Kretzer, J.P., Jakubowitz, E., Reinders, J., Lietz, E., Moradi, B., Hofmann, K. *et al.* (2011). Wear analysis of unicondylar mobile bearing and fixed bearing knee systems: A knee simulator study, *Acta Biomateria*, **7**, 710–715.

Kretzer, J.P., Jakubowitz, E., Sonntag, R., Hofmann, K., Heisel, C. and Thomsen, M. (2010a). Effect of joint laxity on polyethylene wear in total knee replacement, *J Biomech*, **43**, 1092–1096.

Kretzer, J.P., Krachler, M., Reinders, J., Jakubowitz, E., Thomsen, M. and Heisel, C. (2010b). Determination of low wear rates in metal-on-metal hip joint replacements based on ultra trace element analysis in simulator studies, *Tribol Lett*, **37**, 23–29.

Kretzer, J.P., Zietz, C., Schroder, C., Reinders, J., Middelborg, L., Paulus, A. *et al.* (2012). Principles of tribological analysis of endoprostheses, *Orthopade*, **41**, 844–852.

Langton, D.J., Jameson, S.S., Joyce, T.J., Hallab, N.J., Natu, S. and Nargol, A.V. (2010). Early failure of metal-on-metal bearings in hip resurfacing and large-diameter total hip replacement: A consequence of excess wear, *J Bone Joint Surg Br*, **92**, 38–46.

Libouban, H., Massin, P., Gaudin, C., Mercier, P., Basle, M.F. and Chappard, D. (2009). Migration of wear debris of polyethylene depends on bone microarchitecture, *J Biomed Mater Res B Appl Biomater*, **90**, 730–737.

Livermore, J., Ilstrup, D. and Morrey, B. (1990). Effect of femoral head size on wear of the polyethylene acetabular component, *J Bone Joint Surg Am*, **72**, 518–528.

MacDonald, D., Hanzlik, J., Sharkey, P., Parvizi, J. and Kurtz, S.M. (2012). *In vivo* oxidation and surface damage in retrieved ethylene oxide-sterilized total knee arthroplasties, *Clin Orthop Relat R*, **470**, 1826–1833.

MacDonald, D., Sakona, A., Ianuzzi, A., Rimnac, C.M. and Kurtz, S.M. (2011). Do first-generation highly crosslinked polyethylenes oxidize *in vivo*?, *Clin Orthop Relat R*, **469**, 2278–2285.

Malik, A., Maheshwari, A. and Dorr, L.D. (2007). Impingement with total hip replacement, *J Bone Joint Surg Am*, **89**, 1832–1842.

Manson, T.T., Kelly, N.H., Lipman, J.D., Wright, T.M. and Westrich, G.H. (2010). Unicondylar knee retrieval analysis, *J Arthroplasty*, **25**, 108–111.

Martell, J.M. and Berdia, S. (1997). Determination of polyethylene wear in total hip replacements with use of digital radiographs, *J Bone Joint Surg Am*, **79**, 1635–1641.

McCalden, R.W., Naudie, D.D., Yuan, X. and Bourne, R.B. (2005). Radiographic methods for the assessment of polyethylene wear after total hip arthroplasty, *J Bone Joint Surg Am*, **87**, 2323–2334.

McEwen, H.M., Barnett, P.I., Bell, C.J., Farrar, R., Auger, D.D., Stone, M.H. *et al.* (2005). The influence of design, materials and kinematics on the *in vitro*wear of total knee replacements, *J Biomech*, **38**, 357–365.

McKellop, H.A. (2007). The lexicon of polyethylene wear in artificial joints, *Biomaterials*, **28**, 5049–5057.

Morlock, M.M., Bishop, N., Zustin, J., Hahn, M., Ruther, W. and Amling, M. (2008). Modes of implant failure after hip resurfacing: Morphological and wear analysis of 267 retrieval specimens, *J Bone Joint Surg Am*, **90**(Suppl 3), 89–95.

Niedzwiecki, S., Klapperich, C., Short, J., Jani, S., Ries, M. and Pruitt, L. (2001). Comparison of three joint simulator wear debris isolation techniques: Acid digestion, base digestion, and enzyme cleavage, *J Biomed Mater Res*, **56**, 245–249.

Pedersen, D.R., Brown, T.D., Hillis, S.L. and Callaghan, J.J. (1998). Prediction of long-term polyethylene wear in total hip arthroplasty, based on early wear measurements made using digital image analysis, *J Orthop Res*, **16**, 557–563.

Purdue, P.E., Koulouvaris, P., Potter, H.G., Nestor, B.J. and Sculco, T.P. (2007). The cellular and molecular biology of periprosthetic osteolysis, *Clin Orthop Relat R*, **454**, 251–261.

Raimondi, M.T., Sassi, R. and Pietrabissa, R. (2000). A method for the evaluation of the change in volume of retrieved acetabular cups, *Proc Inst Mech Eng H*, **214**, 577–587.

Revell, P.A. (2008). The combined role of wear particles, macrophages and lymphocytes in the loosening of total joint prostheses, *J R Soc Interface*, **5**, 1263–1278.

Scholes, S.C. and Unsworth, A. (2006). The effects of proteins on the friction and lubrication of artificial joints, *Proc Inst Mech Eng H*, **220**, 687–693.

Sieber, H.P., Rieker, C.B. and Kottig, P. (1999). Analysis of 118 second-generation metal-on-metal retrieved hip implants, *J Bone Joint Surg Br*, **81**, 46–50.

Sieving, A., Wu, B., Mayton, L., Nasser, S. and Wooley, P.H. (2003). Morphological characteristics of total joint arthroplasty-derived ultra-high molecular weight polyethylene (UHMWPE) wear debris that provoke inflammation in a murine model of inflammation, *J Biomed Mater Res A*, **64**, 457–464.

Underwood, R., Matthies, A., Cann, P., Skinner, J.A. and Hart, A.J. (2011). A comparison of explanted articular surface replacement and birmingham hip resurfacing components, *J Bone Joint Surg Br*, **93**, 1169–1177.

Utzschneider, S., Becker, F., Grupp, T.M., Sievers, B., Paulus, A., Gottschalk, O. *et al.* (2010). Inflammatory response against different carbon fiber-reinforced PEEK wear particles compared with UHMWPE *in vivo*, *Acta Biomater*, **6**, 4296–4304.

Utzschneider, S., Harrasser, N., Schroeder, C., Mazoochian, F. and Jansson, V. (2009a). Wear of contemporary total knee replacements — a knee simulator study of six current designs, *Clin Biomech*, **24**, 583–588.

Utzschneider, S., Paulus, A., Datz, J.C., Schroeder, C., Sievers, B., Wegener, B. *et al.* (2009b). Influence of design and bearing material on polyethylene wear particle generation in total knee replacement, *Acta Biomater*, **5**, 2495–2502.

Walter, W.L., Insley, G.M., Walter, W.K. and Tuke, M.A. (2004). Edge loading in third generation alumina ceramic-on-ceramic bearings: Stripe wear, *J Arthroplasty*, **19**, 402–413.

Wooley, P.H., Morren, R., Andary, J., Sud, S., Yang, S.Y., Mayton, L. *et al.* (2002). Inflammatory responses to orthopaedic biomaterials in the murine air pouch, *Biomaterials*, **23**, 517–526.

Chapter 4

Metal Bearings

Catherine Van Der Straeten
Research Department Orthopaedics and Traumatology;
Biobank, Ghent University Hospital,
Ghent, Belgium

1. Metallurgy of Metal Orthopaedic Joint Arthroplasty Devices

Metal devices used for joint arthroplasty consist of different metal alloys. A common alloy is cobalt–chromium–molybdenum (CoCrMo) consisting of $\geq$60% Co, $\pm$30% Cr, $\pm$6% Mo, <0.5% Ni, Fe, and Carbon (C). CoCrMo alloy is widely used in orthopaedic applications as it is the hardest known biocompatible alloy featuring a high wear and corrosion resistance, with all metal bearing components being made of CoCrMo alloy. The manufacturing process used on these alloys strongly influences the features produced. To a large extent, these are associated with the addition of carbon in the alloy, causing the formation of carbides in the microstructure. There are two types of CoCrMo alloys used for biomedical applications depending on the amount of carbon added in the casting process (Yan *et al.*, 2007). Low carbon CoCrMo alloy contains 0.05–0.08 wt% C, while high carbon alloy contains 0.20–0.25 wt% C. Carbon additions between 0.1 and 0.3 wt% have been shown to enhance the formation of carbides which increase wear resistance (Kauser, 2007; Varma *et al.*, 2002). Carbides are complex micron-size molecules which form at the surface of the alloys during the solidification process. They combine several atoms of metal (usually Mo and/or Cr) and several atoms of carbon.

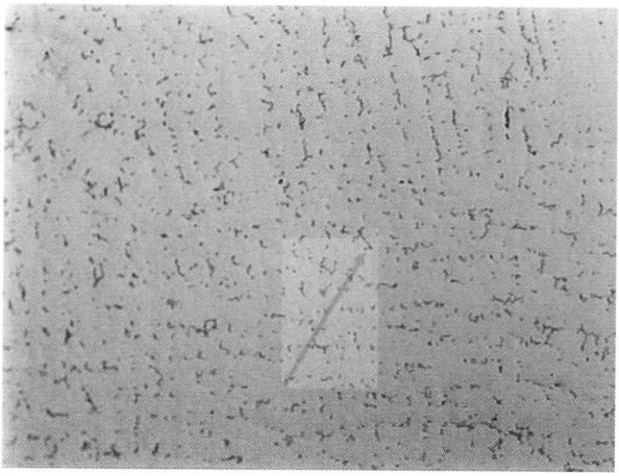

Figure 4-1. 100X magnification: Cast CoCrMo alloy: Carbides M23C6 (arrow).

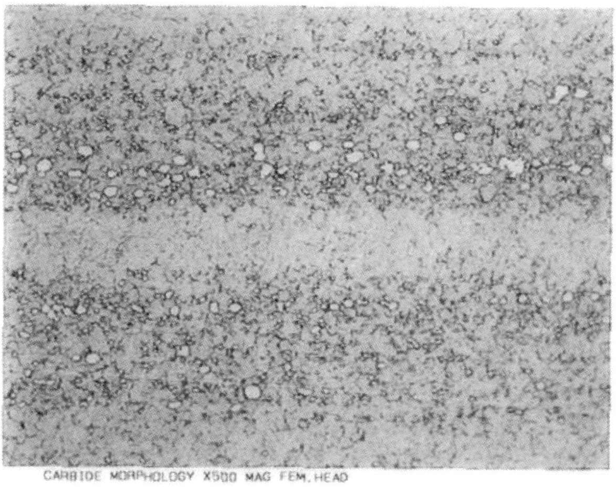

Figure 4-2. 500X magnification: Forged CoCrMo alloy: Carbides M7C3 (arrow).

Figure 4-1 shows a typical cast structure with the surface carbides extending from the surface. In the forgings, carbides are typically smaller (Figure 4-2). Carbides are ceramic in nature and thus much harder than the alloys' matrix and protect the surface from wear (Bowsher *et al.*, 2006). They form hard asperities sticking out of the surface of the alloy (Figure 4-3). Experiments using cast low carbon

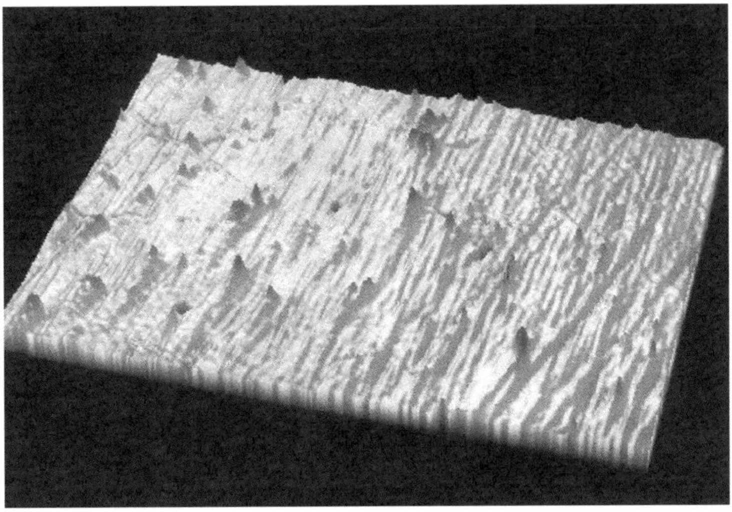

Figure 4-3. Carbides asperities (arrow).

Table 4-1. Characteristics of cast and wrought/forged CoCrMo alloys (McKellop *et al.*, 1998).

	Cast alloy	Wrought/forged alloy
Grain size	1–3 mm	15 μm
Carbide size	Up to 200 μm	2–8 μm
Hardness	310 H_v	470 H_v

CoCrMo have been associated with higher wear rates compared with cast high carbon material (Kunbrum*et al.*, 2008; Yan *et al.*, 2007). Since high carbon content CoCrMo alloy wears a lot less than low carbon content alloy, it is a better option for bearing surfaces such as in metal-on-metal (MoM) hip prostheses.

CoCrMo alloys may be cast or wrought/forged with similar chemical compositions based on American Society for Testing and Materials (ASTM) standards. The casting or forging process has an influence on the microstructure and the hardness of the material (Table 4-1).

Cast alloys are mostly used for complicated shapes which are difficult to machine, such as acetabular components of total hip replacements. However, the casting process may lead to inhomogeneous microstructures as a result of unequal cooling. The hot forging of alloys, on the other hand, results in refining of the microstructure as possible shrinkage voids are closed up. Overall, because of the smaller carbides, smaller grain size, and higher hardness, the wrought/forged metal bearings may have a slight advantage in terms of wear characteristics (Vendittoli *et al.*, 2007). Cast implants with the larger carbides are sometimes heat treated. Heat treatment causes carbides to dissolve back into their original elements, metal and carbon, a phenomenon which is supposed to lead to smoother surfaces, although this claim is controversial (Daniel *et al.*, 2010; Kamali *et al.*, 2010). Hot isostatic pressing (HIPping) is sometimes used to reduce microporosity resulting from casting, thus improving the fatigue strength (McMinn, 2003; Wang *et al.*, 1999). Double heat treatment involves solution treatment (ST) followed by HIPping. However, the concern is that HIP-ST may lead to increased metal wear due to the decrease in size and area fraction of carbides (Daniel *et al.*, 2010; Kamali *et al.*, 2010).

Other metals and alloys are also used for a variety of related purposes:

- **Stainless steel** is also used for orthopaedic devices and contains Cr and Nickel (Ni) but no Co. It is weaker and less wear resistant compared to CoCrMo. It is therefore not advocated for use in metal bearings.
- **Titanium-Aluminum-Vanadium (TiAlV)** alloys are used for hip and knee implants for non-cemented fixation, and in porous coatings. This alloy is less resistant to friction and therefore again not suitable for articulating surfaces.
- **Tantalum (Ta)** is used in porous form. Porous Ta has low modulus of elasticity, which allows for more physiologic load transfer and relative preservation of bone stock (Levine *et al.*, 2006). Because of its bioactive nature and ingrowth properties, Ta augments are also used as structural bone graft substitutes in arthroplasty revision surgery.

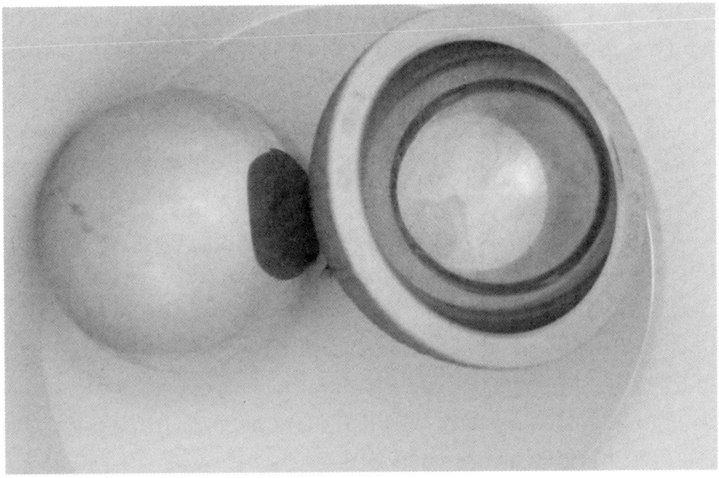

Figure 4-4. Retrieved TiNb-nitride surface engineered MoM hip resurfacing prosthesis. Wear patch is visible on outer surface of femoral component (head) and inner surface of acetabular component (cup).

- **Ceramisized metals** like **oxidized zirconium (Zr)** are now used in hip and knee arthroplasty (Bourne *et al.*, 2005). The hard ceramic surface is more resistant to abrasive wear but is not available for MoM articulating surfaces yet. Surface engineering with hard **ceramisized Titanium-niobium-nitride** has been used in MoM bearings. It increases the corrosion resistance of MoM bearing surfaces (Thull, 1991) but does not protect them from abrasive wear during the run-in phase of the wear cycle (Figure 4-4).

2. Tribology of Metal Bearings

As explained in Chapter 1, tribology is the study of friction, wear, and lubrication. The word has been used since the mid 1960s to describe the phenomena when surfaces in engineering machines interact in relative motion. The tribological interactions of a solid exposed metal surface with interfacing materials may result in loss of metal material from the surface. The process leading to loss of material is called 'wear' (Kretzer *et al.*, 2009; Williams *et al.*, 2006). With metal bearings, major types of wear include abrasive wear, friction or adhesive wear, and erosive wear which is caused by impingement of particles that remove fragments from the surface. At the areas of contact, friction, i.e. rubbing of one contact surface against another, may lead to material failure and the formation of material debris. When two metal surfaces articulate as in the case of a MoM hip implant, two-body grooving can occur where hard asperities (carbides) make contact with their opposite surface to cause deep grooves. This can lead to the release of metal ions and particulate wear debris. The wear particles lead to third-body wear where the released particle rolls in the middle of the two articulating surfaces causing further damage. The whole wear process especially occurs during the first 9 to 12 months (the so-called 'running in' period) till the articulating surfaces have been smoothened out and the wear decreases.

Wear can be minimized by modifying surface properties with surface engineering or finishing processes, or by use of lubricants. Lubricants are fluid and semi-fluid materials which minimize component contact or eliminate contact altogether. In our natural joints, synovial fluid acts as a lubricant between articulating surfaces. When an artificial joint is implanted, it is important that the articulating surfaces are separated and protected by a small film of synovial fluid during motion, in order to reduce the wear.

When two surfaces are separated by a lubricant, three situations can exist. When a lubricant is present between two articulating surfaces, a pressurized fluid film can be generated by the movement of the surfaces. The non-compressible nature of this film separates the surfaces and prevents contact. The thickness of the lubrication film and the surface roughness determine the lubrication regime (McKellop *et al.*, 1998) (Figure 4-5). When two surfaces are completely separated by a continuous fluid film, a hydrodynamic or fluid film lubrication condition is created (Figure 4-5). Although hydrodynamic lubrication is the ideal situation, in many situations it cannot be maintained. An increase in load will decrease the fluid film thickness. Boundary lubrication is a condition in which the lubricant film becomes too thin to provide total surface separation, leading to contact between surface asperities. The third type of lubrication condition is a mixed lubrication regime.

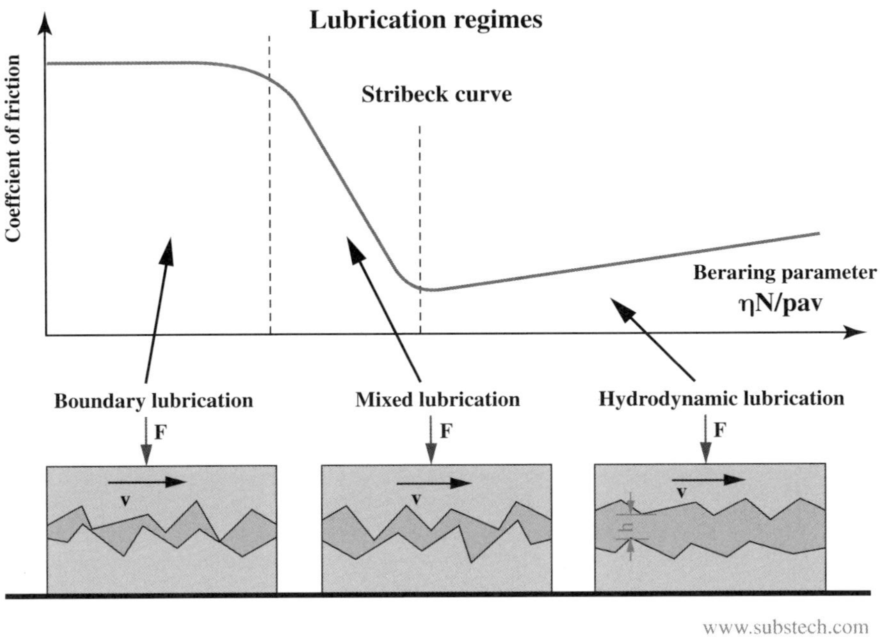

Figure 4-5. Lubrication regimes (courtesy of Dr Dmitri Kopeliovich. Available at: http://www.substech.com).

In MoM hip arthroplasty, an important factor influencing the lubrication is the clearance (Kretzer *et al.*, 2009). Diametral clearance is twice the radial clearance (Figure 4-6) and is defined as the difference between the inner diameter of the cup and the diameter of the head. When the clearance is too large, the contact area between the femoral head and the acetabular cup during loading will be small (polar loading), leading to high contact stresses and increased wear. When the clearance is too small, equatorial contact may occur during loading and both components will be jammed together which also leads to increased wear (equatorial loading). In the ideal situation a small wedge exists between the acetabular and femoral component via which a fluid film will be entrained during motion (Figure 4-6, arrow).

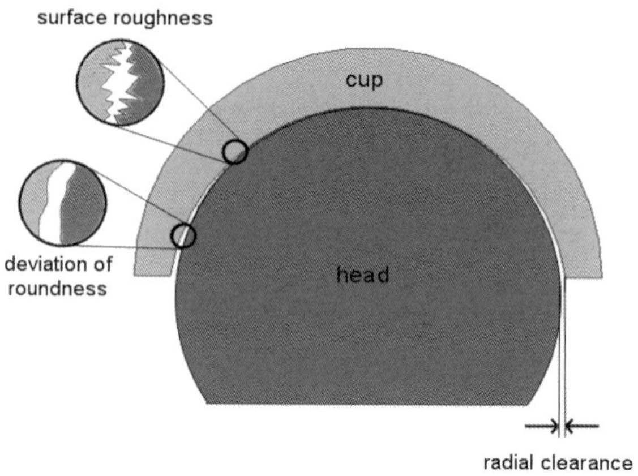

Figure 4-6. Radial clearance between acetabular and femoral components of a MoM hip (Kretzer *et al.*, 2009).

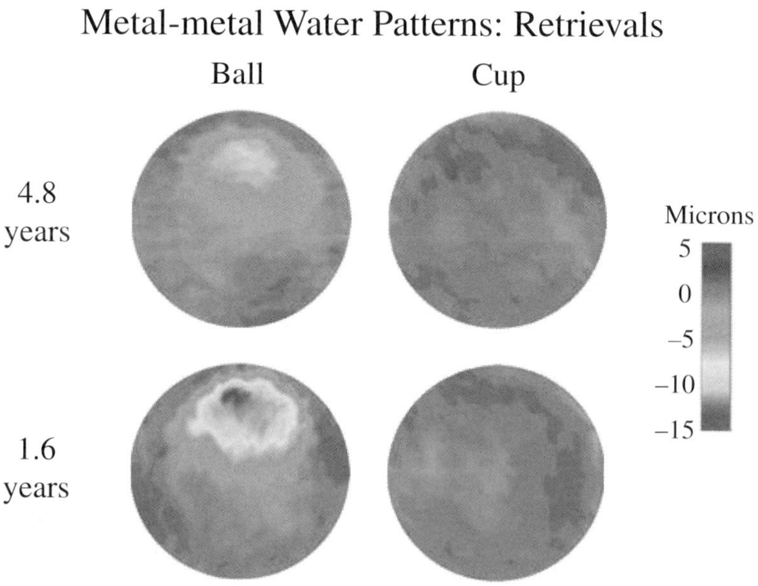

Figure 4-7. Higher wear at the femoral component of MoM hip bearings (Barnes *et al.*, 2008).

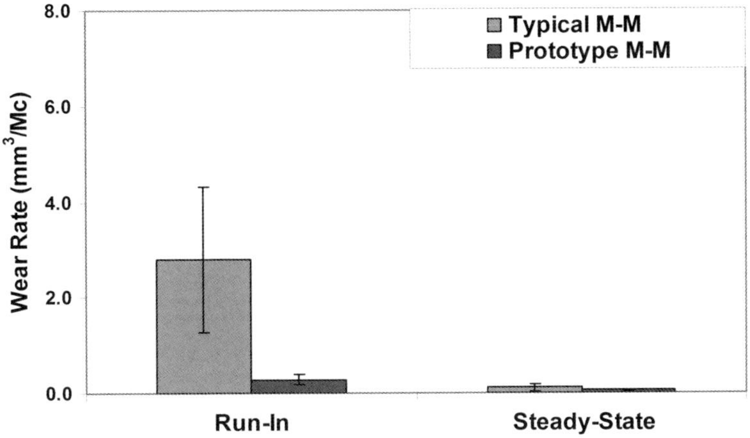

Figure 4-8. *In vitro* hip simulator studies showed lower wear rate in differential hardness bearings (prototype) compared to standard MoM bearing couples (Hanawa, 2004).

With MoM hip arthroplasty, both *in vitro* and *in vivo* studies have demonstrated that the femoral head wears more than the acetabular component (Barnes *et al.*, 2008) (Figure 4-7). Hence, differential hardness bearing MoM or ceramic-on-metal articulations have been designed where the femoral head is manufactured in harder, more friction (adhesion) resistant metal by changing the microstructure of the metal alloy (or ceramic, which is harder than metal). The aim was to reduce the wear on the femoral side. *In vitro* studies showed that differential hardness couples produced ten times less wear debris during the initial run-in period of wear and only half of the debris during the steady state. The typical standard MoM bearing couples run-in rate (2.8 mm^3/Mc) is ten times greater than differential hardness bearing couples (0.28 mm^3/Mc) (Hanawa, 2004) (Figure 4-8).

Besides metallurgic characteristics, a number of design features of hip resurfacing arthroplasty (HRA) have been identified as being decisive with regard to articulating surface wear characteristics. The diametrical clearance is important for lubrication, but the most critical design feature discerning successful from failing HRA has been the subtended articular arc and the coverage angle. In order to avoid impingement with the anatomical femoral neck, acetabular HRA

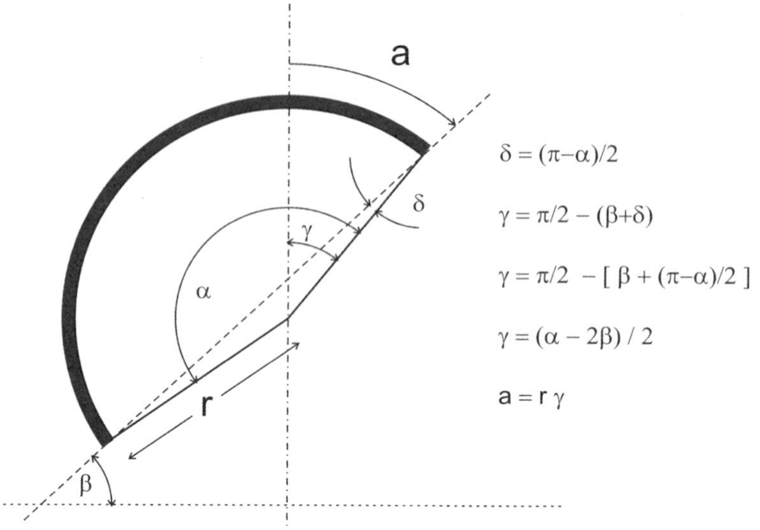

Figure 4-9. Coverage arc (a), abduction angle (β), and subtended articular surface angle (α) (Gill *et al.*, 2013).

components are not fully hemispherical. This may lead to reduced coverage of the femoral component by the acetabular component. The coverage from the proximal pole of the femoral component to the lateral edge of the cup is particularly important, as this will indicate the risk of edge loading. The coverage arc is given by the product of the component radius (r) and angle (in radians) subtended between the vertical and the lateral cup edge (γ): $\mathrm{a} = \mathrm{r} \cdot \gamma$. This angle, γ, is dependent on the cup inclination angle β and the angle δ subtended between the chord of the cup arc and the radial line from the cup edge to the centre of curvature of the cup (Gill *et al.*, 2013). This is related to the included or subtended articular surface angle of the cup, α (Figure 4-9). The coverage arc is directly related to the contact patch-to-rim distance (CPR), defined by Bergmann *et al.* (2001) as the distance between the point of intersection of the hip reaction force with the cup and the closest point on the inner side of the cup rim (Figure 4-10). The CPR is computed from the cup abduction and anteversion angles, the subtended articular surface angle α, and the cup size (Van Der Straeten *et al.*, 2013; Yoon *et al.*, 2013).

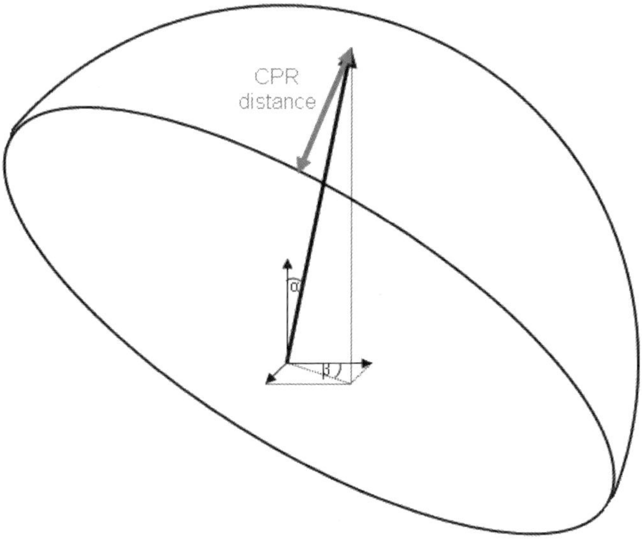

Figure 4-10. Contact patch-to-rim (CPR) distance (Yoon *et al.*, 2013).

A smaller coverage arc or CPR distance will lead to so-called edge loading where most of the load exerted on the hip is concentrated on a small area of contact of the acetabular rim area with the femoral head. This has been associated with a substantial increase of wear (Gill *et al.*, 2013; Van Der Straeten *et al.*, 2013; Yoon *et al.*, 2013).

3. Corrosion of Metal Bearings

Corrosion is the deterioration of materials by a chemical reaction with their environment. The term corrosion generally refers to metals and consists of an electrochemical redox reaction which occurs when metal surfaces come into contact with fluid. Abrasive wear may be accelerated by corrosion (oxidation) of the rubbing surfaces. Increased temperature during motion and removal of the protecting oxide films from the surface during the initial wear promote the oxidation process. Friction provides continuous removal of the passive layer or oxide film followed by continuous formation of a new oxide film (repassivation) (Yan *et al.*, 2013). Passivation refers to a material becoming passive, i.e. less affected by its environment. A shielding outer layer of oxides (e.g. Cr2O3 in CoCrMo alloys) is formed, which preserves the deeper layers from further corrosion (Yan *et al.*, 2006, 2013). This layer is thought to be 1–4 nm thick and gives very good corrosion resistance (Contu *et al.*, 2003; Sinnett-Jones *et al.*, 2005).

During the corrosion process, metal ions are generated which may either form oxides or hydroxides and may be reused for the passive film on the metal surface. This is what occurs mostly with Cr ions. Other ions which are more soluble may continue to float around as ions and bind with biomolecules such as proteins or pass the cell membrane and bind with RNA and DNA. Co is known to bind preferentially to proteins (Hanawa, 2004). It is noteworthy that metal ions generated by corrosion are not only derived from the articulating surfaces but also from the small wear particles which have a large cumulative surface and may account for substantial metal ion generation in high wear conditions. It is thought that one third of the metal ion production from MoM Hip arthroplasty is generated by corrosion (Yan *et al.*, 2006).

4. Tribocorrosion of Metal Bearings

In increased wear conditions such as edge loading, hard oxide particles removed from the surface and trapped between the sliding/rolling surfaces may additionally increase the wear rate by third-body abrasive wear mechanism. Tribocorrosion describes the cumulative interaction of abrasion with corrosion, which accelerates the degradation of an alloy (Sinnett-Jones *et al.*, 2005; Yan *et al.*, 2006). When excessive load and/or motion is applied to the bearing surfaces, the corrosion potential will shift from a passive area to an active area as the passive film is removed from the surface during sliding under load, resulting in accelerated corrosion (Sinnett-Jones *et al.*, 2005; Yan *et al.*, 2006). As metal ions are released, their hydrolysis can lower the pH locally, leading to anodic dissolution and more corrosion. The underlying active bare metal is then exposed to an electrochemical reaction with the tissue fluid, which results in more material loss. After the run-in period and provided there is no excessive edge loading, it is assumed that a repassivation process can occur with the reformation of a protective oxide layer (Rashidi *et al.*, 2007).

Crevice corrosion is a localized corrosion in confined spaces (crevices) where a stagnant solution is present (Langton *et al.*, 2011; Paganelli *et al.*, 2002). Crevices allow for a different chemical environment compared to freely exposed surfaces by keeping fluid and excluding oxygen. In addition, corrosion products are concentrated and particles and third bodies may be trapped. Fontana demonstrated that once the oxygen inside the crevice is consumed, the cathodic reaction prevails with formation of metal chlorides and lowering of the pH by hydrolysis of the metal chlorides (Paganelli *et al.*, 2002). This will accelerate the metal dissolution (fretting corrosion) with more creation of metal ions forming more metal chlorides and further lowering the pH. The low pH and degradation products create a highly toxic environment. Crevice corrosion is one of the most harmful types of corrosion and is now recognized as one of the failure mechanisms at the taper/trunnion modular connection of MoM THA with large diameter heads (Figure 4-11). The term 'trunnion' refers

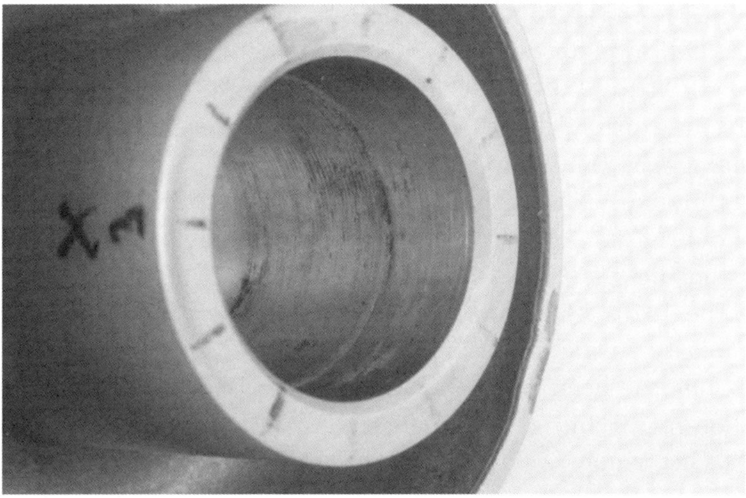

Figure 4-11. Crevice corrosion at the taper (without sleeve adaptor) of a large diameter MoM femoral head. The patient had a soft tissue reaction around the femoral neck. (Photo courtesy of Dr Philippe Kretzer.)

to the proximal conal extremity of the femoral stem or the 'male' component of the modular junction. The term 'taper' describes the area inside the femoral head, which receives the trunnion or 'female' component of the modular junction. It may refer to either a sleeve which is inserted into the femoral head (metal or ceramic) or to the internal cone of the head in systems not using a sleeve adaptor (Langton *et al.*, 2011) (Figure 4-11).

The biocompatibility of CoCrMo alloy is closely linked to its high resistance to corrosion, which is attributed to the spontaneous formation of a passive oxide film. The integrity of this oxide film has been strongly correlated with the chemical and mechanical stability of the alloy once implanted into the body (Metikos-Hukovic and Babic, 2007).

5. Clinical Implications

In recent years, substantial research has been undertaken in an attempt to optimize materials and design of orthopaedic bearings. In the early days of hip arthroplasty, MoM bearings were used, developed mostly in the United Kingdom by surgeons such as McKee and Farrar, and implanted mainly between 1960 and 1975. The McKee–Farrar MoM total hip arthroplasty (THA) produced varying clinical results, due primarily to inappropriate design and manufacturing. Loosening was the main cause of failure, due to inadequate cementing techniques. Although metallosis (black colouring of tissues by metal debris) was observed during revisions, adverse effects of metal debris on the soft tissues or the bone were not described.

In the 1970s, Sir John Charnley's technique for low friction hip arthroplasty, using metal-on-polyethylene (MoP) bearings with a small femoral head diameter (22 mm), became widely used and metal-on-metal hip replacements were abandoned (Mellon *et al.*, 2013). The primary causes of failure of these 22 mm low friction MoP THAs were dislocation and component loosening. Loosening was often associated with extensive bone destruction (osteolysis) caused by an immunological macrophage response to particles of polyethylene debris released from the bearing surface (Mellon *et al.*, 2013). In the younger, more active patient group, the wear process was accelerated, leading to earlier failure of the THA, substantial bone loss, and difficult revision procedures.

Therefore, since 1988, MoM articulations were reintroduced as a bearing surface for hip arthroplasty to solve the problem of particle-induced osteolysis secondary to conventional polyethylene wear (Rieker, 2010). *In vitro* hip simulator studies demonstrated much less volumetric wear and much smaller particles with MoM compared to MoP (Jacobs *et al.*, 2009). This finding was confirmed *in vivo* with 28 mm and 32 mm MoM THA (Jacobs *et al.*, 2009; Weber and Rieker, 2002) using wrought, high-carbon CoCrMo alloys such as the Metasul® MoM bearings which were highly polished to reduce surface roughness (Weber and Rieker, 2002). In addition, the use of larger-diameter femoral heads ($\geq$32 mm) as a solution to post-operative dislocation became possible with the development of MoM bearings with less apparent wear compared to MoP. Larger heads have effectively reduced the dislocation rate (Plate *et al.*, 2012). MoM HRA was reintroduced to address the inferior survivorship and unsatisfactory clinical results with THA in young and active patients (Dorr *et al.*, 2000; Swedish Hip Arthroplasty Registry, 2010). Following the early success of MoM HRA, large diameter MoM THAs consisting of the same acetabular component articulating with a CoCrMo large diameter head on a cemented or non-cemented prosthetic femoral stem were introduced. These large diameter metal heads on a femoral stem were initially only meant as a hip resurfacing revision option after a fractured femoral neck which was the main reason for failure of MoM HRA in the early days. Because of the reduced dislocation rate and the theoretically more anatomical reconstruction with a large diameter head, orthopaedic surgeons started to use these implants as primary hip replacements.

Approximately 1 million MoM hip prostheses, including all current HRA prostheses, have been implanted worldwide (Mellon *et al.*, 2013). These implants contain femoral and acetabular bearing surfaces made of CoCrMo alloys. Although the majority of MoM hip replacements have been successful, multiple recent reports have documented markedly increased Co and Cr concentrations in the joint synovial fluid, periprosthetic tissue, blood, and even peripheral tissues of some patients with MoM hip prostheses even with small diameter MoM bearings (Metasul® 28 mm) (Bjorgul *et al.*, 2013). Higher metal ion levels have been found in whole blood, serum, and urine of patients with MoM hip arthroplasties (THA and HRA) compared to preoperative values, and to THA with other bearing surfaces (MoP, ceramic-on-polyethylene, ceramic-on-ceramic) (MacDonald *et al.*, 2004). Higher levels of Co and Cr ions are also found in bilateral MoM hip replacement compared to unilateral. Although MoM hip arthroplasty has been shown to produce less volumetric wear compared to MoP, the wear debris consists of more numerous, small, nanometre size particles which are ingested by macrophages (Kwon *et al.*, 2009). Contrary to polyethylene, metal particles and ions are not chemically inert but may have directly toxic, biological effects and may elicit hypersensitivity reactions in addition to the macrophage-driven, innate, foreign-body immune responses to particulate debris of any material. Adverse soft tissue reactions to large diameter MoM THA in particular have been associated with extensive tissue necrosis. In a number of recent case reports, very high cobalt ion levels were also linked with systemic symptoms of neurotoxicity, cardiac, and thyroid toxicity (Tower, 2010). Consequently, concerns have been raised about the physiological consequences of metal release from MoM hip prostheses into the periprosthetic tissue and systemic circulation. The measurement of systemic levels of metal ions gives an insight into the wear occurring (i.e. state of the bearing couple) (Van Der Straeten *et al.*, 2013) and is advocated by regulatory bodies as routine practice in the assessment of MoM hips since 2010 (Medical Device Alert, 2010; FDA, 2011). Co and Cr concentrations in the serum and hip joint fluid correlate with the degree of MoM implant wear and are increased in individuals with an accumulation of metal debris in the periprosthetic tissue (De Smet *et al.*, 2008). Metal ions are mainly excreted via the kidneys but intracellular uptake in red blood cells and lymphocytes and tissue accumulation in the reticulo-endothelial system (lymph nodes, liver, spleen) has been demonstrated in at least a third of patients with well-functioning MoM (Mao *et al.*, 2011). Similarly, elevated systemic levels of Co and Cr and liver and spleen accumulation have been noted with failed conventional THA (Bjorgul *et al.*, 2013). After revision and elimination of the metal wear source, the levels decreased rapidly (De Smet *et al.*, 2011).

The analysis of consecutive ion levels demonstrated a statistically significant overall decrease of Cr and Co levels with time. In 25% of patients with a well-functioning HRA at more than ten years post-operatively, ion levels were undetectable at ten years or more post-operatively (Van Der Straeten *et al.*, 2013). These findings are in accordance with tribocorrosion studies indicating a lower-wear bedding-in phase after the initial running-in phase of higher wear (Kamali *et al.*, 2010). An increase in ion levels after the run-in phase was demonstrated to be an indication of continued surface wear, which may eventually lead to implant failure potentially associated with soft tissue and bone destruction. Hence, metal ion measurements were confirmed to be a valuable diagnostic tool for the early detection of wear of MoM HRA (Van Der Straeten *et al.*, 2013).

The difference in ion levels between different resurfacing designs may reflect differences in clearance, metallurgy, and coverage angle. In general, metal ion levels below the proposed acceptable limits are found with all HRA designs. Outliers occurred more often with designs with a smaller coverage angle, leading to an increased risk of edge loading especially in the smaller size range.

Monitoring of metal ions is now generally advocated as a screening tool for implant performance in order to detect increased wear at an early stage and perform a hip revision before extensive tissue destruction has occurred.

References

Barnes, C.L., Nambu, S., Carroll, M., Timmerman, I. and Svarczkopf, T. (2008). Differential hardness bearings in hip arthroplasty, *J Surg Orthop Adv*, **17**(1), 40–44.

Bergmann, G., Deuretzbacher, G., Heller, M., Graichen, F., Rohlmann, A., Strauss, J. and Duda, G.N. (2001). Hip contact forces and gait patterns from routine activities, *J Biomech*, **34**, 859–871.

Bjorgul, K., Novicoff, W.N., Andersen, S.T., Ahlund, O.R., Bunes, A., Wiig, M. and Brevig, K. (2013). High rate of revision and a high incidence of radiolucent lines around Metasul metal-on-metal total hip replacements: Results from a randomised controlled trial of three bearings after seven years, *Bone Joint J*, **95-B**(7), 881–886.

Bourne, R.B., Barrack, R., Rorabeck, C.H., Salehi, A. and Good, V. (2005). Arthroplasty options for the young patient: Oxinium on cross-linked polyethylene, *Clin Orthop Relat R*, **441**, 159–167.

Bowsher, J.G., Nevelos, J., Williams, P.A. and Shelton, J.C. (2006). 'Severe' wear challenge to 'as-cast' and 'double heat-treated' large-diameter metal-on-metal hip bearings, *Proc Inst Mech Eng H*, **220**(H2), 135–143.

Contu, F., Elsener, B. and Bohni, H. (2003). Electrochemical behavior of CoCrMo alloy in the active state in acidic and alkaline buffered solutions, *J Electrochem Soc*, **150**(9), B419–B424.

Daniel, J., Ziaee, H., Kamali, A., Pradhan, C., Band, T. and McMinn, D.J. (2010). Ten-year results of a double-heat-treated metal-on-metal hip resurfacing, *J Bone Joint Surg Br*, **92**(1), 20–27.

De Smet, K., De Haan, R., Calistri, A., Campbell, P.A., Ebramzadeh, E., Pattyn, C. and Gill, H.S. (2008). Metal ion measurement as a diagnostic tool to identify problems with metal-on-metal hip resurfacing, *J Bone Joint Surg Am*, **90**(Suppl 4), 202–208.

De Smet, K.A., Van Der Straeten, C., Van Orsouw, M., Doubi, R., Backers, K. and Grammatopoulos, G. (2011). Revisions of metal-on-metal hip resurfacing: Lessons learned and improved outcome, *Orthop Clin N Am*, **42**, 259–269.

Dorr, L.D., Wan, Z., Longjohn, D.B., Dubois, B. and Murken, R. (2000). Total hip arthroplasty with use of Metasul metal-on-metal articulation. Four to seven-year results, *J Bone Joint Surg Am*, **82**(6), 789–798.

Food and Drug Administration (FDA). 2011. *Guidance for Industry and FDA Staff — Postmarket Surveillance Under Section 522 of the Federal Food, Drug and Cosmetic Act.* [Online]. Available at: http://www.fda.gov/downloads/medicaldevices/deviceregulationandguidance/guidancedocuments/ucm072564.pdf [Accessed 16 August 2011].

Gill, R., Campbell, P.C. and De Smet, K.A. (2013). The use of metal ion levels to evaluate hip resurfacing, in De Smet, K.A., Campbell, O.C. and Van Der Straeten, C. (eds), *The Hip Resurfacing Handbook*, Woodhead Publishing Ltd, Oxford, 267–278.

Hanawa, T. (2004). Metal ion release from metal implants, *Mat Sci Eng C*, **24**, 745–752.

Jacobs, J.J., Urban, R.M., Hallab, N.J., Skipor, A.K., Fischer, A. and Wimmer, M.A. (2009) Metal-on-metal bearing surfaces, *J Am Acad Orthop Sur*, **17**(2), 69–74.

Kamali, A., Hussain, A., Li, C., Pamu, J., Daniel, J., Ziaee, H., Daniel, J. and McMinn, D.J. (2010). Tribological performance of various CoCr microstructures in metal-on-metal bearings: The development of a more physiological protocol *in vitro*, *J Bone Joint Surg Br*, **92**(5), 717–725.

Kauser, F. (2007). *Corrosion of CoCrMo alloys for biomedical applications*, Department of Metallurgy and Materials, School of Engineering, University of Birmingham. 4–285.

Kinbrum, A. and Unsworth, A. (2008). The wear of high-carbon metal-on-metal bearings after different heat treatments, *Proc Inst Mech Eng H*, **222**(H6), 887–895.

Kretzer, J.P., Kleinhans, J.A., Jakubowitz, E., Thomsen, M. and Heisel, C. (2009). A meta-analysis of design- and manufacturing-related parameters influencing the wear behavior of metal-on-metal hip joint replacements, *J Orthop Res*, **27**(11), 1473–1480.

Kwon, Y.M., Xia, Z., Glyn-Jones, S., Beard, D., Gill, H.S. and Murray, D.W. (2009). Dose-dependent cytotoxicity of clinically relevant cobalt nanoparticles and ions on macrophages *in vitro*, *Biomed Mater*, **4**(2), 025018.

Langton, D.J., Jameson, S.S., Joyce, T.J., Gandhi, J.N., Sidaginamale, R., Mereddy, P., Lord, J. and Nargol, A.V. (2011). Accelerating failure rate of the ASR total hip replacement, *J Bone Joint Surg Br*, **93**(8), 1011–1016.

Levine, B., Della Valle, C.J. and Jacobs, J.J. (2006). Applications of porous tantalum in total hip arthroplasty, *J Am Acad Orthop Sur*, **14**(12), 646–655.

MacDonald, S.J., Brodner, W. and Jacobs, J.J. (2004). A consensus paper on metal ions in metal-on-metal hip arthroplasties, *J Arthroplasty*, **19**(8 Suppl 3), 12–16.

Mao, X., Wong, A.A. and Crawford, R.W. (2011). Cobalt toxicity — an emerging clinical problem in patients with metal-on-metal hip prostheses?, *Med J Australia*, **194**(12), 649–651.

McKellop, H., Lu, B. and Wiser, H. (1998). The effect of specimen orientation and lubricant concentration on the wear of metal/metal hip implants in a wear simulator, *Proc 24th Ann Meet Soc Biomater*, 422.

McMinn, D. (2003). Development of metal-on-metal hip resurfacing, *Hip Int*, **13,** S41–S53.

Medicines and Healthcare products Regulatory Agency (MHRA) (2010). Medical device alert of the on all metal-on-metal (MoM) hip replacements. MDA/2010/033. [Online] (Issued April 22, 2010). Available at: http://www.mhra.gov.uk/Publications/Safetywarnings/MedicalDeviceAlerts/CON079157 [Accessed 22 April 2010].

Mellon, S.J., Liddle, A.D. and Pandit, H. (2013). Hip replacement: Landmark surgery in modern medical history, *Maturitas*, **75**(3), 221–226.

Metikos-Hukovic, M. and Babic, R. (2007). Passivation and corrosion behaviours of cobaltand cobalt–chromium–molybdenum alloy, *Corros Sci*, **49**(9), 3570–3579.

Paganelli, C., Salgarello, S., Mensi, M., Fontana, P., Visconti, L. and Sapelli, P.L. (2002). *In vitro* study of amalgam corrosion, *Med Lav*, **93**(3), 286–289.

Plate, J.F., Seyler, T.M., Stroh, D.A., Issa, K., Akbar, M. and Mont, M.A. (2012). Risk of dislocation using large versus small-diameter femoral heads in total hip arthroplasty, *BMC Res Notes*, **5**, 553.

Rashidi, N., Alavi-Soltani, S. and Asmatulu, R. (2007). Crevice corrosion theory, mechanisms and prevention methods, *Proc 3rd Ann GRASP symp*, 215–216.

Rieker, C.B. (2010). Large metal-on-metal bearings. Current situation in 2010. *Eur Cells Mater*, **19**(Suppl 2), 17.

Sinnett-Jones, P.E., Wharton, J.A. and Wood R.J.K. (2005). Micro-abrasion-corrosion of a CoCrMo alloy in simulated artificial hip joint environments, *Wear*, **259**, 898–909.

Swedish Hip Arthroplasty Registry (2010). *Annual Report 2010*, Göteborg, Sweden. Available at: http://www.shpr.se.

Thull, R. (1991). Corrosion behavior of dental alloys coated with titanium niobium oxinitride, *Deut Zahnaerztl Z*, **46**(11), 712–717.

Tower, S.S. (2010). Arthroprosthetic cobaltism: Neurological and cardiac manifestations in two patients with metal-on-metal arthroplasty: A case report, *J Bone Joint Surg Am*, **92**, 2847–2851.

Van Der Straeten, C., Grammatopoulos, G., Gill, H.S., Calistri, A., Campbell, P. and De Smet, K.A. (2013). The 2012 Otto Aufranc Award. The Interpretation of metal ion levels in unilateral and bilateral hip resurfacing, *Clin Orthop Relat R*, **471**(2), 377–385.

Van Der Straeten, C., Van Quickenborne, D., De Roest, B., Calistri, A., Victor, J. and De Smet, K. (2013). Metal ion levels from well-functioning Birmingham hip resurfacings decline significantly at ten years, *Bone Joint J*, **95-B**(10), 1332–1338.

Van Der Straeten, C. and De Smet, K.A. (2013). The practical application of metal ion level measurement in evaluating hip resurfacing of metal ion levels to evaluate hip resurfacing, in De Smet, K.A., Campbell, O.C. and Van Der Straeten, C. (eds), *The Hip Resurfacing Handbook*, Woodhead Publishing Ltd, Oxford, 279–318.

Varma, A., Li, B. and Mukasayan, A. (2002). Novel synthesis of orthopedic implant materials, *Adv Eng Mat*, **4**(7), 482–486.

Vendittoli, P.A., Mottard, S., Roy, A.G., Dupont, C. and Lavigne, M. (2007). Chromium and cobalt ion release following the Durom high carbon content, forged metal-on-metal surface replacement of the hip, *J Bone Joint Surg Br*, **89**(4), 441–448.

Wang, K.K., Wang, A. and Gustavson, L.J. (1999). Metal-on-metal wear testing of Co-Cr alloys, in Disegi, J.A., Kennedy, R.L. and Pilliar, R. (eds), Cobalt-Base Alloys for Biomedical Applications, Special Technical Publication 1365, American Society for Testing and Materials, 135–144.

Weber, B.G. and Rieker, B.C. (2002). The history of Metasul, *Acta Chir Orthop Tr*, **69**(5), 277–284.

Williams, S., Jalali-Vahid, D., Brockett, C., Jin, Z., Stone, M.H., Ingham, E. and Fisher, J. (2006). Effect of swing phase load on metal-on-metal hip lubrication, friction and wear, *J Biomech*, **39**(12), 2274–2281.

Yan, Y., Dowson, D. and Neville, A. (2013) *In situ* electrochemical study of interaction of tribology and corrosion in artificial hip prosthesis simulators, *J Mech Behav Biomed Mater*, **18**, 191–199.

Yan, Y., Neville, A. and Dowson, D. (2006). Understanding the role of corrosion in the degradation of metal-on-metal implants, *Proc Inst Mech Eng H*, **220**(2), 173–180.

Yan, Y., Neville, A. and Dowson, D. (2007). Tribo-corrosion properties of cobalt-based medical implant alloys in simulated biological environments, *Wear*, **263**, 1105–1111.

Yoon, J.P., Le Duff, M.J., Johnson, A.J., Takamura, K.M., Ebramzadeh, E., Amstutz, H.C. (2013). Contact patch to rim distance predicts metal ion levels in hip resurfacing, *Clin Orthop Relat R*, **471**(5), 1615–1621.

Chapter 5

Ceramic-on-Ceramic Bearings: Simulator Wear Compared to Clinical Retrieval Data

Ian C. Clarke[a], Jean Y. Lazennec[b], Evert J. Smith[c], Nobuhiko Sugano[d], Bryan J. McEntire[e] and Giuseppe Pezzotti[f]

[a]*Peterson Tribology Laboratory, Department of Orthopedics, Loma Linda University, Loma Linda, USA*

[b]*Orthopedic Department, Anatomy Department, La Pitie Hospital, Assistance Publique de Paris, Université Pierre et Marie Curie, Paris, France*

[c]*Musculoskeletal Department, North Bristol NHS Trust, Southmead Hospital, University of Bristol, Bristol, UK*

[d]*Department of Orthopaedic Medical Engineering, Osaka University Graduate School of Medicine, Suita, Japan*

[e]*Research & Development, Amedica Corporation, Salt Lake City, USA*

[f]*Ceramic Physics Laboratory, Kyoto Institute of Technology, Kyoto, Japan*

1. Introduction to Bioceramics

Ceramics represent an abrasion-resistant class of materials suitable for use in environments that would be considered adverse for other materials. The benefits ceramics bring to orthopedic devices such as the total hip arthroplasty (THA) is primarily that of having a bearing surface that is dimensionally stable, chemically inert, and has ultra-high wear resistance (Table 5-1). The obvious limitation is that implants must be designed around ceramic materials that

Table 5-1. Physical and mechanical properties of ceramics compared to CoCr alloy.

Property or performance	Units	Alumina	Zirconia		Zirconia–Alumina composites			Silicon nitride	Cobalt chromium
Composition	N/A	Al_2O_3	Mg-PSZ	Y-TZP	ZTA	AMC	ATZ	Si_3N_4	ASTM F799
Density	g/cc	3.98	5.65–5.77	6.00–6.05	4.25	4.37	5.51	3.24–3.35	8.29–8.50
Grain size	μm	<1.8 Equiaxed	50 Equiaxed	0.1–0.6 Equiaxed	0.4–0.7 Equiaxed	0.54 Equiaxed	0.4 Equiaxed	0.5 × 5.0 Equiaxed	~62 Equiaxed
Flexural strength	MPa	400–580	450–700	900–1200	1200–1300	1400	790–1500	900–1000	827 Tensile
Elastic modulus	GPa	380	200–250	210	340–390	358	240–250	296–313	197–210
Poisson's ratio	N/A	0.23	0.30	0.30	~0.24	0.24	~0.28	0.27	0.27–0.32
Compressive strength	MPa	4100–5000	2000–3000	2000–2200	4000–4500	4300	~2600	4000	600–1800
Weibull modulus	N/A	5–10	22	8–12	N/A	>10	6–17	8–19	N/A
Fracture toughness	MPa·m$^{1/2}$	4.0–4.2	8.0–15.0	5.0–10.0	4.2	6.4	8.0–12.0	5.7–10.6	50–100
Toughening mechanism	N/A	Grain size	t → m-ZrO_2	t → m-ZrO_2	t → m-ZrO_2 Platelet	t → m-ZrO_2 Platelet	t → m-ZrO_2	Acicular grains	Elastic deformation
Hardness	GPa	18.0–23.0	10.0–12.0	11.0–12.5	15.7–20.8	19	13.7–15.0	15.0	3.0–4.0
Wear rate PE	mm^3/MC	20–58	1.8–5.1	11–63	N/A	1–20	17–32	17–25	14–201
HXLPE		0.0–6.9	N/A	5.0–6.0		0.1–4.4	5.6–6.1	3.7–6.3	0.0–11.7
Hard-on-Hard		0.02–4.71		Catastrophic		0.00–0.45	0.02–0.06	0.18–0.98	0.18–25.00
Thermal conductivity	W/m°K	30	2	2–3	~17	17	~6	30–50	12.7
Corrosion and LTD susceptibility	N/A	Stable	Marginal	Unstable	Stable	Marginal	Unstable	Stable	Marginal

Key: LTD = low-temperature hydrothermal degradation.

Table 5-2. Comparison of ceramic properties considered for THA.

ID	Parameter	Low-rank		Mid-rank		High-rank
1	Flexural Strength	Al_2O_3	<	S_3N_4	<	ZTA
2	Fracture Toughness	Al_2O_3	<	ZTA	<	S_3N_4
3	LTD Susceptibility	Al_2O_3	=	S_3N_4	<	ZTA
4	Thermal Conductivity	ZTA	<	Al_2O_3	<	S_3N_4
5	Hardness	S_3N_4	<	ZTA	<	Al_2O_3

Table 5-3. Tribological issues for CoC bearings.

#	THA parameters	CoC details	CoC commentary
1	Severe articular wear	Mainly one-piece pioneering designs	Believed patients ambulated on loose cups
2	Steep cups	Risk common to all hip designs	To be avoided at surgery
3	Stripe wear	Consequence of cup edge wear	Seldom perceived as clinical risk
4	Metal debris	Ceramic hardness (sapphire) close to diamond	Least risk of any bearing material
5	Squeaking	Incidence varies greatly	Believed multifactorial (lubricant failure)
6	Alternative ceramics	ZTA, Si_3N_4, DHOxZr	Pre-clinical testing and clinical history

are both brittle and much stiffer than commonly used metal alloys. Thus, in making the choice of optimal ceramic bearings one must consider both the benefits and the clinical risks that it may enhance or mitigate (Tables 5-2 and 5-3). Use of ceramic bearings with high modulus of elasticity raises the issue of very small contact areas common to HOH counterfaces. Higher shear and contact stresses between microdisparities can raise local temperature and result in surface degradation. High stresses may also reduce or obviate lubrication mechanisms in the hip, thereby implying the risk of surface cracking with grain pullout. The various chemical and mechanical phenomena interacting at the microstructural level will also result in acidic attacks that weaken grain boundaries and create oxygen vacancies. Application of cyclic hip-loading will fracture weakened ceramic grains with consequent pullout and formation of abrasive wear particles (Table 5-3). Thus, superior fracture resistance combined with ultra-low wear and high reliability are stringent requirements for ceramic bearings (Table 5-1).

The literature with respect to hip simulators has been successful in establishing phenomenological correlations between run-in and steady-state wear phases and the difference between standard (ASTM F1714, 2008; ISO 14242-2, 2000; ISO 14242-3, 2008) and microseparation test modes (Clarke *et al.*, 2006; Nevelos *et al.*, 2000). However, the physical and chemical phenomena driving degradation by friction and wear mechanisms have virtually been ignored. It can be anticipated that various patient activities will offer potential for implant impingement and subluxation maneuvers quite unpredictable in the activities of daily life (Table 5-4). Depending on

Table 5-4. Clinical risks for COC bearings.

Item	Features	Risks and benefits	Commentary
1	Fracture	Heads and cups	Incidence reduced with AMC designs
2	Rim chipping	Intra-operatively and in service	Requires extra care at surgery
3	Revision post-fracture	Can be problematic	Retained ceramic debris affects revision implants
4	Adverse wear	Observed rarely	May be unique to pioneering monoblock cup design
5	Ceramic transformation	Observed problem in some zirconia heads	No longer on market
6	Head design	Head diameter and neck length	Fewer options than other designs
7	Cup design	Cup rim-extension options	Generally not available
8	Resurfacing hip design	Risk of fracture with current material concepts	Currrently not available
9	Implant costs	Higher than non-ceramic options	Varies country by country

implant orientations and patient activities, the ceramic femoral head may alternate between subluxing and impinging on the rim of the ceramic cup. Thus a scientific understanding of THA bearing performance in laboratory simulations is absolutely necessary for advancement of clinically relevant test regimes. The question is how ceramic bearings should be studied in the laboratory so that the test is relevant to surface degradation, wear, and fatigue mechanisms. This chapter will review features that are most relevant for a tribological understanding of ceramic performance.

2. Ceramics as THA Bearings

Pure alumina (Al_2O_3) has been the gold standard for hip bearings for four decades. Alternative ceramics for hip bearings include magnesia partially stabilized zirconia (Table 5-2: Mg-PSZ), and yttria-stabilized, tetragonal polycrystalline zirconia (Y-TZP). While the Mg-PSZ bearings continue to feature in clinical use, the Y-TZP ceramic was taken off the market due to an unacceptable incidences of fractures in femoral heads (Clarke and Gustafson, 2008; Clarke *et al.*, 2003a) and will not be discussed further. Silicon nitride (Si_3N_4) is currently used for spinal devices and is under investigation for use in THA bearings (Bal *et al.*, 2007a, 2009; Bal and Rahaman, 2012). There is also a new HOH application using a zirconium oxide surface (monoclinic zirconia) overlying a diffusion-hardened (DH) zone of zirconium metal alloy (DHOxZr^{TM}) (Parikh, 2013a).

2.1. *Alumina*

Many THA designs have incorporated Al_2O_3 since the 1970s (Boutin, 1972, Christel *et al.*, 1988, Griss *et al.*, 1975, Mittelmeier and Harms, 1979). However, it was not until the pioneering monoblock ceramic cups were replaced by modular designs featuring an alumina liner in a metal shell (Furlong, 1993) that one could say the modern era of ceramic hips had begun. This bioceramic has gone through a development comprising three distinct and successive generations, concurrently undergoing profound evolutions in density, purity, and

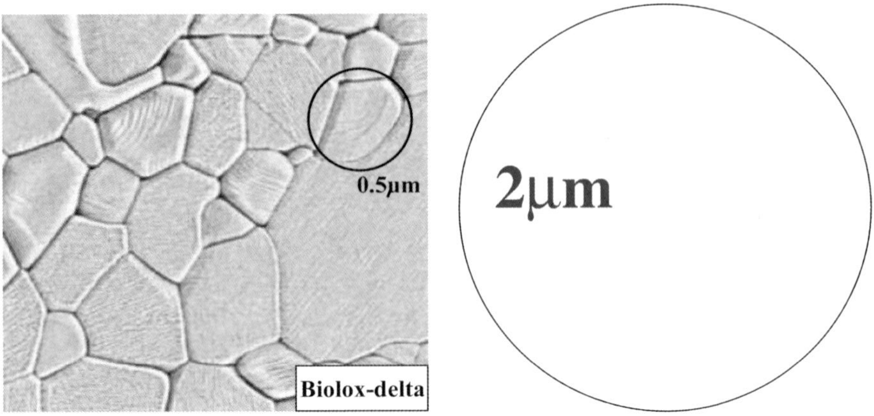

Figure 5-1. Microstructure of alumina grains depicted from sub-micron to 2 μm size as depicted to scale by large circle on the right (micrograph provided courtesy of CeramTec, Plochingen, Germany).

microstructural size/morphology. Modern alumina biomaterials are processed with a combination of conventional sintering and hot isostatic press sintering, which conspicuously eliminates abnormal grain growth and keeps the average grain size at around 1 μm (Figure 5-1). Despite the significant improvement that this evolutional course has brought to the structural reliability of alumina bioceramics, this material intrinsically remains quite brittle. In order to counteract this brittleness, biomaterials technologists have designed alumina-matrix composite microstructures in an attempt to combine the positive properties of monolithic alumina with an improved toughness. Alumina hip bearings have been the subject of much investigation and will not be discussed further here (Christel *et al.*, 1988; Clarke *et al.*, 2013a; Clarke and Willmann, 1994; Hannouche *et al.*, 2005, Nevelos *et al.*, 2001b; Pezzotti *et al.*, 2013c; Sedel *et al.*, 2003).

2.2. *Zirconia-Toughened Alumina*

Zirconia-toughened alumina (ZTA) for hip bearings was first developed in Europe when CeramTec obtained regulatory approval to market its ZTA products (CPE, ceramic-on-ceramic [CoC] bearings) in 2000 (Biolox-delta^{TM}, Plochingen, Germany). For CoC THA systems, CeramTec gained FDA approval for Biolox-delta and

Kyocera Medical gained Japanese approval for AZ209^{TM}, both in 2010. The ZTA composites represented a significant development in alumina technology. ZTA ceramics have much-improved strength and toughness compared to monolithic alumina (De Aza *et al.*, 2002; Pezzotti, 2013a). These are to be contrasted with monolithic zirconia (Y-TZP) in which polymorphic transformation can easily spread from one grain to neighboring grains, thus leading to faster monoclinic growth both in plane and in depth (Clarke *et al.*, 2003a). Such a zirconia ($t \rightarrow m$) proliferation process is minimized in ZTA composites by the presence of surrounding alumina grains.

ZTA ceramics use the polymorphic transformation-toughening mechanism uniquely provided by addition of partially stabilized zirconia (ZrO_2). The alumina matrix utilizes a reinforcing phase consisting of zirconia combined with a low percentage of Y_2O_3 stabilizing phase with other minor fractions of oxides that include chromia. The main toughening mechanism is the transformation of partially stabilized tetragonal zirconia into its monoclinic polymorph under the action of tensile stress fields induced by a propagating crack. The amount of toughening depends upon the fraction of tetragonal phase freshly transformed at the crack tip and around the crack path into the monoclinic phase.

There is also a strict requirement to control grain size and keep the size range as fine as possible. The presence of zirconia particles in the ZTA ceramic represents a considerable refinement controlling grain size in the alumina microstructure. In addition, the thermal expansion coefficient of the alumina matrix is smaller (by approximately 20%) than that of the tetragonal zirconia particle. Thus, when a ZTA ceramic cools from sintering temperature, the zirconia particle contracts more than the alumina matrix. This results in a tensile stress field in the zirconia particle and, for maintaining static equilibrium, in a compressive stress field in the surrounding alumina matrix. Accordingly, the residual stresses in the alumina matrix are compressive in nature when zirconia dispersoids are retained in their tetragonal phase. Such high compressive stresses in the alumina matrix lead to increased resistance to crack propagation with increasing crack extension. This mechanism is additive to the toughening effect produced by the polymorphic transformation of the tetragonal zirconia dispersoids. An apparent increase in hardness/wear resistance with respect to monolithic alumina can also be related to compressive stresses in the Al_2O_3 phase.

ZTA ceramics offer the advantage that their microstructure can be custom designed to optimize properties desirable in a ceramic bearing. The occurrence of polymorphic tetragonal-to-monoclinic ($t \rightarrow m$) transformation during cooling from sintering temperature can be seen as a degree of freedom in designing the ZTA microstructure. For example, the residual stress state in the alumina matrix phase could conceivably be set to nearly zero magnitude by suitably balancing the ratio of tetragonal to monoclinic fractions. An increase in the fraction of monoclinic zirconia phase in the ZTA composite can be obtained by limiting or eliminating the addition of Y_2O_3 stabilizing phase, thus destabilizing the zirconia dispersion during cooling from sintering temperature. This would increasingly push the residual hydrostatic stress fields in the alumina matrix towards the tensile side. It is to be noted that an important aspect of microstructure in ZTA design is to obtain an increase in structural reliability from the transformation toughening effect ($t \rightarrow m$) during crack propagation, while avoiding any tendency to produce the negative effect that can lead to spontaneous surface transformations during exposure to a hydrothermally activated environment. The presence of fully unstabilized zirconia particles creates a higher fraction of monoclinic phase in as-received ZTA components. Increasing the amount of monoclinic fraction in a ZTA ceramic after sintering would obviously reduce the amount of ZrO_2 potentially available for crack-tip transformation and toughening. It would also enhance the magnitude of the tensile residual stresses stored in the residual tetragonal phase. It is therefore possible to make the residual tetragonal phase more prone to transformation during crack propagation by reducing the fraction of stabilizing agent and thus enhancing the tensile residual stress. Such micromechanical enhancement may improve the efficiency of the transformation toughening effect by promoting a more intense although less extensive shielding effect around a propagating crack.

The two well-known ZTA hip bearings are the Biolox-delta^{TM}, as produced by CeramTec (Plochingen, Germany), and the AZ209^{TM}

Table 5-5. Principal oxide content and grain size of ZTA-C and ZTA-K materials.

Parameter	ZTA-C	ZTA-K
ZrO_2 vol% (avg. grain size)	17% (0.45 μm)	14% (0.35 μm)
Al_2O_3 (vol%) (avg. grain size)	82% (1.01 μm)	84% (0.43 μm)
Other oxides	1%	2%

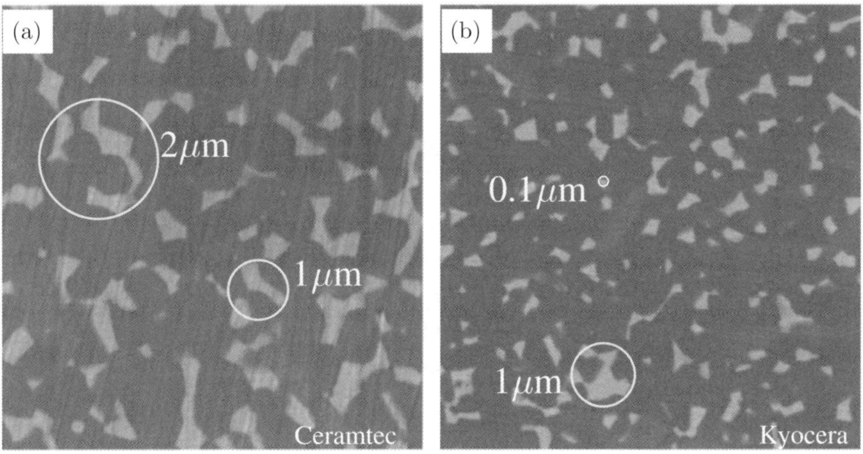

Figure 5-2. Comparison of ZTA microstructures (a) Biolox-forte^{TM}, Ceramtec and (b) AZ209^{TM}, Kyocera Medical (micrographs provided courtesy of M. Boffelli, Kyoto Institute of Technology).

as made by Kyocera Medical (Osaka, Japan). Both contain similar fractions of fine ZrO_2 and Al_2O_3 particles and both have flexural strengths >1 GPa (Table 5-5) (Nakanishi *et al.*, 2007a, 2007b). At the microstructural level the CeramTec material (Figure 5-2a: ZTA-C) has a coarser structure than the Kyocera ceramic (Figure 5-2b: ZTA-K). The amount of stabilizing oxide present in the raw ceramic powder creates the microstructural difference between the ZTA-C (~2 mol% Y_2O_3) and ZTA-K (zero Y_2O_3). The Y_2O_3 oxide has two principal effects in the final ceramic: (i) stabilizing the tetragonal ZrO_2 phase; and, (ii) toughening the bearing surface. This results in a different amount of monoclinic phase in the final

ZTA microstructure. Hence, the ZTA-C material was designed to maximize the toughening effect while keeping phase stability within acceptable limits. In contrast, the ZTA-C material was designed to maximize phase stability at the bearing surface while keeping fracture toughness above an acceptable value (Pezzotti, 2013a). It can be anticipated that the residual stresses on the bearing surfaces will also be quite different as a result of the ZTA-C and ZTA-K microstructures. This topic requires further study.

There are, therefore, two different concepts that depend on microstructural design criterion in ZTA bearings. In the first scenario (composite-A) there can be formation of isolated spots of highly tensile stresses in correspondence with residual tetragonal zirconia dispersoids after long-term hydrothermal loading. In hydrothermal experiments, it was shown that composite-A experienced a continuous increase of monoclinic fraction from 7 up to 70 vol% of the added zirconia fraction. Nevertheless, the experimental results to date with composite-A showed that the impact of transformation on surface morphology was minimal (Pezzotti, 2013a). In the second scenario (composite-B), there can be observed the undesirable presence of pristine, highly compressive stress points at grain boundaries where monoclinic zirconia dispersoids are located. This effect can lead to monoclinic zirconia escaping during articulation with the resulting production of ceramic wear particles. The experimental results with composite-B showed that it possessed an initial 30 vol% fraction of monoclinic in the overall ZrO_2 phase. This controlled the initial amount of the monoclinic phase in the material and ensured surface stability in a hydrothermal environment, which remained unaltered during 300 hours of autoclave exposure (Pezzotti, 2013a).

2.3. *Silicon Nitride*

Silicon nitride (Si_3N_4) is a new ceramic candidate for THA bearings. Silicon nitride (Si_3N_4) is a high-strength, monolithic ceramic (Table 5-6). It has seen application in spinal implants and undergone both CPE and CoC simulator tests (Bal *et al.*, 2008). Silicon nitride has the highest fracture toughness of any ceramic (Table 5-6). Its strength and toughness are comparable with the best values of other

Table 5-6. Benefits of low-wear, stability and crack-propagation resistance in Si_3N_4 bearings.

Item	Parameter	Details
1	Ultra-low wear rates	Comparable to Al_2O_3 and ZTA ceramics
2	Unique acicular grain structure	Highest fracture toughness
3	Phase-stable material	Hydrothermal degradation is not an issue
4	Ceramic wear products	Bioresorbable species
5	Oxygen affinity	May offer beneficial protective mechanism

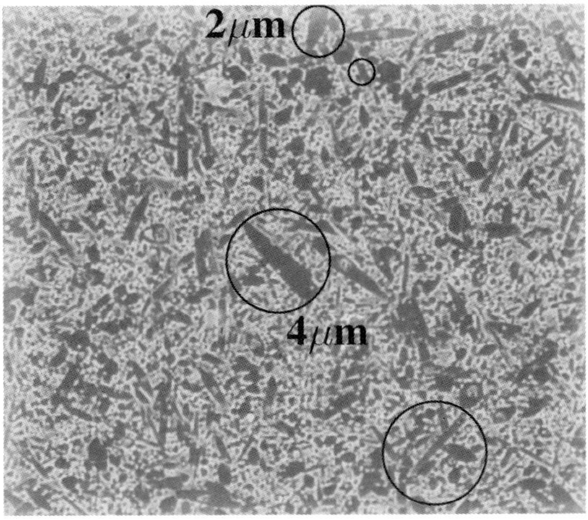

Figure 5-3. Typical fibrous microstructure created by appearance of acicular shaped grains of ß-Si_3N_4 (micrograph provided courtesy of Amedica).

ceramics (Bal and Rahaman, 2012; Mazzocchi and Bellosi, 2008a; Mazzocchi *et al.*, 2008b). Si_3N_4 derives strength and toughness by microstructural engineering and not by phase transformations. Its superior strength and toughness are derived from a unique acicular grain structure (Figure 5-3). This fibrous microstructure is generated during densification via an irreversible dissolution reprecipitation process. The equiaxed α-Si_3N_4 particles are converted into acicular ß-Si_3N_4 grains that are typically 1–4 μm in length (Figure 5-3). The latter architecture imparts high toughness and strength without the need for addition of a metastable phase such as zirconia. Consequently, by avoiding the ZrO_2 toughening mechanism, Si_3N_4 is not susceptible to hydrothermal degradation. Its microstructure is composed of asymmetric needle-like interlocking grains surrounded by a <2 nm refractory grain-boundary glass. This unique fibrous structure provides Si_3N_4 with its exceptional strength and toughness. Two industrial standards have been adopted from its use as an industrial ceramic bearing (ASTM F2094/F2094M-14, 2011; ISO 26602, 2009). Monolithic Si_3N_4 was first utilized 1968 in Australia for clinical trials evaluating a lumbar-spine spacer (Sorrell *et al.*, 2004). Si_3N_4 can also be produced as a coating using physical vapor (PVD) and chemical vapor deposition (CVD) methods. The coated silicon nitrides can be amorphous or nano-crystalline and non-stoichiometric. These coatings can have comparable hardness to the monolithic ceramic but do not have the same strength or toughness. A European consortium was formed in 2013 to develop PVD silicon nitride coatings for application to CoCr hip and knee bearings. Beginning in 2008 in the USA, Si_3N_4 has been used as a fusion cage for arthrodesis of the cervical and thoracolumbar spine. It has also produced exceptionally low wear-rates. Pre-clinical testing has indicated suitability for THA (Clarke and Bowsher, 2007; Jahanmir *et al.*, 2004; Williams *et al.*, 2005; Zhou *et al.*, 1997) but it has yet to be given regulatory clearance for this purpose (Bal *et al.*, 2009, Bal and Rahaman, 2012).

2.4. *Zirconia Ceramic Surface on Zirconium Alloy*

An alternate approach to the use of monoblock ceramic components would be to cover a metal bearing with a ceramic coating, thereby obtaining the benefits of a ceramic surface wedded to the mechanical resiliency of the bulk metallic component. It would be additionally beneficial if indeed such a ceramic structure not only reduced wear but also minimized or eliminated diffusion of metal ions from the bulk metal. While this would appear an intuitively desirable approach, it involves a number of manufacturing issues and imperceptible technical difficulties to achieve such a concept. Hence, no implant system has emerged to date with successful ceramic coatings.

One novel approach that has demonstrated clinical utility in both THA and TKA systems utilizes an intrinsically formed oxidation layer on the bulk metal surface. It is apparent that the combination of properties displayed by the Oxynium^{TM} bearing systems has contributed an effective metal-polyethylene (MPE) system (Smith and Nephew, Memphis TN) (Parikh, 2013b). The Oxynium bearing is not a coating but rather an intrinsically formed oxidation layer on the bulk metal surface. It has been demonstrated that such a grown oxide layer can tolerate localized damage or material loss without risk of catastrophic failure, such as those induced by spalling or delamination. The oxidation surface products consist almost exclusively of monoclinic zirconia polymorph (Pezzotti, 2013b).

A new composition of oxidized zirconium (DHOxZr) has been developed as a potential bearing material for hard-on-hard (HOH) hip arthroplasty (Parikh, 2013a). Beneath the ceramic surfaces is a thick DH zone of zirconium metal. The monoclinic zirconia surface and the underlying DH-zone are expected to produce low wear with minimal release of metal ions. This concept of a zirconia and DH-layered metallic bearing may provide a CoC concept with no fracture risk.

3. What is Normal Ceramic Wear in Patients?

The first point to establish is how much wear occurs in a ceramic hip over time. In this regard, it is necessary to consider all CoC wear reports even if it is suspected that some could be outliers, perhaps due to a combination of ceramic quality, THA design, or possibly confounding clinical parameters. Some early studies noted gross wear in CoC retrieval (Figure 5-4) (Kummer *et al.*, 1990; Nevelos *et al.*, 1999). These appeared limited to the ceramic hip designs of the 1970s that featured wide femoral necks and press-fit, monoblock cups (Figures 5-5–5-7). Volumetric wear varied from <1 to over $200\,mm^3/year$ (Nevelos *et al.*, 1999). With the advantage of hindsight, it would appear that the alumina ceramic used 40 years ago was not optimal

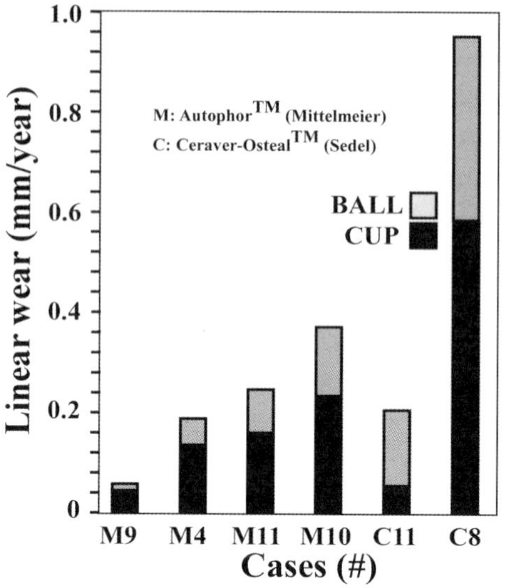

Figure 5-4. Linear wear-rates measured on retrieved THA featuring pioneering design of monoblock ceramic cup (Nevelos *et al.*, 2001b).

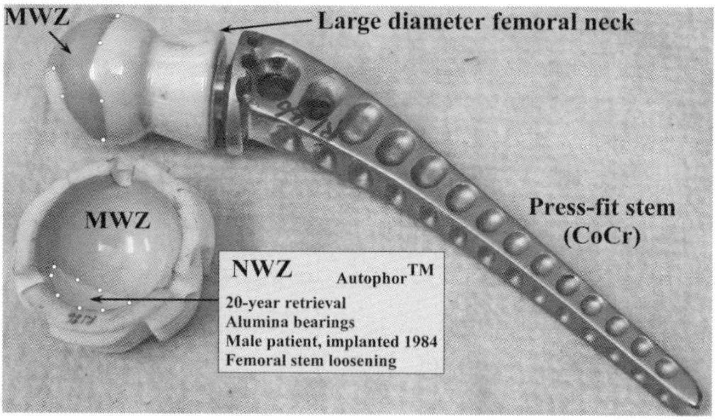

Figure 5-5. Pioneering Autophor™ design featuring a large femoral neck and threaded monoblock alumina cup. Wear patterns on this 20-year retrieval are stained pink and white circles mark the boundaries (THA loaned courtesy of K. Keggi MD).

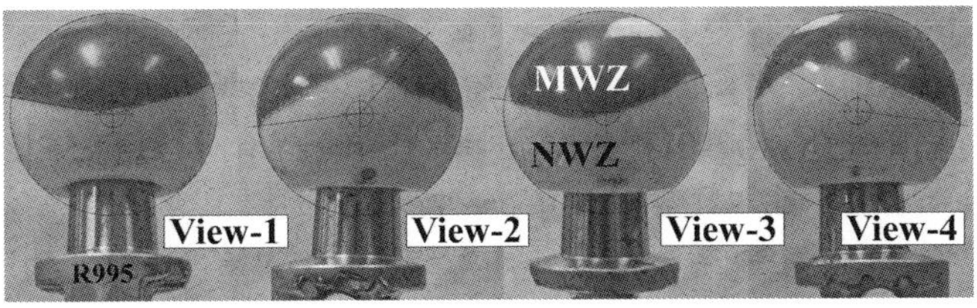

Figure 5-6. Head wear pattern shown in four orthogonal views for Autophor design retrieved at 32 years (THA loaned courtesy of R. Grijalva MD).

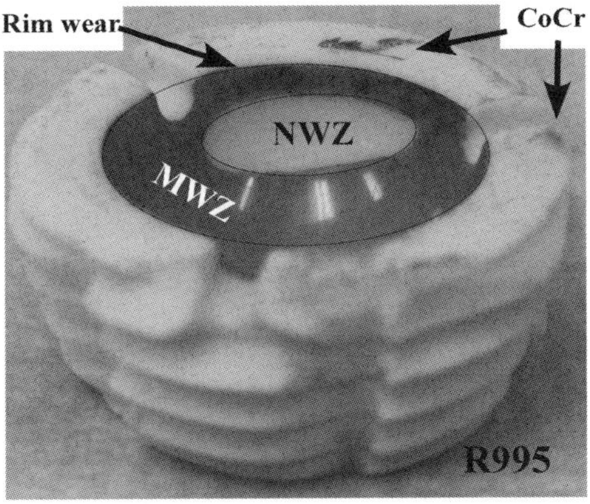

Figure 5-7. Cup main wear zone (for THA in Figure 5-3) with stained MWZ and showing small elliptical non-wear zone (NWZ) located inferiorly. Small patches of CoCr metal stain are also present on the cup rim.

and the early THA concepts clearly had range-of-motion limitations (Figure 5-5), while cup and stem fixation techniques were not as reliable as with contemporary THA. Examples of gross ceramic wear (Figure 5-4) were believed to be due to patients ambulating on loose cups that were in the process of migrating and tilting (Christel *et al.*, 1988; Clarke *et al.*, 1988; Sedel *et al.*, 1990, 2003). From a contemporary perspective, we suspect that such cases represented extreme edge wear, a known risk when the rim of the cup impinges on both the femoral head and against the femoral neck (Clarke *et al.*, 2014b; Harris, 2012; McHugh *et al.*, 2013).

Ceramic performance parameters will be defined here using habitual-wear versus non-wear zones (NWZ), adverse stripe wear, surface roughness, and CoC wear rates. The main-wear zone (MWZ) will be defined as that area of habitual wear created during normal ambulation of the patient. The defined NWZ lies outside the MWZ area but may show wear damage inconsistently due to adverse and unpredictable events. The MWZ pattern on femoral heads generally appears circular and is typically situated close to and somewhat superior to the axis of the femoral neck (Figure 5-6). This will occupy 50–100% of the head's hemispherical area depending on THA design, patient activities, and the duration of follow-up. Cup wear patterns are much more varied in size and shape but typically will show a small NWZ area in the inferior aspect (Figure 5-7).

Comparison of ceramic roughness data can be problematic in both retrieval and simulator studies. Firstly, it is important to separate MWZ from NWZ patterns (Figures 5-5–5-7) and to characterize their roughness parameters separately. Secondly, it is important to note in the field of view that there may be arrays of large scratches, sometimes referred to as 'stripe wear'. This roughness may need to be characterized into fields with stripes and those without stripes (Halim *et al.*, 2014). In general, MWZ roughness can be anticipated to be higher than for the NWZ. For example, the NWZ and MWZ roughness (Ra) in a 32-year CoC retrieval averaged 17 nm and 123 nm, respectively, a seven-fold difference (Table 5-7, Figure 5-8). Surface roughness was also classified into six grades for ease of comparison between the retrieval and simulator studies (Table 5-8). The 30-year CoC retrieval was observed to have a NWZ roughness level of II and a MWZ level of V. However, it is noted that NWZ roughness can be much higher when stripe damage is present.

Table 5-7. Sample roughness 32-year CoC.

Head	Ra (nm)	Rz (nm)	PV (nm)	Rsk
New	5–7			
NWZ	17	1354	1802	−10.4
MWZ	123	3686	4342	−4.6
MWZ/NWZ	7.2	2.7	2.4	0.4

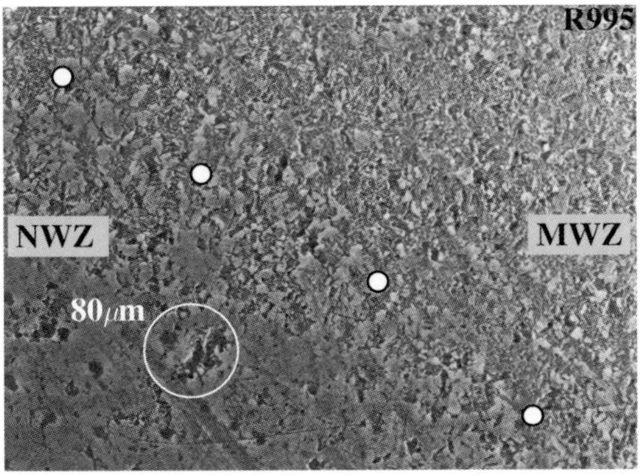

Figure 5-8. SEM imaging of MWZ and NWZ in the head of a 32-year retrieval (see Figure 5-3). Scale of surface damage indicated by 80 μm ring and transition between MWZ and NWZ marked by blank circles.

Table 5-8. Ceramic roughness classification.

Class	Ra (nm)	Classification	Observational
I	<10	Superior	New surface
II	10–24	Excellent	Very fine scratches
III	25–50	Good	Scratches with some pitting
IV	50–100	Mild wear process	Surface polish removed locally, porosity increased
V	100–300	Moderate wear process	Greater loss of surface, more grains exposed
VI	>300	Adverse wear effect	Gross excavation of grains

Stripe wear has been a well-reported phenomenon on retrieved CoC bearings (Dorlot *et al.*, 1992; Esposito *et al.*, 2012; Manaka *et al.*, 2003; Shishido *et al.*, 2003; Walter *et al.*, 2004). A study of 54 revisions of a modern CoC design noted that 83% of retrievals had stripe wear (Esposito *et al.*, 2012). In seven cases the stripes were on the posterior aspect of the heads (cups impinging anteriorly) and in 32 cases the stripes were on the anterior aspects (cups impinging posteriorly). A further six heads featured two stripes, one each on the anterior and posterior aspects. It was noted that the median volumetric wear rates varied from 0.2 to 1.9 mm^3/year for

Table 5-9. Ranking of clinical wear-rates.

Class	Stripe wear	Wear rate (mm^3/Yr)	Stripe risks (RSS)	Squeaking/clicking/grinding
A	None	<0.1	Negligible	Unlikely
B	Negligible	0.1 to 0.5	None or faint stripe wear	Some bearing noise possible
C	Yes	0.5 to <1	Mild stripe wear	Some bearing noise possible
D	Yes	1 to <5	Moderate stripe wear	Bearing noise more likely
E	Multiples	5 to <10	Multiple distinct stripes, elevated wear	Bearing noise likely
F	Surface loss	>10	Aggressive stripe wear	Collateral damage, loose cup

anterior versus posterior stripes, respectively. In three revised cases of bearing-related failures, wear rates were 0.3, 1.9, and 7.2 mm^3/year. Wear was noted to be undetectable in CoC bearings lacking stripe damage. This important CoC retrieval study demonstrated that wear rates could vary from near zero to 0.2 mm^3/year for cases with posterior stripes, 1.9 mm^3/year for cases with anterior stripes, and up to 7.2 mm^3/year in one case revised for squeaking. The authors noted that posterior edge loading (impingement) occurred even with well-positioned cups and could likely be considered a normal occurrence. In summary, this CoC retrieval study offered for the first time an extremely useful set of *in vivo* wear rates for comparison with laboratory data. Therefore, six wear grades have been defined for ease of comparison between retrieval and simulator studies (Table 5-9). Note that wear classes D and E were included for completeness, i.e. encompassing runaway wear phenomenon as described in the early CoC literature (Figure 5-4, Table 5-10).

4. What is Abnormal Ceramic Wear *In Vivo*?

Impingement of the cup rim against the metal femoral neck cannot be designed against and also cannot be predicted in any THA patient

Table 5-10. Comparison of clinical and simulator wear-rates.

Wear class	Retrievals (Esposito *et al.*, 2012)	Wear in retrievals (mm^3/Yr) (Esposito *et al.*, 2012)[2]	Simulator wear rate (mm^3/Mc)	Simulator test mode
A	No stripe damage	0	0.05	Standard (average)
B	Posterior stripe cases	0.2	0.19	Mild micro-separation
C	Anterior stripe cases	1.9	1.8	Severe micro-separation
D	Worst stripe (revision, squeak)	7.2	6.3	Run-in wear rate (average)

population. Notching of titanium alloy (Ti_6Al_4V) femoral necks has resulted in metal transfer onto both CoCr and ceramic bearing surfaces (Bowsher *et al.*, 2008; Clarke *et al.*, 2013b, 2014b; Eickmann *et al.*, 2003; Iida *et al.*, 1999; McMurtrie *et al.*, 2009). Bal *et al.* (2007b) reported on ten ceramic heads that had undergone multiple dislocations. The 28 mm heads had black articular areas indicative of metal contamination, notably Ti_6Al_4V. Six of the ten acetabular shells revealed damage due to impingement by metal femoral necks. Murali *et al.* (2008) presented two revision cases that had 32 mm alumina CoC. In the female patient the Ti_6Al_4V femoral neck had been excessively anteverted. The patient was active and performed yoga regularly. Revision was undertaken at seven years for osteolysis. It was noted that the Ti_6Al_4V neck had impinged at three locations on the Ti_6Al_4V fence surrounding the cup rim (anteriorly, posteriorly, and laterally). A similar CoC impingement case was previously reported by Eickmann *et al.* (2003). The clicking/squeaking noises were created at hip extension during walking and it was found that the femoral neck had destroyed the Ti_6Al_4V fence on the cup rim and suffered two notches in consequence. Murali's second case was a 48-year-old male carpenter who complained of squeaking noises at six months. The hip was painful and began to squeak, clunk, and click at every step. CT imaging identified osteolysis, and posterior

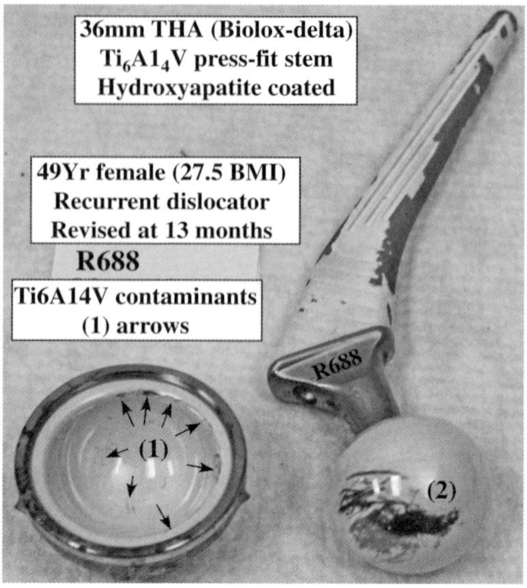

Figure 5-9. Biolox-delta™ retrieval showing black metallic staining (revised at 13 months for multiple dislocations). The stem and metal shell were Ti_6Al_4V alloy and the black stains were identified as containing Ti, Al, and V metals.

impingement was noted at revision. The tissues showed abundant black granular Ti_6Al_4V debris. Therefore, a common pathway exists in such cases with impingement or subluxation bringing the femoral neck into contact against the cup rim resulting in the production of metal debris. This cloud of metal particles can then migrate around the joint space and into the bearing areas (Figures 5-9 and 5-10). Black staining with titanium alloy elements has been identified frequently on CoC revisions. Co and Cr contamination has also been noted in designs with press-fit CoCr stems (Shishido *et al.*, 2003; Tateiwa *et al.*, 2007).

5. What is Normal Simulator Wear?

There are many misconceptions regarding the efficacy of hip simulator studies used to predict wear in ceramic bearings. It is quite common to find published arguments that laboratory wear studies were flawed because they produced wear rates consistently lower than

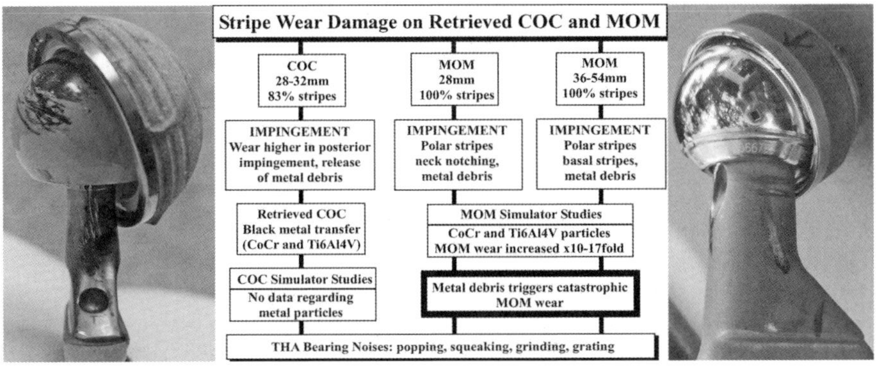

Figure 5-10. Stripe wear algorithm depicting the progression that can result from impingement and subluxation, releasing metal debris that invades the joint space and stains ceramic surfaces black. In the case of metal-on-metal (MoM) this can produce catastrophic wear. Note the notching on the femoral neck.

those measured in retrieval studies (Kamali *et al.*, 2010). First, it must be appreciated that artificial hip joints have to perform in a wide variety of patients whose performance levels will vary from pedestrian to high-impact sporting activities. It is also apparent that bearing wear can vary depending on factors such as patient age, surgical positioning of implants, range of motion in the hip joint, and job set (e.g. a clerical worker versus a farmer's regular activities). It should be no surprise that laboratory test methods cannot possibly encompass such a variety of patient performance. Second, there is a major difference between a simulator research project and a document published as a standard guideline. The latter represents a consensus document assembled by experts in the field to support well-defined test methodologies. It provides consistency in implant evaluations, which benefits tribology science, but also greatly assists implant reviews by the various regulatory bodies. A standards document therefore typically provides guidance for one set of well-prescribed test conditions (ISO 14242-1, 2002; ISO 14242-3, 2008). In contrast, a simulator publication may represent an exploratory project to further tribological science and thus may have departed considerably from established methodology. Those involved in the regulatory approval process rely more on published standards and much less on individual research publications.

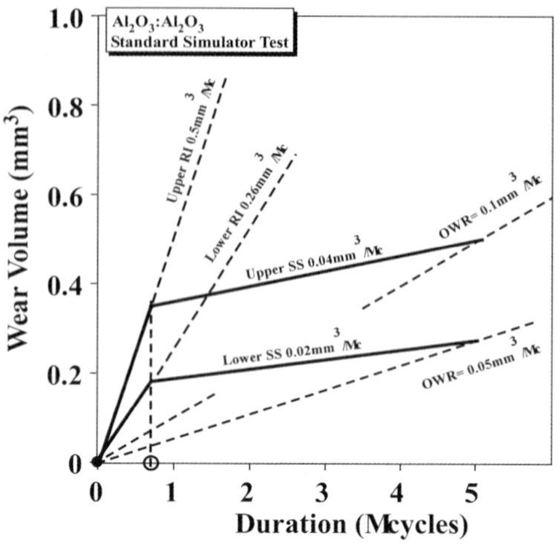

Figure 5-11. Assemblage of data regarding alumina wear trends in standard hip simulator studies (Clarke *et al.*, 2003b, 2011, 2013a). Upper and lower ranges are indicated for run-in and steady-state wear phases typical of the standard simulator test mode.

Simulator wear studies (ASTM F1714, 2008; ISO 14242-1, 2002; ISO 14242-3, 2008) of CoC bearings have demonstrated that there was an initial run-in wear phase followed by a steady-state phase with wear reduced (Figure 5-11). Reviews in the literature have indicated that CoC run-in wear rates were typically in the range 0.26–0.5 mm^3/Mc (Clarke *et al.*, 2003b, 2011, 2013a; Oonishi *et al.*, 2004). Steady-state wear was immeasurably low in some studies but appeared to range 0–0.04 mm^3/Mc. For comparison with retrieval studies, the overall wear rates (average over 5 Mc duration) would be 0.05–0.1 mm^3/Mc (Figure 5-11). It is to be noted that the standard simulator test does not produce microseparation or edge wear in the bearings (ISO 14242-1, 2002; ISO 14242-3, 2008). Therefore, such wear studies should represent the normal spectrum anticipated for patients with minimal impingement risk, i.e. no stripe wear (Tables 5-9, 5-10) (Esposito *et al.*, 2012).

6. Simulator Wear with Steep Cups

It is assumed in simulator standards that the acetabular cup will be inclined at 45° to the horizontal plane (Figure 5-12) (ISO 14242-1,

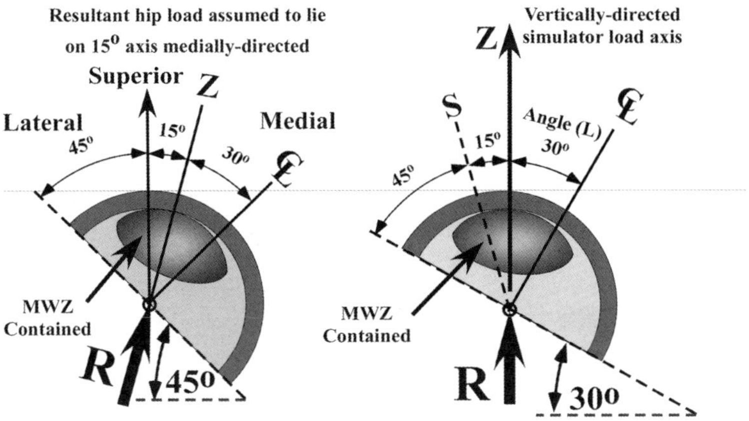

(a) AP-view in-vivo (b) Simulator (ISO 14242-1)

Figure 5-12. Cup mounting as depicted in standard simulator guideline ISO-14242-1, (a) as viewed in AP-radiograph image of patient and (b) as mounted in hip simulator.

2002; ISO 14242-3, 2008). It is also assumed that the resultant load vector in the human hip will be inclined 15° medial to the vertical plane. However, in the simulator the resultant load vector will generally lie in the vertical plane (Figure 5-12b). A 30° inclined simulator cup is thus defined analogous to a 45° cup in the patient. The desired result creates a wear pattern fully contained within the cup rim, i.e. no edge wear (Bowsher *et al.*, 2009).

Simulator studies have analyzed wear in cups inclined at angles steeper than the 30° inclination stipulated in guidelines (ISO 14242-1, 2002). The objective was to simulate the edge wear seen in certain retrievals (Esposito *et al.*, 2012; Underwood *et al.*, 2012; Walter *et al.*, 2004). Two parameters need to be ascertained for a successful test: (i) the diameter of the wear patch; and, (ii) a criterion to define degree of edge wear. Such details have been presented in standard simulator studies (Figure 5-13) but not in tests with steep cups. What is known from simulator tests of metal-on-metal (MoM) bearings is that wear patterns in cups varied from 400 to 600 mm^2 in area (Figure 5-13) (Bowsher *et al.*, 2009; Lee *et al.*, 2008; Leslie *et al.*, 2008). Normalizing for bearing diameters (39–60 mm

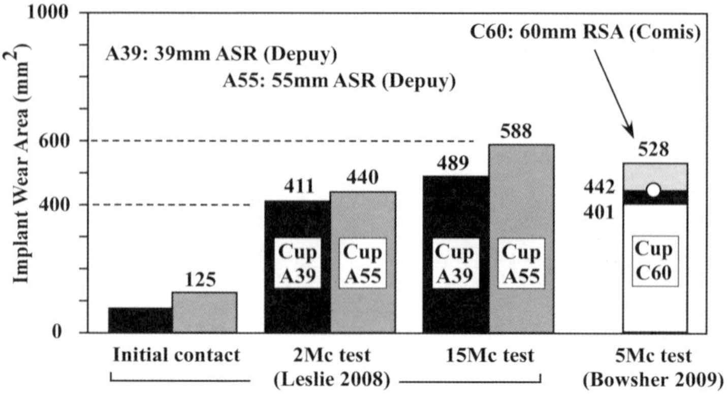

Figure 5-13. Wear patterns in acetabular cups as mounted in anatomic simulator mode for MoM studies (Bowsher *et al.*, 2009; Leslie *et al.*, 2008).

diameters), such wear patterns represented 8–18% of the hemispherical cup area (Figure 5-14a–5-14c) (Clarke *et al.*, 2013b). One 28 mm MoM study estimated the circular wear pattern to have a half-width of 8 mm (Firkins *et al.*, 2001). This would correspond to a wear pattern of 221 mm^2 and a hemi-area ratio of 18%. The data from Korduba *et al.* (2014) for wear areas at various cup inclinations in 28 mm MPE provided the same ratio (Figures 5-14d–5-14g). Plotting these MoM data (anatomical tests) provided the first demonstration of an algorithm relating cup wear patterns to THA diameters (Figure 5-15) (ISO 14242-1, 2002).

Nevelos *et al.* (2001) ran 28 mm CoC bearings with cups at 40° and 60° inclinations and found no difference in wear rates, with an overall average of 0.9 mm^3/Mc (Table 5-9: Class A). From consideration of MoM cup geometry (Figures 5-13–5-15), it would appear that a 40° inclined 28 mm cup would cover the MWZ area of a 28 mm head (Figure 5-15a), whereas the 60° cup would leave the MWZ slightly uncovered (Figure 5-15b). Given the rigidity and high wear resistance of alumina, it is likely that the MWZ pattern in CoC bearings would be at least 20% smaller than with MoM. Thus, the 60° CoC cup likely could not experience edge wear and this may explain why the wear rates were unaffected by 40° and 60° cup inclinations (Nevelos *et al.*, 2001).

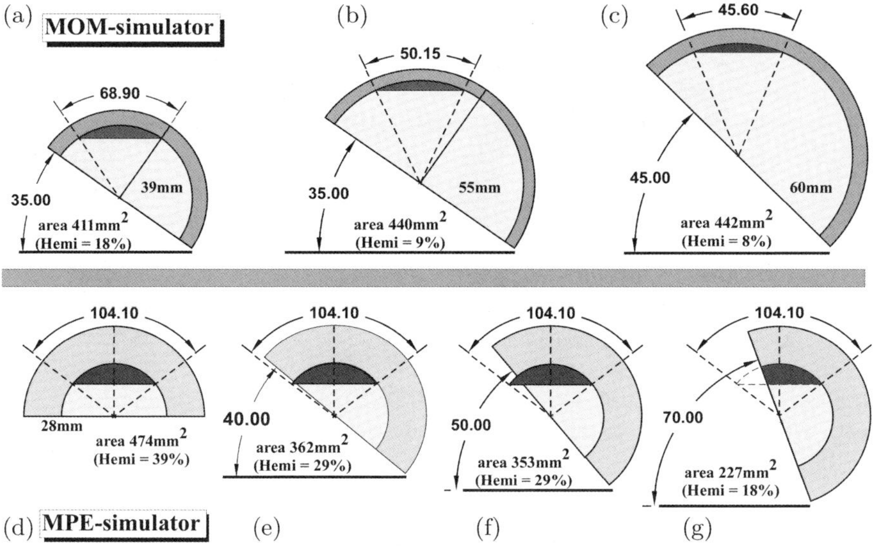

Figure 5-14. Comparison of cup wear patterns for metal-polyethylene (MPE) bearings and metal-on-metal (MoM) bearings: (a–c) MoM bearings diameter 39–60 mm diameter (see Figure 5-13); and, (d–g) 28 mm MPE bearings run with cups at different inclinations (Korduba *et al.*, 2014).

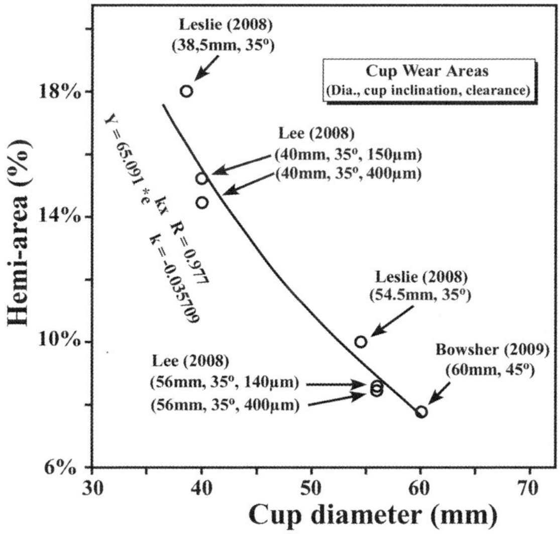

Figure 5-15. Algorithm relating areas of cup wear patterns (hemi-area ratios from Figure 5-14) that decreased with respect to increasing THA diameters.

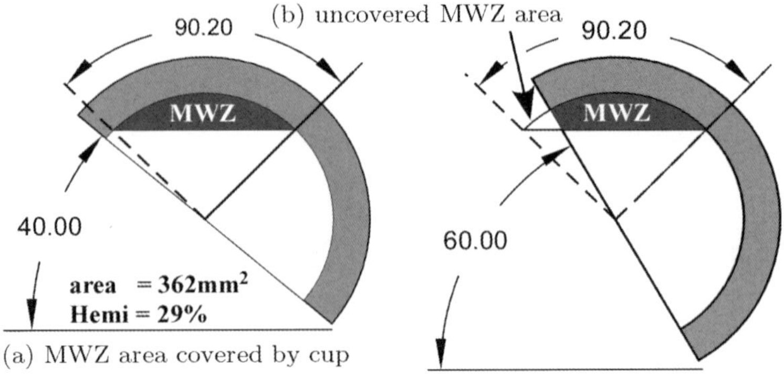

Figure 5-16. Estimated wear patterns (MWZ) depicted for 28 mm MoM here with cup inclinations of 40° and 60° in an anatomical simulator test (Nevelos *et al.*, 2001a).

7. Wear with Simulator Microseparation

The microseparation test (MSX) was developed by the Biomedical Engineering Group (BME) at Leeds University (UK) to create stripe damage similar to that seen on Al_2O_3 retrievals (Nevelos *et al.*, 1999, 2000). The MSX test raised CoC wear rates by an order of magnitude and for the first time enabled discrimination between Al_2O_3 and ZTA bearings (Figure 5-18a). Alumina wear rates with 28 mm CoC bearings increased 3-fold and 30-fold in mild and severe MSX tests, respectively (Figure 5-17). At Loma Linda University (LLU), the four combinations of 36 mm Al_2O_3 and ZTA bearings in MSX test mode demonstrated the stripe wear phenomenon within first 100,000 cycles (Clarke *et al.*, 2006; Green *et al.*, 2007). Perhaps coincidentally, the LLU wear average of 1.84 mm^3/Mc with 36 mm Al_2O_3 was identical to the BME study with 28 mm Al_2O_3 (Figure 5-18a). Thus, despite many experimental differences between the BME and LLU studies, the CoC wear-rates were comparable.

It was noted that with similar ceramic pairings (Al_2O_3/Al_2O_3 and ZTA/ZTA), the heads contributed ~50% of total CoC wear. However, in the hybrid pairs the Al_2O_3 heads in ZTA liners contributed 33% of total wear. Similarly, when combined with ZTA heads the Al_2O_3 cups contributed only 33% to total wear. Thus, the ZTA components were preferentially compared to their mating Al_2O_3

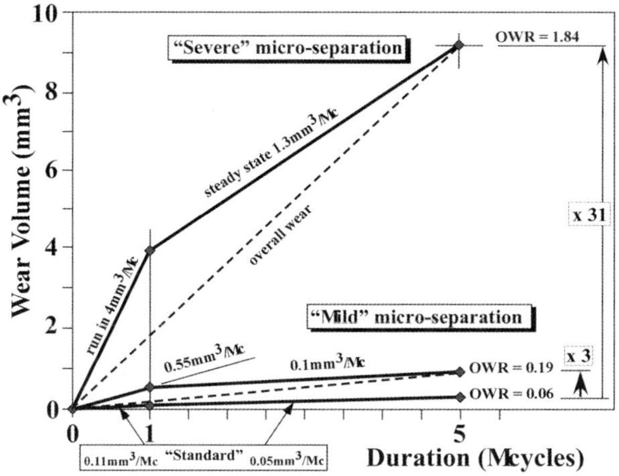

Figure 5-17. Wear trends for 28 mm Al_2O_3/Al_2O_3 bearings run with (a) standard simulator test, (b) mild microseparation test, and (c) severe microseparation test. Here overall wear rates are indicated for comparison with CoC retrieval studies.

bearings. This illustrated the difference the harder Al_2O_3 surface made, even while the ZTA hybrid pairs contributed to a three-fold wear reduction overall (Figure 5-18b).

The new CoC combination of oxidized zirconium (DHOxZr) has also been run in the MSX simulator mode. This ceramic has a thick DH zone beneath the oxide layer (Parikh *et al.*, 2013). The DHOxZr steady-state wear rate increased from 0.02 mm^3/Mc estimated in the standard test to 0.07 mm^3/Mc with microseparation (Figure 5-19). While this represented a three-fold increase, the wear rate was still so low as to correspond to class A (Table 5-10). Nevertheless, this MSX study discovered that stripe damage had worn through the zirconia surface to expose the DH metal zone.

8. CoC Simulator Wear with Debris Contamination

Despite abundant retrieval evidence of contamination risk by third-body metal particles (Bal *et al.*, 2007b; Eickmann *et al.*, 2003; Heiner *et al.*, 2008; Iida *et al.*, 1999; Lundberg *et al.*, 2007; McMurtrie *et al.*, 2009; Murali *et al.*, 2008), wear studies with metal particles have been

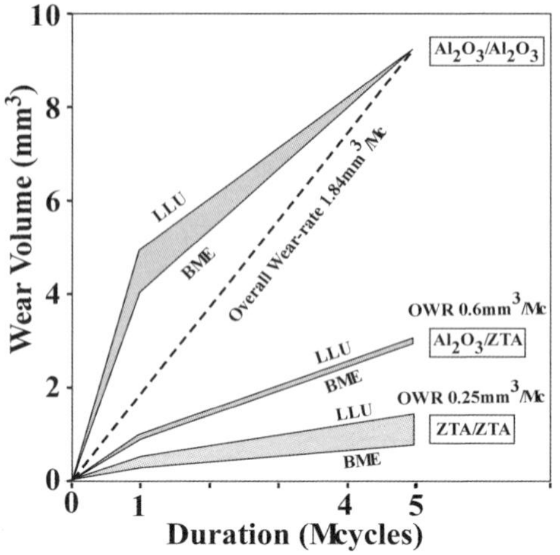

(a)

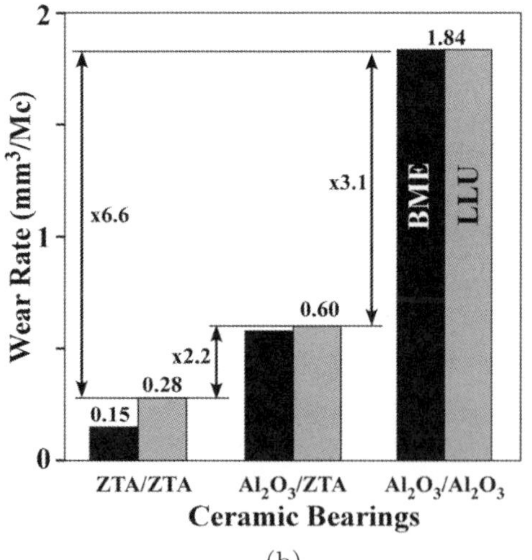

(b)

Figure 5-18. (a) Al_2O_3 and ZTA wear data run in simulators at severe microseparation mode in the Biomedical Engineering Group (BME, Leeds University) and the Peterson Tribology Laboratory (LLU: Loma Linda University). BME studies used 28 mm and LLU studies used 36 mm CoC, showing (a) run-in, steady-state, and overall-wear trending, and (b) comparison of overall wear rates for the three ceramic combinations. (b) Comparison of overall wear rates for Al_2O_3 and ZTA combinations.

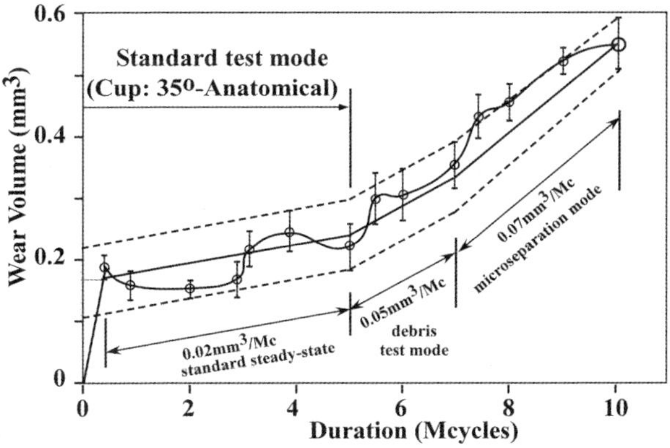

Figure 5-19. Simulator wear trending with the new ceramic DHOxZr run in standard, abrasive, and microseparation modes. (Graph redrawn from Parikh *et al.*, 2013a.)

scant, appearing only in a few MoM simulator studies (Halim *et al.*, 2013, 2014; Lu *et al.*, 2000). Particles of bone cement, CoCr, and Ti6Al4V were compared, running in abrasive tests with 36 mm MoM bearings (Clarke *et al.*, 2014; Halim *et al.*, 2014). Bone cement had no affect on CoCr surfaces but both CoCr and Ti6Al4V particles created black lubricants and raised wear rates by an order of magnitude. One CoC simulator study used bone cement for abrasion studies (PMMA: Versabond^{TM}, Smith & Nephew) (Parikh *et al.*, 2013a). The bearing was the new composition of oxidized zirconium (DHOxZr) with a thick DH zone beneath the oxide layer. With a PMMA concentration of 10 mg/ml in lubricant, the DHOxZr steady-state wear rate increased from the 0.02 mm^3/Mc estimate to 0.05 mm^3/Mc (Figure 5-19). While this represented a doubling of the DHOxZr wear-rate, this remained within class A (Table 5-10).

9. Discussion

The role of pre-clinical test methods is to provide insight into biomaterial and tribological interactions *in vivo*. Indeed, many test methods could be envisaged and developed by individual research laboratories but the question is which ones will have clinical relevance

Table 5-11. Comparison of squeaking parameters–surgical and design.

Item	Parameter	Risk	Details
1	Brand mismatches	Surgical	Off-label use
2	CoC material mismatch	Unlikely	ZTA head/Al_2O_3 cup
3	CoM material mismatch	Surgical	ZTA head/CoCr cup
4	Cup steeply inclined	Surgical	Frequently reported
5	Cup anteversion too low/high	Surgical	Frequently reported
6	Contact area too conforming/too large	Unlikely	Due to high wear?
7	Stripe wear	Possible	Biomechanics study
8	Metal contamination on ceramic bearing	Likely	Biomechanics study
9	Debris interposed between bearings	Possible	Biomechanics study
10	High friction/ lubrication failure	Possible	Biomechanics study
11	Edge loading	Possible	Common?
12	Impingement (patient driven)	Possible	Common?

and utility? It is therefore necessary to carefully interrogate the clinical and retrieval records to deduce what type of failure mechanism should be simulated. Clearly the CoC simulator studies have produced both successes and failures. In this review it has been observed that the role of hip impingement has been seriously underestimated and only now is it becoming apparent that the secondary effects created by the release of metal particles can be significant. This also includes the phenomena termed 'squeaking' in CoC arthroplasty. Explanations for noise production, such as popping, clicking, squeaking, grinding, and grating, have been varied (Table 5-11) (Chevillotte *et al.*, 2010; Ecker *et al.*, 2008; Eickmann *et al.*, 2003; Esposito *et al.*, 2012; Restrepo *et al.*, 2008, 2010; Walter *et al.*, 2007, 2008). For example, formation of stripe wear was once thought to initiate squeaking (Taylor *et al.*, 2007). However, clinical and retrieval studies have clearly documented stripe wear in CoC bearings retrieved from patients with no history of squeaking (Walter *et al.*, 2004, 2008). Biomechanical studies also confirmed that CoC bearings with stripe wear did not squeak under lubricated conditions (Chevillotte *et al.*, 2010). While ceramic squeaking has been referred to as a problem of high friction and lubrication failure (Chevillotte *et al.*, 2010; Esposito *et al.*, 2012; Imbuldeniya *et al.*, 2013; Murali *et al.*, 2008), seldom discussed has been the role of hip impingement,

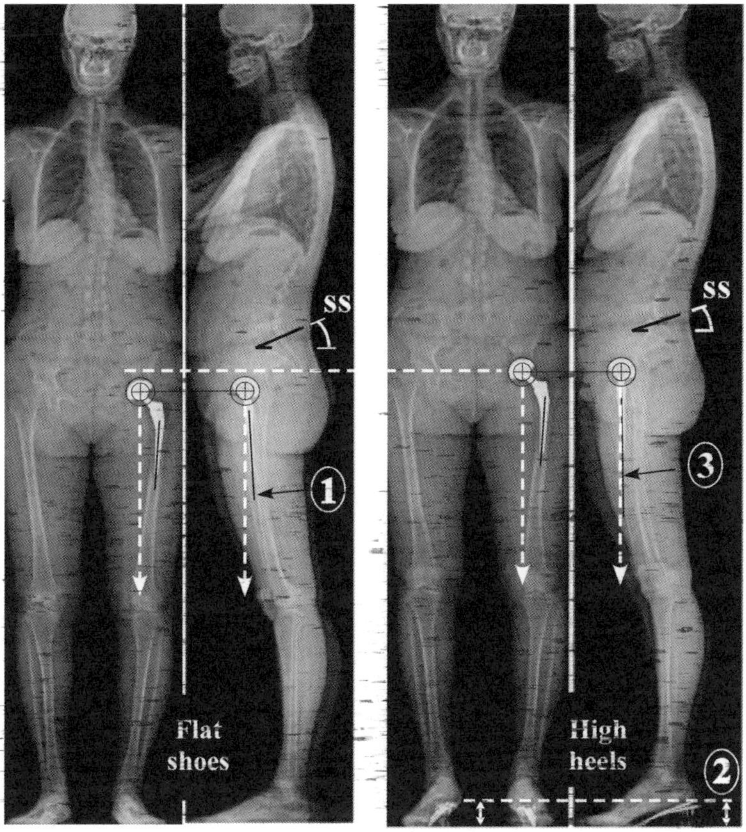

(a) (b) (c) (d)

Figure 5-20. Anterior and lateral EOS views of female patient revealing her standing posture while wearing either flat or high-heeled shoes: (a) AP view in flat shoes, demonstrating femoral stem inclined posteriorly from vertical plane, revealing hyperextension of THA; (b) Lateral view in flat shoes and femoral stem (1) inclined 3.4° posteriorly; (c) AP view in high-heeled shoes (2) with femoral stem inclined similarly to view 5-20a; (d) Lateral view in high-heeled shoes with femoral stem (3) now virtually aligned in the vertical plane. Posterior pelvic tilt was also reduced in high heels, indicated by reduction of sacral-slope angle (SS).

i.e. when the rim of a metal or ceramic cup slides across the metal femoral neck in repetitive, functional hip motions (Figures 5-9, 5-10, 5-22) (Clarke *et al.*, 2014; Eickmann *et al.*, 2003; Iida *et al.*, 1999). Dr. Lazennec collected eleven CoC cases at La Pitie Hospital (Paris, France) with documented squeaking. Using the EOS imaging system

(Lazennec *et al.*, 2011, 2012, 2013), hip impingement was demonstrated in each patient's functional 'squeaking' posture. In addition, some patients could demonstrate squeaking, or not, as they chose. In the first example, a female patient squeaked routinely while wearing flat shoes (Figure 5-20a, 5-20b). However, she noted that when wearing high heels the squeaking disappeared. The lateral EOS view with the patient in stance position wearing high-heeled shoes revealed that the femoral stem had approximately 3° less hyperextension (Figure 5-20c). The three-dimensional 'sky-view' reconstruction of her pelvis and femurs showed that her femur became more internally rotated when wearing high-heeled shoes (Figure 5-21b). These quite subtle angular shifts in implant positions changed her CoC hip from one of squeaking to one of non-squeaking. A similar effect was recorded in a male patient who squeaked consistently while walking uphill but not at all walking downhill. In both cases squeaking was a consequence of femoral neck and cup impingement, regardless of whether or not metal debris had penetrated the ceramic bearing. Thus the belief is that the primary cause of CoC squeaking is hip impingement (Figure 5-10), i.e. a repetitive sub-clinical subluxation (RSS) mechanism that patients are generally unaware of (McPherson *et al.*, 2012). All THA procedures carry the risk of the metal neck impinging against either the ceramic or metallic cup rim, thereby releasing clouds of metal debris (Clarke *et al.*, 2014b). It is to be noted that impingement can produce both cup damage and notching of femoral necks regardless of the THA design in question (Figure 5-22). The resulting circulating cloud of metal particles then ingresses the ceramic bearing and stains surfaces black (Figures 5-9 and 5-10) (Bal *et al.*, 2007b; Bowsher *et al.*, 2008; Eickmann *et al.*, 2003; Shishido *et al.*, 2003). Hence, squeaking and other noises can result (i) during impingement and (ii) as and when the metal particles ingress the ceramic bearing. This fits with the biomechanical evidence of squeaking in lubricated CoC bearings (Chevillotte *et al.*, 2010). Certainly the presence of metal debris with metal contamination of articular surfaces could result in a lubrication failure. However, in the French studies, it was apparent that patient functionality controlled whether squeaking occurred or not. CoC squeaking could thus be defined as a problem

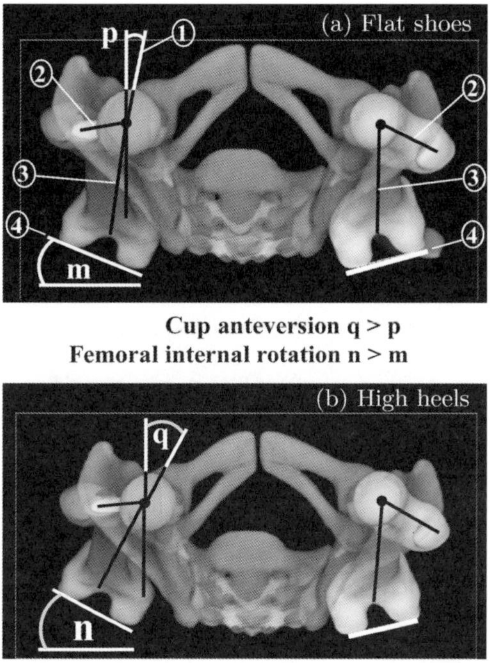

Figure 5-21. Reconstructed three-dimensional pelvic and femoral models from EOS images (as in Figure 5-20). The 'sky view' images present this patient's pelvis as would be viewed from a superior to inferior direction: (1) In her posture with no heels, the cup anteversion is indicated by angle (p) and with high heels by angle (q). Note the increased acetabular anteversion due to the enhanced posterior pelvic tilt; (2) Axis of femoral neck; (3) Femoral axis; (4) In her posture with no heels, the axis of posterior condyles is indicted by angle (n) and with high heels by angle (m). Note with heels she obtained an increase in internal rotation of the femur.

of component positioning and patient postural adaption. It is to be noted that it is still unproven whether ingress of metal debris and metal contamination will be deleterious to Al_2O_3 or ZTA bearings (Table 5-12).

Retrieval studies have indicated that impingement, as indicated by production of stripe damage, was a common finding in retrieved CoC and MoM bearings. In 28 mm and 32 mm CoC bearings, the incidence was noted to be 83% (Esposito *et al.*, 2012). In addition, almost 100% evidence of stripe damage was found in retrieved MoM

Table 5-12. OC simulator ceramic chapter.

Item	Simulator test mode	Details	Results
1	5-Mc duration standard test	Al_2O_3	Not effective (class A wear)
2	14-Mc duration standard test	Al_2O_3	Not effective (class A wear)
3	Stop-and-go mechanics	With reversal	Not effective (class A wear)
4	Steep cup effect	Edge wear	Not effective (class A wear)
5	Severe micro-separation	Al_2O_3	Wear corresponded to class B
6	Severe micro-separation	Al_2O_3, ZTA-C	Excellent discrimination with class D wear
7	Debris	PMMA	Not effective (class A wear)
8	Debris	CoCr	None
9	Debris	Ti64	None
10	Debris	Al_2O_3	None
11	Surface contamination	Ti6Al4V	None
12	Physico-chemical changes	Microstructure	Some data, minimalistic

with diameters ranging 28–54 mm (Clarke *et al.*, 2013b, 2014b). Thus, while stripe wear does not appear to result in squeaking, it does indicate that repetitive subclinical subluxations (McPherson *et al.*, 2012; Pelt *et al.*, 2013) with concomitant risk of cup-on-neck impingement is likely a common pathway leading to revision of THA (Figure 5-10) (Clarke *et al.*, 2013b, 2014b).

The retrieval study by Esposito *et al.* (2012) presents the first published clinical perspectives of impingement risks combined with CoC wear rates. Based on the nature of cup impingement and stripe damage, 54 cases were stratified into retrievals with (i) no stripes, (ii) posterior stripes, and (iii) anterior stripes. With follow-up extending from one to ten years, CoC wear was immeasurable in cases that displayed no stripe wear (Table 5-10). Thus, early concepts of THA designs that achieved well-fixed and well-positioned implants have performed well for over 30 years (Figure 5-23). In contrast, the CoC retrievals with stripe wear on posterior and anterior head sites averaged 0.2 and 1.9 mm^3/year, respectively, virtually one order of magnitude difference. The highest recorded wear rate was 7.2 mm^3/year in a case revised for squeaking.

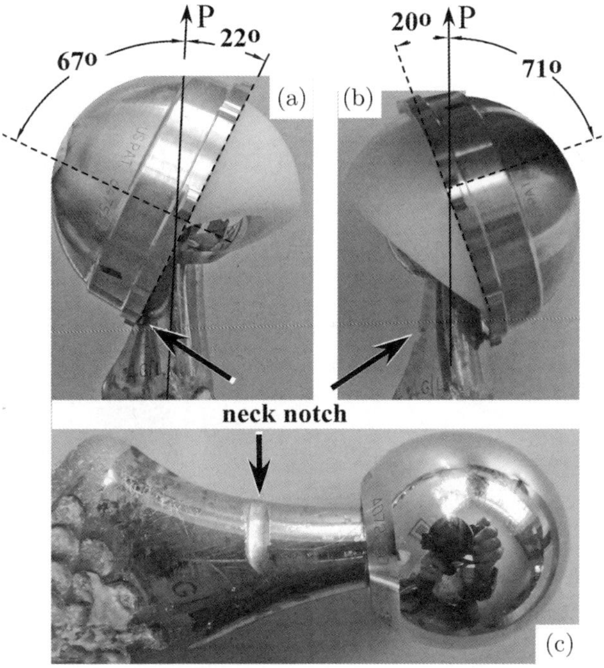

Figure 5-22. Example of dual-modular design with a notched Ti_6Al_4V femoral neck that was cut by cup rim over hundreds of thousands of cycles in approximately one year to revision. This illustrates that hip impingement is the conundrum for all THA procedures.

Standard simulator test guidelines (ISO14242-1,2,3) used with Al_2O_3 bearings produced overall wear rates of 0.1 mm^3/Mc or less. For comparative purposes, it will be assumed here that a wear rate of 1 mm^3 per million cycles in a hip simulator (1 mm^3/Mc) is analogous to a patient wear rate of 1 mm^3 per year (1 mm^3/year). Some studies argue for higher numbers of cycles per year of patient use (Silva *et al.*, 2002) and some for lower (Kamali *et al.*, 2010). It is left to the reader to increase or decrease the ratio of patient activity levels as deemed relevant. Thus, the standard simulator test would likely correspond to clinical cases without stripe damage and immeasurable wear (Table 5-10: Class A). In the mild MSX test mode (Figure 5-17), overall wear rates for Al_2O_3 averaged 0.19 mm^3/Mc. This corresponded well to CoC retrievals with posterior stripe damage

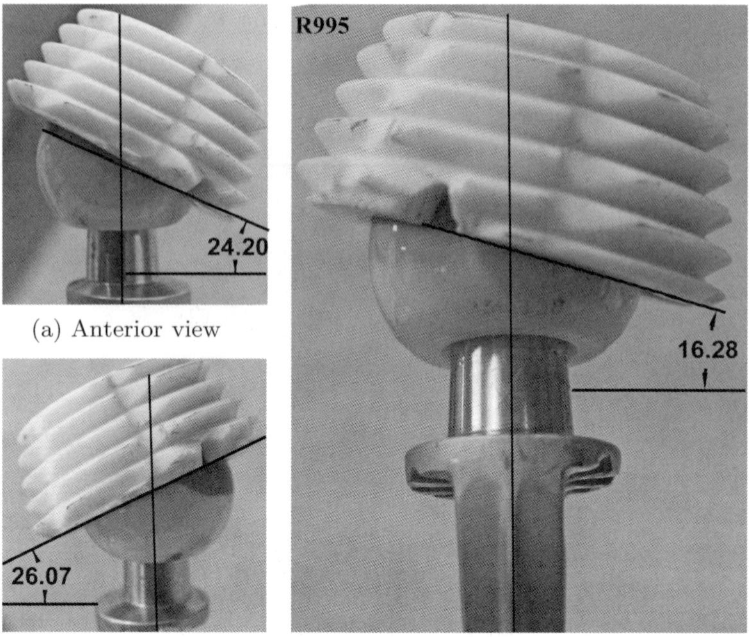

(a) Anterior view

(b) Posterior view

(c) Superior view

Figure 5-23. A 30-year successful result with a pioneering CoC design that had centralized wear patterns, satisfactory range of motion, no neck notching, and no stripe wear (see Figures 5-5–5-8).

(Table 5-10: Class B). In the severe MSX mode, Al_2O_3 averaged wear an order of magnitude higher at 1.8 mm^3/Mc (Figure 17). This corresponded well to CoC retrievals featuring anterior stripe damage (Table 5-10: Class D). Therefore, there appears to be a workable correlation relationship between clinical and simulator data. It was noted in the study by Esposito *et al.* (2012) and others (Hannouche *et al.*, 2005; Nevelos *et al.*, 2001b; Nizard *et al.*, 2008; Prudhommeaux *et al.*, 2000) that such levels of ceramic wear did not result in adverse tissue reactions around the hip joint (osteolysis).

The severe MSX simulator mode was valuable in that it provided clear discrimination between ZTA and Al_2O_3 combinations not apparent in the standard simulator test mode (ISO-14242-1). It was also notable that the BME and LLU studies were in complete agreement regarding MSX wear rates (Figure 5-18). This was additional evidence to support the claim that the zirconia-reinforced alumina combination (ZTA/ZTA) was at least six times more resistant to stripe wear mechanisms than Al_2O_3/Al_2O_3. The MSX mode also discriminated against implants with a zirconia ceramic overlying a metal substrate. Parikh *et al.* (2013a) demonstrated stripe formation within 3 million cycles with concomitant cracking of the oxide surface and exposure of the DH zirconium substrate.

The standard test guidelines (ISO 14242-1 and -3) appear to have little relevance for ultra wear-resistant CoC bearings. In one 28 mm CoC study, alumina bearings were run out to 14 million cycles to better assess run-in and steady-state wear phases. This test, which included interrupted test intervals with machine rotation reversals, averaged 0.27 and 0.007 mm^3/Mc, respectively (Figure 5-24). The latter value represented only 2.6% of the run-in rate, barely contributing to the overall wear rate assessment of 0.04 mm^3/Mc (Oonishi *et al.*, 2004). This test consumed a lot of resources over an 18-month period to ascertain such a ceramic wear rate so close to zero (Table 5-10: Class A). Clearly the mild and severe MSX tests raised CoC wear rates by a factor of 3 and 30, respectively (Figure 5-17).

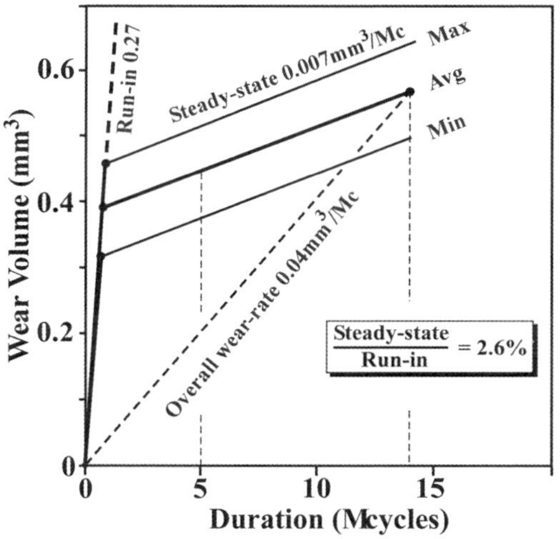

Figure 5-24. Wear trending (maximum, average, minimum) with 28 mm CoC bearings (N = 9) that were run to 14 million cycles to more adequately assess the steady-state wear phase.

The severe MSX test mode thus offered good clinical relevance with matching wear rates produced within a typical 5-million cycle test.

From this review of ceramic tribology it was apparent that the standard simulator test (ISO142420) was successful in documenting CoC wear rates during the run-in phase but had great difficulty in assessing the ultra-low wear rates in the steady-state phase (Table 5-12: Class A). In fact, one conclusion is that the standard simulator test has been of minimal value for CoC bearings. In addition, some alternative methods, such as (i) extended test durations, (ii) stop-and-go/reversing tests, and (iii) steep cups, all remained with class A wear, i.e. the anticipated adverse wear rates did not materialize (Table 5-12). Similarly, one CoC abrasion study with bone cement also produced a class A wear rate. Clearly lacking were abrasion studies with clinically relevant particles, such as CoCr, Ti_6Al_4V, or Al_2O_3 (Table 5-12). In addition, it was not possible to find any CoC wear study with ceramic surfaces contaminated by layers of titanium alloy (Figure 5-9: Blackened heads and cups). In addition, minimal attention has been given to physic-chemical interactions at the ceramic surfaces and how these are resisted by different microstructures (Al_2O_3, ZTA, S_3N_4, etc). Clearly the microseparation test modes have proved of considerable utility (Table 5-10). However, to the best of the authors' knowledge, only two ceramic types (Biolox-forte, Biolox-delta) have been assessed in such tests. More detailed information is greatly needed.

10. Summary

1. A few studies of pioneering ceramic THA from the 1970s reported volumetric wear $>5\,mm^3/Mc$ (class E). These reports of gross wear appeared confined to pioneering designs with monoblock cups. These were easily loosened and could impinge on the femoral neck during patient activities. However, it is noted that a retrieval study of contemporary THA designs reported one case with a $7.2\,mm^3/Mc$ wear-rate, also class E wear.
2. Squeaking in ceramic hips has been attributed to various patient and THA characteristics but has particularly been described as

lubrication failure. Biomechanical studies indicated that causation was most likely metal contamination on ceramic surfaces. Such metal debris in CoC cases would indicate that the metal femoral neck had impinged on either the ceramic or metal rim of the acetabular cup. Squeaking was thus either directly or indirectly attributable to repetitive hip impingement in particular patient postures, and as such should not be reported as lubrication or bearing failure *per se*.

3. Clinical retrieval studies (Al_2O_3/Al_2O_3) indicated CoC wear rates could be classified into three groups: (i) those with femoral heads with no stripe damage; (ii) those with posterior stripes; and, (iii) those with anterior stripes. Corresponding wear rates were zero (class A), $0.2\,mm^3$/year (class B), and $1.9\,mm^3$/year (class D), respectively.
4. Overall wear rates (Al_2O_3/Al_2O_3) in the standard simulator test were $<0.05\,mm^3$/Mc (class A). This method (ISO-14242) was of little value because it could not differentiate between ceramic types. Even a longer-term standard test (>10 million cycles) offered little benefit.
5. Overall wear rates (Al_2O_3/Al_2O_3) in the mild and severe microseparation tests averaged 0.19 and $1.84\,mm^3$/Mc (classes B and C).
6. The severe microseparation simulator test in two independent laboratory studies successfully differentiated between Al_2O_3 and ZTA wear performance. The ZTZ/ZTA combination reduced wear six-fold compared to the Al_2O_3/Al_2O_3 combination.
7. The severe microseparation test also differentiated between the hybrid combinations of Al_2O_3 and ZTA. Compared to Al_2O_3/Al_2O_3, the Al_2O_3/ZTA hybrids reduced CoC wear by two-fold. It was notable that as either the head or cup, the Al_2O_3 component contributed only 33% to the total CoC wear. The hybrids thus demonstrated that there were two ceramic wear mechanisms present as follow: (i) fatigue wear due to cup rim impinging against the femoral head; and, (ii) abrasive wear following release of ceramic particles. The ZTA toughness offered protection against mechanical damage and the Al_2O_3 hardness

offered protection against abrasive wear. Both hybrid combinations were effective but not as beneficial as the ZTZ/ZTA combination.

8. There was one microseparation study of a new bearing defined as a monoclinic-zirconia surface (DHOxZr). This proved of discriminatory ability by cracking the ceramic surface within 3 million cycles.
9. There is minimal data available on microseparation tests and therefore this mode cannot truly be considered a proven and clinically relevant method of testing. Fortuitously, it has provided good discrimination between Al_2O_3, ZTA, and the DHOxZr ceramics within the standard 5-million cycle duration. The CoC simulator tests run under (i) standard, (ii) mild microseparation, and (iii) severe microseparation test modes provided wear rates that matched contemporary retrieval data. The case was made here for this strong correlation, which now invalidates prior arguments that simulator wear rates were not clinically relevant. The three levels of wear rate correlations outlined here may be fortuitous but will certainly stimulate simulator studies of ceramic systems in development.
10. Data on available on steep cup test modes appears minimal and further studies are needed for a better definition of edge wear effects in CoC bearings.
11. The review of clinical and retrieval literature indicated that subluxation and impingement were likely to be the main risks in all THA designs. However, the concomitant risk of metal debris released during recurrent impingement events has not been adequately recognized or studied. While one CoC simulator study did introduce bone-cement particles, that test mode did not challenge CoCr surfaces and would be unlikely to damage harder ceramic surfaces.
12. It may be assumed that metal particles have little effect against the hard ceramic surfaces. Nevertheless, this appears to be an obvious omission from pre-clinical wear studies.
13. In all of the foregoing it is noted that there exists a paucity of information on the physico-chemical interactions present at

the microstructural level of ceramic bearings in such pre-clinical testing.

Acknowledgments

Thanks are due to the companies who have donated ceramic components and funded our CPE and CoC research programs over the years, including Amedica (Salt Lake City, UT), CeramTec (Plochingen, Germany), DJO Global (Austin, TX), Kyocera Medical (Osaka, Japan), Norton St. Gobain (Paris, France), and Smith and Nephew (Memphis, TN).

References

ASTM F1714. (2008). *Standard Guide for Gravimetric Wear Assessment of Prosthetic Hip Designs in Simulator Devices*, ASTM.

ASTM F2094/F2094M-14. (2011). *Standard Specification for Silicon Nitride Bearing Balls*, ASTM.

Bal, B.S. and Rahaman, M.N. (2012). Orthopedic applications of silicon nitride ceramics, *Acta Biomater*, **8**(8), 2889–2898.

Bal, B.S., Garino, J., Ries, M. and Rahaman, M.N. (2007a). A review of ceramic bearing materials in total joint arthroplasty, *Hip Int*, **17**(1), 21–30.

Bal, B.S., Khandkar, A., Lakshminarayanan, R., Clarke, I., Hoffman, A.A. and Rahaman, M.N. (2008). Testing of silicon nitride ceramic bearings for total hip arthroplasty, *J Biomed Mater Res B Appl Biomater*, **87**(2), 447–454.

Bal, B.S., Khandkar, A., Lakshminarayanan, R., Clarke, I.C., Hoffman, A.A. and Rahaman, M.N. (2009). Fabrication and testing of silicon nitride bearings in total hip arthroplasty, *J Arthroplasty*, **24**(1), 110–116.

Bal, B.S., Rahaman, M.N., Aleto, T., Miller, F.S., Traina, F. and Toni, A. (2007b). The significance of metal staining on alumina femoral heads in total hip arthroplasty, *J Arthroplasty*, **22**(1), 14–19.

Boutin, P. (1972). Total arthroplasty of the hip by fritted aluminum prosthesis. Experimental study and 1st clinical applications, *Rev Chir Orthop*, **58**(3), 229–246.

Bowsher, J.G., Clarke, I.C., Williams, P.A. and Donaldson, T.K. (2009). What is a "normal" wear pattern for metal-on-metal hip bearings?, *J Biomed Mater Res B Appl Biomater*, **91**(1), 297–308.

Bowsher, J.G., Donaldson, T.K., Williams, P.A. and Clarke, I.C. (2008). Surface damage after multiple dislocations of a 38-mm-diameter, metal-on-metal hip prosthesis, *J Arthroplasty*, **23**(7), 1090–1096.

Chevillotte, C., Trousdale, R.T., Qingshan, C., Guyen, O. and An, K.N. (2010). Hip squeaking. A biomechanical study of ceramic-on-ceramic bearing surfaces, *Clin Othop Rel R*, **468**, 345–350.

Christel, P., Meunier, A., Dorlot, J.M., Crolet, J.M., Witvoet, J., Sedel, L. *et al.* (1988). Biomechanical compatibility and design of ceramic implants for orthopedic surgery, *Ann NY Acad Sci*, **523**, 234–256.

Clarke, I., Green, D., Williams, P., Donaldson, T. and Pezzotti, G. (2006). US perspective on hip simulator wear testing of Biolox delta in 'severe' test modes, in Benazzo, F., Falez, F. and Dietrich, M. (eds), *Bioceramics and Alternative Bearings in Joint Arthroplasty: 11th Biolox Symp Proc*, Stienkopff, Rome, 189–205.

Clarke, I.C. and Bowsher, J. (2007). Thermal conductivity of femoral ball strongly influenced UHMWPE wear in a hip simulator study, *53rd Ann Orthop Res Soc*, 278.

Clarke, I.C. and Gustafson, A. (2008). The design of ceramics for joint replacement, in Kokubo, T. (ed), *Bioceramics and their Clinical Applications*, JMM, Osaka, 106–132.

Clarke, I.C. and Willmann, G. (1994). Structural ceramics in orthopedics, in Cameron, H.U. (ed), *Bone Implant Interface*, Mosby, St. Louis, 203–252.

Clarke, I.C., Pezzotti, G. and Sugano, N. (2013a). Materials in hip surgery: Mechanical properties that influence the design and performance of ceramic hip bearings, in Berry, D. and Lieberman, J. (eds), *Surgery of the Hip*, Elsevier, Saunders, 102–118.

Clarke, I.C., Donaldson, T.K., Burgett, M.D., Smith, E.J., Bowsher, J., Savisaar, C. *et al.* (2013b). Normal and adverse wear patterns created in-vivo on MOM surfaces — a retrieval study representing four vendors, in Kurtz, S.M., Greenwald, S.A., Mihalko, W.M. and Lemons, J.A. (eds), *STP1560: Metal-on-Metal Total Hip Replacement Devices*, ASTM, West Conshohocken, 157–192.

Clarke, I.C., Donaldson, T.K., Kubo, K., Lazennec, J.Y., McPherson, E., Peters, C. *et al.* (2011). Wear performance of MOM and COC bearings — a correlation of laboratory and retrieval studies', in Wang, A. and Streicher, R. (eds), *Tribology and Bearing Surfaces in Total Joint Replacements*, Transworld Research Network, 211–244.

Clarke, I.C., Dorlot, J.M., Graham, J., Levine, D.J., Oonishi, H., Rieu, J. *et al.* (1988). Biomechanical stability and design. Wear, *Ann NY Acad Sci*, **523**, 292–296.

Clarke, I.C., Halim, T., Burgett, M., Bowsher, J.G., Savisaar, C. and Donaldson, T.K. (2014a). Severe Metal-on-Metal bearing wear triggered by 3rd body metal particulates in hip simulator study, *Hip Int*, **24**, 513.

Clarke, I.C., Lazennec, J.Y., Brusson, A., Savisaar, C., Bowsher, J.G., Burgett, M. *et al.* (2014b). Risk of impingement and third-body abrasion with 28-mm metal-on-metal bearings, *Clin Orthop Relat R*, **472**(2), 497–508.

Clarke, I.C., Manaka, M., Green, D.D., Williams, P., Pezzotti, G., Kim, Y.H. *et al.* (2003a). Current status of zirconia used in total hip implants, *J Bone Joint Surg Am*, **85**(Suppl 4), 73–84.

Clarke, I.C., Manaka, M., Shishido, T., Oonishi, H., Gustafson, A. and Boehler, M. (2003b). Tribological and material properties for all-alumina THR–convergence with clinical retrieval data, in Zippel, H. and Dietrich, M. (eds), *Bioceramics in Joint Arthroplasty*, Steinkopff, Berlin, 3–18.

De Aza, A.H., Chevalier, J., Fantozzi, G., Schehl, M. and Torrecillas, R. (2002). Crack growth resistance of alumina, zirconia and zirconia toughened alumina ceramics for joint prostheses, *Biomaterials*, **23**(3), 937–945.

Dorlot, J.M., Christel, P. and Meunier, A. (1992). Long-term effects of alumina components in total hip prostheses, *Clin Orthop Relat R*, **282**, 47–52.

Ecker, T.M., Robbins, C., van Flandern, G., Patch, D., Steppacher, S.D., Bierbaum, B. *et al.* (2008). Squeaking in total hip replacement: No cause for concern, *Orthopedics*, **31**(9), 875–876.

Eickmann, T.H., Clarke, I.C. and Gustafson, A. (2003). Squeaking in a ceramic on ceramic total hip, in Zippel, H. and Dietrich, M. (eds), *Bioceramics in Joint Arthroplasty*, Steinkopff, Darmstadt, 187–192.

Esposito, C.I., Walter, W.L., Roques, A., Tuke, M.A., Zicat, B.A., Walsh, W.R. *et al.* (2012). Wear in alumina-on-alumina ceramic bearings. A retrieval analysis of edge loading, *J Bone Joint Surg Am*, **7**, 901–907.

Firkins, P.J., Tipper, J.L., Ingham, E., Stone, M.H., Farrar, R. and Fisher, J. (2001). Influence of simulator kinematics on the wear of metal-on-metal hip prostheses, *Proc Inst Mech Eng H*, **215**(1), 119–121.

Furlong, R. (1993). Six years use of the unmodified Furlong hydroxyapatite ceramic coated total hip replacement, *Acta Orthop Belg*, **59**(Suppl 1), 323–325.

Green, D.D., Donaldson, T.K., Williams, P., Pezzotti, G. and Clarke, I.C. (2007). Long term stripe wear rates of 3rd and 4th generation ceramic-on-ceramic under microseparation, *53rd Ann Orthop Res Soc*, 1776.

Griss, P., Heimke, G., Von Andrian-Werburg, H., Krempien, B., Reipa, S., Lauterbach, H.J. *et al.* (1975). Morphological and biomechanical aspects of Al2O3 ceramic joint replacement. Experimental results and design considerations for human endoprostheses, *J Biomed Mater Res*, **9**(4), 177–188.

Halim, T., Burgett, M.D., Clarke, I.C. and Donaldson, T.K. (2013). Ten-fold increase in MOM wear rates resulting from 3rd body metal particulates: A simulator model, *J Bone Joint*, **95-B**(Suppl 34), 340.

Halim, T., Burgett, M., Donaldson, T.K., Savisaar, C., Bowsher, J.G. and Clarke, I.C. (2014). Profiling the third-body wear damage produced in CoCr surfaces by bone cement, CoCr, and Ti6A14V debris: A 10-cycle metal-on-metal simulator test, *Proc Inst Mech Eng H*, **228**, 703–713.

Hannouche, D., Hamadouche, M., Nizard, R., Bizot, P., Meunier, A. and Sedel, L. (2005). Ceramics in total hip replacement, *Clin Orthop Relat R*, **430**, 62–71.

Harris, W.H. (2012). Edge loading has a paradoxical effect on wear in metal-on-polyethylene total hip arthroplasties, *Clin Orthop Relat R*, **470**, 3077–3082.

Heiner, A.D., Lundberg, H.J., Baer, T.E., Pedersen, D.R., Callaghan, J.J. and Brown, T.D. (2008). Effects of episodic subluxation events on third body ingress and embedment in the THA bearing surface, *J Biomech*, **41**(10), 2090–2096.

Iida, H., Kaneda, E., Takada, H., Uchida, K., Kawanabe, K. and Nakamura, T. (1999). Metallosis due to impingement between the socket and the femoral neck in a metal-on-metal bearing total hip prosthesis. A case report, *J Bone Joint Surg Am*, **81**(3), 400–403.

Imbuldeniya, A.M., Pearce, S.J., Walter, W.L., Zicat, B.A. and Walter, W.K. (2013). Squeaking: Current knowledge and how to avoid it, *Curr Rev Musculoskelet Med*, **6**(4), 342–349.

ISO 14242-2. (2000). *Implants for surgery — wear of total hip-joint prostheses — Part 2: Methods of measurement*, International Organization for Standardization.

ISO 14242-1. (2002). *Implants for surgery — wear of total hip-joint prostheses — Part 1: Loading and displacement parameters for wear-testing machines and corresponding environmental conditions for test*, International Organization for Standardization.

ISO 14242-3. (2008). *Implants for surgery — wear of total hip joint prostheses– Part 3: Loading and displacement parameters for orbital bearing type wear testing machines and corresponding environmental conditions for test*, International Organization for Standardization.

ISO 26602. (2009). *Fine Ceramics (Advanced Ceramics, Advanced Technical Ceramics) — Silicon Nitride Materials for Rolling Bearing Balls*, International Organization for Standardization.

Jahanmir, S., Ozmen, Y. and Ives, L. (2004). Water lubrication of silicon nitride in sliding, *Tribol Lett*, **17**(3), 409–417.

Kamali, A., Hussain, A., Li, C., Pamu, J., Daniel, J., Ziaee, H. *et al.* (2010). Tribological performance of various CoCr microstructures in metal-on-metal bearings — The development of a more physiological protocol *in vitro*, *J Bone Joint Surg Br*, **92**, 717–725.

Korduba, L., Essner, A., Pivec, R., Lancin, P., Mont, M., Wang, A. *et al.* (2014). Effect of acetabular cup abduction angle on wear of ultrahigh-molecular-weight polyethylene in hip simulator testing, *Am J Orthop*, **43**, 466–471.

Kummer, F.J., Stuchin, S.A. and Frankel, V.H. (1990). Analysis of removed autophor ceramic-on-ceramic components, *J Arthroplasty*, **5**(1), 28–33.

Lazennec, J.Y., Clarke, I.C., Brusson, A. and Donaldson, T.K. (2013). Correlating MOM retrieval wear maps with functional "*in vivo*" implant positioning in 28 mm MOM patients, *59th Ann Orthop Res Soc*, San Antonio.

Lazennec, J.Y., Rousseau, M.A., Brusson, A. and Catonne, Y. (2012). THA patients in standing and sitting positions: A prospective evaluation using the EOS imaging system.

Lazennec, J.Y., Boyer, P., Gorin, M., Catonne, Y. and Rousseau, M.A. (2011). Acetabular anteversion with CT in supine, simulated standing, and sitting positions in a THA patient population, *Clin Orthop Relat R*, **469**(4), 1103–1109.

Lee, R., Essner, A. and Wang, A. (2008). Tribological considerations in primary and revision metal-on-metal arthroplasty, *J Bone Joint Surg Am*, **90**(Suppl 3), 118–124.

Leslie, I., Williams, S., Brown, C., Isaac, G., Jin, Z., Ingham, E. *et al.* (2008). Effect of bearing size on the long-term wear, wear debris, and ion levels of large diameter metal-on-metal hip replacements — An *in vitro* study, *J Biomed Mater Res B*, **87**(1), 163–172.

Lu, B., Marti, A. and McKellop, H. (2000). Wear of a second-generation metal-on-metal hip replacement effect of third-body abrasive particles, *World Biomat Congr*, Hawaii, 183.

Lundberg, H.J., Liu, S.S., Callaghan, J.J., Pedersen, D.R., O'Rourke, M.R., Goetz, D.D. *et al.* (2007). Association of third body embedment with rim damage in retrieved acetabular liners, *Clin Orthop Relat R*, **465**, 133–139.

Manaka, M., Clarke, I.C., Shishido, T., Gustafson, A., Shoji, H. and Imakiire, A. (2003). Analysis of ceramic-ceramic THA wear comparison of short term and long term retrievals, *Soc Biomater*.

Mazzocchi, M. and Bellosi, A. (2008a). On the possibilty of silicon nitride as a ceramic for structural orthopaedic implants. Part I: Processing, microstructure, mechanical properties, cytotoxicity, *J Mater Sci Mater Med*, **19**(8), 2881–2887.

Mazzocchi, M., Gardini, D., Traverso, P.L., Faga, M.G. and Bellosi, A. (2008b). On the possibility of silicon nitride as a ceramic for structural orthopaedic implants. Part II: Chemical stability and wear resistance in body environment, *J Mater Sci Mater Med*, **19**(8), 2889–2901.

McHugh, D., Currier, J., Kennedy, F., Collier, J., Van Critters, D. (2013). Plastic deformation from edge loading is common on retrieved metal-on-metal hips and can be predicted with finite element analysis, in Kurtz, S.M., Greenwald, S.A., Mihalko, W.M. and Lemons, J.A. (eds), *STP1560: Metal-On-Metal Total Hip Replacement Devices*, ASTM, 235–250.

McMurtrie, A., Abhijit, R., Guha, A.R. and Wootton, J.R. (2009). Loose Metasul liner causing partial amputation of the neck of the femoral component, *J Arthroplasty*, **24**(1), 159.e1–3.

McPherson, E.J., Clarke, I.C. and Donaldson, T.K. (2012). Lesson learned from retrieval analysis of a dislocating, large diameter MoM revision THA — A case report, *Reconstr Rev*, **2**(2), 10–14.

Mittelmeier, H. and Harms, J. (1979). Treatment of post-traumatic hip joint disease by total replacement with a ceramic endoprosthesis (author's transl), *Unfallheilkunde*, **82**(2), 67–75.

Murali, R., Bonar, S.F., Kirsh, G., Walter, W.K. and Walter, W.L. (2008). Osteolysis in third-generation alumina ceramic-on-ceramic hip bearings with severe impingement and titanium metallosis, *J Arthroplasty*, **23**(8), 1240.e13–19.

Nakanishi, T., Sasaki, M., Ikeda, J., Miyaji, F. and Kondo, M. (2007a). Mechanical and phase stability of zirconia toughened alumina, *Key Eng Mat*, **330**, 1267–1270.

Nakanishi, T., Sasaki, M., Ikeda, J., Miyaji, F. and Kondo, M. (2007b). Mechanical and phase stability of zirconia toughened alumina, *Key Eng Mat*, **330**, 1267–1270.

Nevelos, J., Ingham, E., Doyle, C., Streicher, R., Nevelos, A., Walter, W. *et al.* (2000). Microseparation of the centers of alumina–alumina artificial hip joints during simulator testing produces clinically relevant wear rates and patterns. *J Arthroplasty*, **15**(6), 793–795.

Nevelos, J.E., Ingham, E., Doyle, C., Fisher, J. and Nevelos, A.B. (1999). Analysis of retrieved alumina ceramic components from Mittelmeier total hip prostheses. *Biomaterials*, **20**(19), 1833–1840.

Nevelos, J.E., Ingham, E., Doyle, C., Nevelos, A.B. and Fisher, J. (2001a). The influence of acetabular cup angle on the wear of "BIOLOX Forte" alumina ceramic bearing couples in a hip joint simulator. *J Mater Sci Mater Med*, **12**(2), 141–144.

Nevelos, J.E., Prudhommeaux, F., Hamadouche, M., Doyle, C., Ingham, E., Meunier, A. *et al.* (2001b). Comparative analysis of two different types of alumina-alumina hip prosthesis retrieved for aseptic loosening. *J Bone Joint Surg Br*, **83**(4), 598–603.

Nizard, R., Pourreyron, D., Raould, A., Hannouche, D. and Sedel, L. (2008). Alumina-on-alumina hip arthroplasty in patients younger than 30 years old. *Clin Orthop Relat R*, **466**(2), 317–323.

Oonishi, H., Clarke, I.C., Good, V., Amino, H. and Ueno, M. (2004). Alumina hip joints characterized by run-in wear and steady-state wear to 14 million cycles in hip-simulator model. *J Biomed Mater Res*, **70A**(4), 523–532.

Parikh, A., Hill, P., Pawar, V. and Sprague, J. (2013a). Hip simulator wear testing of modular diffusion hardened oxidized zirconium couples, *Orthop Res Soc*, San Antonio, 298.

Parikh, A., Hill, P., Pawar, V. and Sprague, J. (2013b). Long-term simulator wear performance of an advanced bearing technology for THA, *Orthop Res Soc*, San Antonio, 1028.

Pelt, C.E., Erickson, J., Clarke, I.C., Donaldson, T.K., Layfield, L. and Peters, C.L. (2013). Histologic, serologic, and tribologic findings in failed metal on metal total hip arthroplasty: AAOS exhibit selection, *J Bone Joint Surg Am*, **95**(21), e.163.1–11.

Pezzotti, G. (2013a). Alumina-zirconia composites for joint replacement, in Pezzotti, G. (ed), *Advanced Materials for Joint Implants*, Pan Stanford Publishing, 207–286.

Pezzotti, G. (2013b). Future trends in joint arthroplasty, in Pezzotti, G. (ed), *Advanced Materials for Joint Implants*, Pan Stanford Publishing, 415–495.

Pezzotti, G. (2013c). Polycrystalline alumina for joint replacement, in Pezzotti, G. (ed), *Advanced Materials for Joint Implants*, Pan Stanford Publishing, 71–136.

Prudhommeaux, F., Hamadouche, M., Nevelos, J., Doyle, C., Meunier, A. and Sedel, L. (2000). Wear of alumina-on-alumina total hip arthroplasties at a mean 11-year followup, *Clin Orthop Relat R*, **379**, 113–122.

Restrepo, C., Matar, W.Y., Parvizi, J., Rothman, R. and Hozack, W.J. (2010). Natural history of squeaking after total hip arthroplasty, *Clin Othop Relat R*, **468**, 2340–2345.

Restrepo, C., Parvizi, J., Kurtz, S.M., Sharkey, P.F., Hozack, W.J. and Rothman, R.H. (2008). The noisy ceramic hip: Is component malpositioning the cause?, *J Arthroplasty*, **23**(5), 643–649.

Sedel, L., Hamadouche, M., Bizot, P. and Nizard, R. (2003). Long term data concerning the use of alumina on alumina bearings in total hip replacements, in Ben-Nissan, B., Sher, D. and Walsh, W. (eds), *Bioceramics 15*, Trans Tech Publications, New Hampshire, 769–772.

Sedel, L., Kerboull, L., Christel, P., Meunier, A. and Witvoet, J. (1990). Alumina-on-alumina hip replacement. Results and survivorship in young patients, *J Bone Joint Surg Br*, **72**(4), 658–663.

Shishido, T., Clarke, I.C., Williams, P., Boehler, M., Asano, T., Shoji, H. *et al.* (2003). Clinical and simulator wear study of alumina ceramic THR to 17 years and beyond, *J Biomed Mater Res B*, **67**(1), 638–647.

Silva, M., Shepherd, E.F., Jackson, W.O., Dorey, F.J. and Schmalzried, T.P. (2002). Average patient walking activity approaches 2 million cycles per year: Pedometers under-record walking activity, *J Arthroplasty*, **17**(6), 693–697.

Sorrell, C., Hardcastle, P., Druitt, R., Howlett, C. and McCartney, E. (2004). Results of 15-year clinical study of reaction-bonded nitride intervertebral spacers, *7th World Biomater Conf*, 1872.

Tateiwa, T., Clarke, I.C., Pezzotti, G., Sedel, L., Kumakura, T., Shishido, T. *et al.* (2007). Surface micro-analyses of long-term worn retrieved "Osteal (TM)" alumina ceramic total hip replacement, *J Biomed Mater Res B*, **83**(2), 562–570.

Taylor, S., Manley, M. and Sutton, K. (2007). The role of stripe wear in causing acoustic emissions from alumina ceramic-on-ceramic bearings, *J Arthroplasty*, **22**(7), 47–51.

Underwood, R.J., Zografos, A., Sayles, R.S., Hart, A. and Cann, P. (2012). Edge loading in metal-on-metal hips: Low clearance is a new risk factor, *Proc Inst Eng H*, **226**(3), 217–226.

Walter, W.L., Insley, G.M., Walter, W.K. and Tuke, M.A. (2004). Edge loading in third generation alumina ceramic-on-ceramic bearings: Stripe wear, *J Arthroplasty*, **19**(4), 402–413.

Walter, W.L., O'Toole, G.C., Walter, W.K., Ellis, A. and Zicat, B.A. (2007). Squeaking in ceramic-on-ceramic hips: The importance of acetabular component orientation, *J Arthroplasty*, **22**(4), 496–503.

Walter, W.L., Waters, T.S., Gillies, M., Donohoo, S., Kurtz, S.M., Ranawat, A.S. *et al.* (2008). Squeaking hips, *J Bone Joint Surg Am*, **90**(Suppl 4), 102–111.

Williams, P.A., Lakshminarayanan, R., Kandkar, A., Green, D.D. and Clarke, I.C. (2005). Wear debris morphology of silicon-nitride generated from a hip simulator model, *Ann Meet Soc Biomat*, Pittsburg, **29**, 553.

Zhou, Y.S., Ikeuchi, K. and Ohashi, H. (1997). Comparison of the friction properties of four ceramic materials for joint replacements, *Wear*, **210**(1-2), 171–177.

Chapter 6

Crosslinked Polyethylene

Ebru Oral and Orhun K. Muratoglu
Massachusetts General Hospital,
Department of Orthopaedic Surgery,
Harris Orthopaedic Biomechanics and Biomaterials Laboratory,
Massachusetts, USA

1. Background

Ultra-high molecular weight polyethylene (UHMWPE) is the polymeric material of choice in total joint reconstructions. The most widely used bearing couple is a hard-on-soft articulation comprising a metal femoral head and an UHMWPE acetabular component in total hip reconstruction or a metal femoral chondylar piece and an UHMWPE tibial component in total knee reconstruction. In recent years, with the advances in the processing and performance of ceramic materials used in total joint implants (Chapter 5), ceramic heads are also widely used in total hip implants and ceramicized metallic components are introduced in total knee arthroplasties.

Currently, there are over 1 million total hip and knee reconstruction operations in the US annually (Kurtz *et al.*, 2007) and over 3 million worldwide. The advent of crosslinked UHMWPEs has resulted in a great improvement in the clinical performance of total joint implants, especially in the hip, in their first decade of use (Kurtz *et al.*, 2011). In total hip arthroplasties, approximately 70–80% of bearing surface couples using UHMWPE now comprise a crosslinked UHMWPE formulation (Canadian Institute for Health Information, 2013). The result is an 87% reduction in incidences of periprosthetic osteolysis compared to historical conventional UHMWPE based on a number of clinical studies. Despite ongoing concerns about their resistance to fatigue damage and delamination under high stress (Rodriguez, 2008), the lack of such events after almost a decade has also increased the usage of crosslinked UHMWPEs in the knee (Hodrick *et al.*, 2008). There is still a great need for methods of measuring *in vivo* wear in the knee as well as well-designed, comprehensive clinical studies to determine the clinical performance improvements, if any, afforded by crosslinked UHMWPE in this joint.

Recent advances in crosslinking technology have focused on incorporating antioxidants into crosslinked UHMWPE to improve its oxidative stability (Bracco and Oral, 2011) and to decrease revisions associated with oxidative damage of the material. Crosslinked UHMWPE incorporating the antioxidant vitamin E has been available clinically in the US in hips since 2007 and in knees since 2008 (E1^{TM}, Biomet, Inc). Early clinical results show good wear rates comparable to those observed with first generation crosslinked UHMWPEs (Greene *et al.*, 2013) that resulted in significant decreases in osteolysis (Kurtz *et al.*, 2011; Leung *et al.*, 2007). It is expected that newer formulations of crosslinked UHMWPEs will include phenolic antioxidants; in fact, a crosslinked UHMWPE using a medical grade synthetic antioxidant has been introduced in total knees (AOX^{TM}, DePuy) (Green *et al.*, 2013; King *et al.*, 2009; Narayan *et al.*, 2009) as well as new formulations of crosslinked UHMWPEs incorporating vitamin E (E-Plus^{TM}, DJO Surgical; Vivacit-E^{TM}, Zimmer). This chapter will also include a summary of published information on the properties of these newer generation antioxidant-containing crosslinked UHMWPEs.

Research and development efforts center on reducing the risk of adverse events by improving methods of surgical placement as well as designing more anatomical and high performance implants to satisfy the increasing demands of joint reconstruction. While there have been significant improvements in the wear resistance and oxidative stability of crosslinked UHMWPEs, further improvements in the fatigue resistance and general mechanical strength of the material may be needed. In younger patients, it is especially desirable to preserve as much good bone stock as possible as it is more likely that these patients will require a revision operation in their lifetime. In addition, in order to prevent dislocation in the hip, it is desirable to use thinner acetabular liners allowing the use of larger femoral heads, perhaps those comparable to those previously used in metal-on-metal implants. Both of these goals can be accomplished by enabling the use of thinner UHMWPE components, which in turn can be realized by increasing the fatigue toughness of the UHMWPE.

The first part of this chapter will give general information about the chemistry, the structure, and processing of UHMWPE and the second part will detail different crosslinking technologies and data on the clinical performance of implants fabricated from these materials wherever possible. The chapter will conclude with a brief discussion on the future of crosslinked UHMWPE.

2. Material and Processing

While work in the current century has focused on decreasing the size of or nanosizing the manufacturing of technologies, the most important advances of the last century were based on the development of manufacturing methods for newly developed synthetic chemicals, which we take for granted today in almost every aspect of our lives. Polyethylene as a polymer family is a great example; with a great deal of focus on its manufacturing methods, polyethylene was prepared in its very low density (VLDPE), low density (LDPE), linear low density (LLDPE), and high density polyethylene (HDPE) forms starting in 1939 in the UK and 1943 in the US (Maibauer and Myers, 1946) and it continues to dominate a large part of our daily life with everything from microwave-safe containers to piping to microwaves themselves. The application of ultra-high molecular weight polyethylene (UHMWPE) to joint reconstruction was only made possible by the invention of the appropriate catalyst systems and the development of a low pressure polymerization process (Peacock, 2000) and thus, the initial manufacture of a polyethylene with more than 1 million g/mol in molecular weight in 1955 by Ruhrchemie AG (later known as Ticona and currently known as Celanese) (Kurtz, 2009).

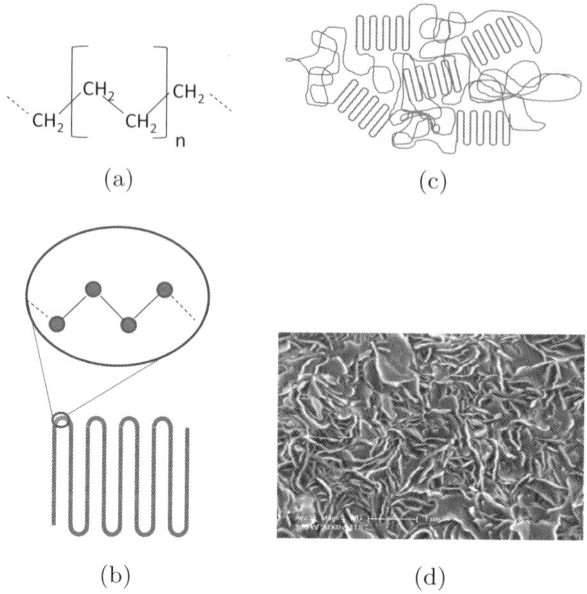

Figure 6-1. The basic chemical composition of polyethylene (a). The formation of folded chain crystals (b). Semi-crystalline macrostructure (c). Visualization of polyethylene crystals after etching lamellar surfaces (d).

This new material replaced polytetrafluoroethylene (PTFE) in Sir Charnley, John clinical application as a bearing surface in 1962, and the rest is history. Despite going through a few revisions in name and operational structure, medical grade UHMWPE is still manufactured and supplied by a single source.

2.1. *Material Structure*

Polyethylene has a simple chemical structure with repeating units of CH2 (Figure 6-1a) resulting in a long backbone with terminal methyl groups. The degree of polymerization can range from 8 to more than 1,400 and results in structures from low molecular weight polyethylene waxes to UHMWPE, which is defined today as a linear polyethylene with an average molecular weight of greater than 3.1 million g/mol by ASTM D4020 and greater than 1 million g/mol by ISO 11542. The size of the molecules is described in terms of molecular weight and the polymeric resin typically contains a distribution of molecular weights. These two properties, i.e. the average molecular weight and the molecular weight distribution, affect macroscopic properties significantly.

The intrinsic viscosity of polyethylene, which increases nonlinearly with increasing molecular weight (Tung, 1957), is a determinant of the bulk impact strength and abrasive wear resistance of the polymer after conversion to bulk/consolidated form. The maximum impact strength of linear polyethylene was found to be at a molecular weight range of 2.4 million to 3.3 million g/mole (Kurtz *et al.*, 1999; Kurtz, 2009). As the intrinsic viscosity increases, abrasive wear resistance also increases, reaching a plateau at about a molecular weight of 3.3 million g/mole. Thus, the wear resistance of UHMWPE is the highest among polyethylenes and in studies using pin-on-disc (PoD) wear testers (Bragdon *et al.*, 2001), the wear of UHMWPE converted into bulk form by compression molding varied between 7–10 mg/million cycles of testing (Gul *et al.*, 2003; Oral *et al.*, 2009).

The macroscopic material properties of different UHMWPE resins may also be affected by the average resin particle size, the size distribution, and morphology of the resin particles (Han *et al.*, 1981), the differences of which have been attributed historically to the use of different catalysts and manufacturing processes (Kurtz, 2009). There are currently two available medical grade resins manufactured by Celanese (GUR 1020 and GUR1050 with molecular weights of 3.5 and 5.5–6 million g/mol, respectively), which have a mean particle size of about 140 μm. The particle morphology of the GUR resins comprises a fine network of sub-micron-sized fibrils which interconnect characteristic microscopic spheroids (Kurtz *et al.*, 1999).

The resilience of UHMWPE as a high performance polymer has been attributed to its semi-crystalline structure. At the nanometer scale, UHMWPE is a semi-crystalline polymer which consists of crystalline lamellae folded rows of carbon (Goldman, 1996), typically 10–50 nm in thickness and on the order of 10–50 μm in length (Figure 6-1b,d). There is a distribution of lamellar sizes within the polymer with the surrounding amorphous phase consisting of randomly oriented polymer chains traversed by tie molecules which interconnect lamellae (Figure 6-1c) and provide resistance to mechanical deformation. Thus, UHMWPE is a complex, viscoplastic composite, which can evolve over time in response to its mechanical, chemical, and thermal history.

The structure of the polymer chains combined with the specific resulting crystalline morphologies possible in different types of resins can affect the tendency of each for further chemical interactions such as crosslinking or oxidation. For example, implants have also been manufactured from a so-called 1900 resin, which was manufactured by Montell Polyolefins and later by Basell Polyolefins. The 1900 resin has had relatively high long-term success; implants which had been fabricated by direct compression molding of this resin showed higher survival rates due to their resistance to oxidation compared to implants fabricated from the conventional GUR resin of similar molecular weight (Currier *et al.*, 2000). The manufacture of this resin was discontinued in 2002 for reasons unrelated to implant performance, but there are still clinical implants manufactured from this type of resin.

The crystallinity and crystal size of UHMWPE are often measured by differential scanning calorimetry (Figure 6-2). Substantial melting of UHMWPE crystals occurs starting at 100°C and continues to around 150°C with a peak melting temperature at 145–147°C in its resin powder form and at 137–140°C in its consolidated form. The breadth of the melting peak is an indication of the polydispersity of the polymer and the imperfections in its crystallization. The mechanical properties of UHMWPE are strongly related to its crystalline content and structure and the amount of interaction between its crystalline and amorphous phases. For example, the mechanical properties of consolidated UHMWPE vary as a function of the cooling rate during consolidation (Truss *et al.*, 1981), which affects the crystallization kinetics and may lead to lower crystallinity at higher cooling rates. In contrast, raising the temperature and pressure during melting to above about 210°C and 290 MPa results in a phase change in UHMWPE where the crystals exhibit hexagonal morphology and the lamellae formation is thought to be less

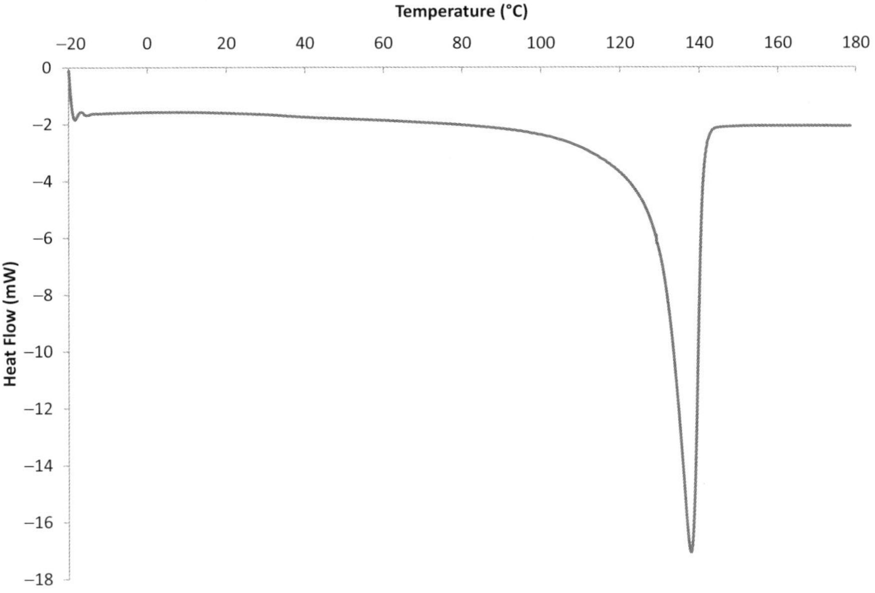

Figure 6-2. The differential scanning calorimeter thermogram of a 0.1 wt% vitamin E-blended UHMWPE showing its melting transition.

inhibited (Bassett *et al.*, 1974; Wunderlich and Davidson, 1969). In this extended chain crystal morphology, the crystal size and the crystalline content increase, resulting in substantially improved mechanical strength up to a yield strength of 27.6 MPa and an ultimate tensile strength of 65 MPa (Bassett *et al.*, 1974; Oral *et al.*, 2009; Wunderlich and Davidson, 1969).

The changes in UHMWPE with radiation exposure have been very important as ionizing radiation is used both for sterilization (25–40 kGy) and for crosslinking (>40 kGy) in most formulations of UHMWPE as a bearing surface. Unlike many other polymers, crosslinking is favored over chain scissioning in polyethylene, especially in its virgin or no additive state. This is presumably because the recombination of free radicals induced by the breaking of C–C bonds on the polymer backbone is energetically favored due to the limited mobility of the high molecular weight chains. The breaking of the C–H bonds, on the other hand, does lead to further free radical reactions as a result of the release of hydrogen. The recombination

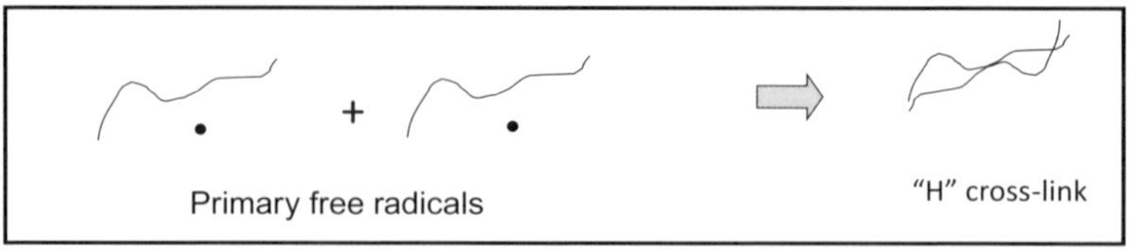

(a)

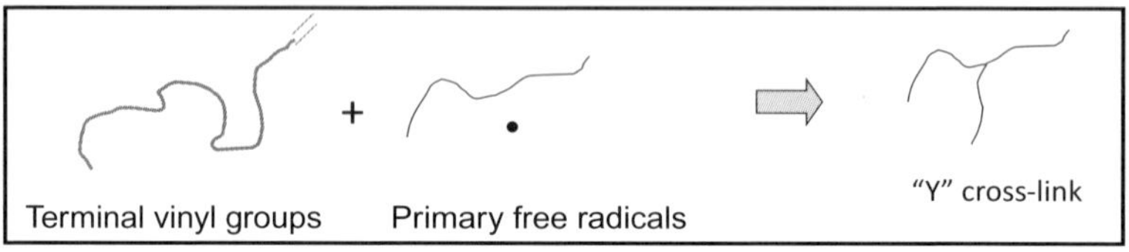

(b)

Figure 6-3. The structure of crosslinks in UHMWPE.

of free radicals formed in this manner on different polymer chains results in so-called 'H-crosslinks' (Figure 6-3a). Alternatively, there is a consistent fraction of vinyl bonds formed at the end of polymer chains, termed 'terminal vinyl groups', which can react with a radiation-induced free radical on a different chain to form a so-called 'Y-crosslink' (Figure 6-3b). While the fraction of each of these types of crosslinks in UHMWPE is not known, the relative changes with different crosslinking environments can result in different crosslinking structures (Parth *et al.*, 2002) and also different material properties (Oral *et al.*, 2013).

Despite the common use of additives such as compatibilizing or stabilizing agents in industrial polymers, their use in medical grade polyethylenes has been limited. This is partly due to the strict requirements for leachable components in implantable devices, but partly also due to the detrimental effect of some additives that have been historically used (Kurtz *et al.*, 1999; Wright *et al.*, 1988). For example, calcium stearate, a catalyst residue found commonly in UHMWPE, appeared to cause increased oxidation at the grain boundaries of the consolidated polymer. Similarly, a carbon-fiber reinforced UHMWPE showed severely deteriorated wear and mechanical resistance due to poor compatibilization of the fibers with the UHMWPE matrix. Despite these concerns, the positive *in vitro* (Jarrett *et al.*, 2010; Oral *et al.*, 2004, 2006, 2008) and *in vivo* results (Greene *et al.*, 2012, 2013) obtained with vitamin E-stabilized UHMWPE as a bearing surface has launched and expanded the use of antioxidant-stabilized UHMWPEs in recent years.

2.2. *Processing*

Due to the high molecular weight and extremely low melt flow index (MFI $<0.1\,g/10\,min$) of UHMWPE, its consolidation and manufacturing is limited to specialized versions of compression molding and ram extrusion. The process in each case involves the heating and pressurizing of resin powder to enable the self-diffusion of the polymer chains to fuse particles and recrystallization under pressure to stabilize the desired large-scale shape such as a rectangular sheet or blocks. The time required for consolidation depends on the thickness of the desired shape and can be up to 24 hours for commercially available sizes.

Consolidation by compression molding requires a press and a mold of a desired shape to contain the resin powder. The powder is packed into the mold and pressure and temperature are applied (usually in a proprietary manner) for a period of time to allow for the sufficient self-diffusion of chains across particle boundaries. The material is then recrystallized by cooling under pressure. The stock material produced in this way can then be machined into implants or other processable parts. In a material produced this way, there are residual stresses in the direction of compression, which should be considered when machining final implants with specific tolerances. Subsequent heating of the material to close to or above its melting point without applying pressure can remove these residual stresses.

A small-scale version of compression molding is termed 'direct' compression molding where the shape of the mold used during consolidation is designed close to or in the final shape of the implant, and thus the compression molding process results directly in a shape usable as a final implant. This process can be costly as there is a dedicated process time for each implant whereas in bulk consolidation, hundreds of implants can be made from the resulting stock material.

The advantage of direct compression molding is that it can be used with specialized processes that do not lend themselves to bulk consolidation such as implants with spatially controlled properties (Oral *et al.*, 2010, 2013).

Another consolidation method is ram extrusion: A specialized extrusion method using a hydraulic ram to pressurize the heated UHMWPE and move it along a horizontal chamber. This process can be used to produce UHMWPE rods of up to 12 inches (30.48 cm) in diameter but processing times have to be slow due to the high melt viscosity of UHMWPE as well as the long cooling time for large material (Kurtz, 2009).

A fourth consolidation method is hot isostatic pressing (HIPping), where the powder is first made into a green body by pressurizing without heating above the melt and then exposing the green body to consolidation temperatures and pressures while packaged in inert gas using a hydrostatic pressure chamber. The advantage of this method is the lack of directional stresses.

2.3. *Material Requirements*

An ASTM standard provides guidelines and requirements for the resin powder and the manufactured properties of bulk/consolidated forms of UHMWPE before implant-specific treatments such as radiation crosslinking, thermal treatments, or antioxidant stabilization (Table 6-1).

Table 6-1. Mechanical properties of consolidated UHMWPE. Test methods are specified in the standard as: ASTM D 792 or D 1505 for density, ASTM D 638 Type IV, 5.08 cm/min for tensile strength and elongation and ASTM F648 Annex A1 for IZOD impact strength.

	GUR1020 (Type 1)	GUR1050 (Type 2)
Density (kg/m^3)	927–944	927–944
Ultimate tensile strength (MPa)	35	27
Yield strength (MPa)	21	19
Elongation (%)	300	300
IZOD impact strength (kJ/m^2)	126	73

While some batch-to-batch variation as well as variation due to consolidation process can be seen in the properties of UHMWPEs, there is little evidence that there is a significant advantage of one processing method over another in terms of structure–property relationships. Therefore, the decision to use one consolidation process over another is usually based on the individual technical and business requirements of the orthopedic manufacturers.

3. Properties as Joint Bearing Surface

While the minimum requirements outlined in ASTM F 648 govern the basic mechanical properties of UHMWPE-fabricated forms after consolidation, there is no established standard for the requirements of UHMWPE as a total joint implant bearing surface. Therefore, an attempt will be made here to provide a thorough discussion of these property requirements and their relationship to processing methods other than consolidation, focusing specifically on crosslinking.

3.1. *Wear Resistance*

Periprosthetic osteolysis has been a major factor limiting the longevity and function of joint implants and was linked to wear particles of the UHMWPE surface over a decade ago (Bragdon *et al.*, 1995; Harris, 1994). The analysis of retrieved acetabular components showed that the highly worn areas contained numerous multidirectional scratches along with fine, drawn-out fibrils oriented parallel to each other (Jasty *et al.*, 1997). Wear of UHMWPE appeared to occur through the break-up of fibrils formed by large-strain plastic deformation and orientation of the surface (Edidin *et al.*, 1999). The fibrils were presumably weakened in the transverse direction to orientation and subsequently ruptured during multidirectional motion of the hip. These findings prompted the development of *in vitro* testing devices that simulate the wear behavior of UHMWPE *in vivo* and subsequently to formulations of UHMWPE with increased wear resistance.

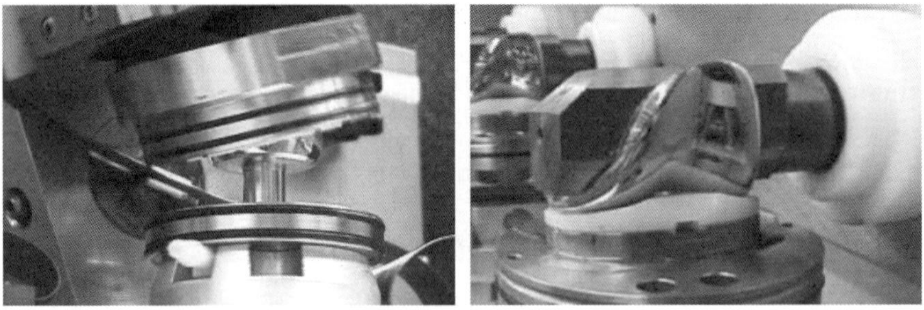

(a) (b)

Figure 6-4. The simulation of *in vivo* gait and kinematics in hip (a) and knee (b) simulators. The environmental chamber to hold the test environment is not shown for clarity.

3.1.1. *In vitro testing*

In vitro testing methodologies of pin-on-flat wear testers (Bragdon *et al.*, 2001; Cooper *et al.*, 1993) and joint simulators for both the hip and knee joints (Figure 6-4) (Burgess *et al.*, 1997; Dumbleton *et al.*, 1972; Ramamurti *et al.*, 1996; Saikko *et al.*, 1992; Scales *et al.*, 1969; Shaw and Murray, 1973; Stallforth and Ungethum, 1977; Walker *et al.*, 1997) were developed to understand and replicate the wear behavior observed on the surfaces of retrievals. The wear behavior was quantified by the linear or volumetric wear rate measured gravimetrically or by analyzing the worn surface and the shape, size, and reactivity of the wear debris.

In vivo factors such as component positioning, temperature, loading, and kinematics of normal gait (Bergmann *et al.*, 1993; Johnston and Smidt, 1969; Paul, 1966; Ramamurti *et al.*, 1996, 1998) are now known to affect the wear rate of UHMWPE. Multidirectional motion was also shown to be an integral part of the mechanism of wear of UHMWPE in reproducing the adhesive/abrasive wear found in retrieval surfaces (Wang *et al.*, 1996; Wang, 2001). Surface roughness of the metal counterface played a role (Cooper *et al.*, 1993), increasing the wear rate of conventional UHMWPEs sterilized by gamma irradiation using low dose (25–40 kGy) and crosslinked using higher doses of irradiation (>50 kGy) (McKellop, 1999a; Muratoglu, 2004;

Wang, 1998b). Another factor affecting wear in the simulator is the testing environment. While bovine serum is the accepted analog for synovial fluid, dilution of bovine serum with water to obtain protein concentrations relevant to *in vivo* conditions is commonly used. However, wear of conventional (gamma sterilized) UHMWPE has been shown to increase with bovine serum dilution (Wang *et al.*, 1998). At high water concentration, non-physiological wear mechanisms can dominate the wear process (Liao *et al.*, 1999). Other factors that may affect the outcome are stress levels and loading mode (dynamic vs. constant) (Haider, 2009).

Because UHMWPE is a dense hydrophobic material, there is no significant diffusion of aqueous-based components during the simulator test. Thus, it is possible to quantify the wear of the bearing surface gravimetrically. Typically, the absorbed species found in UHMWPE are lipophilic or amphiphilic components of the synovial fluid. In order to assess more accurately the wear rate of the test material undergoing simulated *in vivo* loading and kinematic profiles, load soak controls are utilized. These controls are subjected to the same loads as the test components in the absence of the articular motion. Any weight gain in the controls is recorded and subtracted from the weight changes observed in the test components. Typically, there is an initial bedding-in period governed by the removal of the larger macroscopic asperities on the UHMWPE surface and the creep of the polymer, after which a linear, steady-state wear rate can be calculated.

3.1.2. *The development of crosslinked UHMWPE (hips)*

Crosslinking polyethylene by using irradiation doses higher than sterilization dose (>40 kGy) was introduced to decrease the abrasive/adhesive wear of UHMWPE, thus decreasing the incidence of periprosthetic bone loss directly caused by UHMWPE wear debris.

In the early 1970s, acetabular cups which had been irradiated using 600 kGy of gamma irradiation had been implanted (Shikata *et al.*, 1977) and radiographic wear measurements showed 0.006 mm/year compared to 0.98 mm/year for ethylene-oxide sterilized UHMWPE (Oonishi *et al.*, 2006). In addition, crosslinking using 800

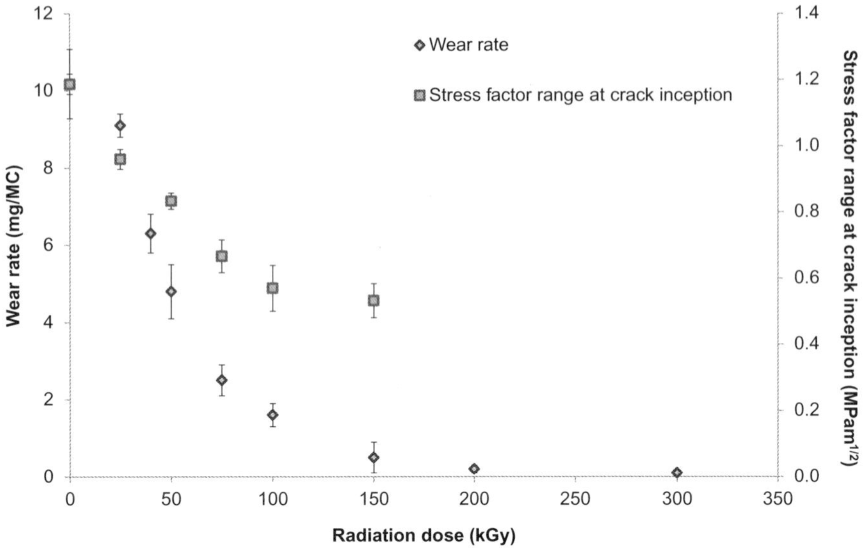

Figure 6-5. The dependence of wear resistance and fatigue toughness (as measured by ΔK_i, the stress factor range at crack inception) of crosslinked virgin UHMWPE as a function of radiation dose.

kGy gamma irradiation in the presence of acetylene gas was also performed (Du Plessis *et al.*, 1977) and showed high wear resistance (Grobbelaar *et al.*, 1999). Current clinical formulations of crosslinked UHMWPEs were developed in the 1990s together with optimization of the wear rate and mechanical properties (Figure 6-5) (McKellop *et al.*, 1999; Muratoglu *et al.*, 1999). While UHMWPEs exposed to radiation doses above 40 kGy are generally described as 'crosslinked', in hips, wear resistance is prioritized, therefore acetabular liner formulations of crosslinked virgin UHMWPEs tend to use radiation doses close to 100 kGy. In contrast, in knees, the fatigue toughness is prioritized, therefore tibial insert formulations of crosslinked virgin UHMWPEs use lower radiation doses, in the range of 50–75 kGy (Kurtz, 2009).

First generation highly crosslinked UHMWPEs were developed in conjunction with two different thermal treatments after radiation crosslinking (Figure 6-6a). The primary goal of these treatments was to eliminate or reduce the radiation-induced free radicals, some

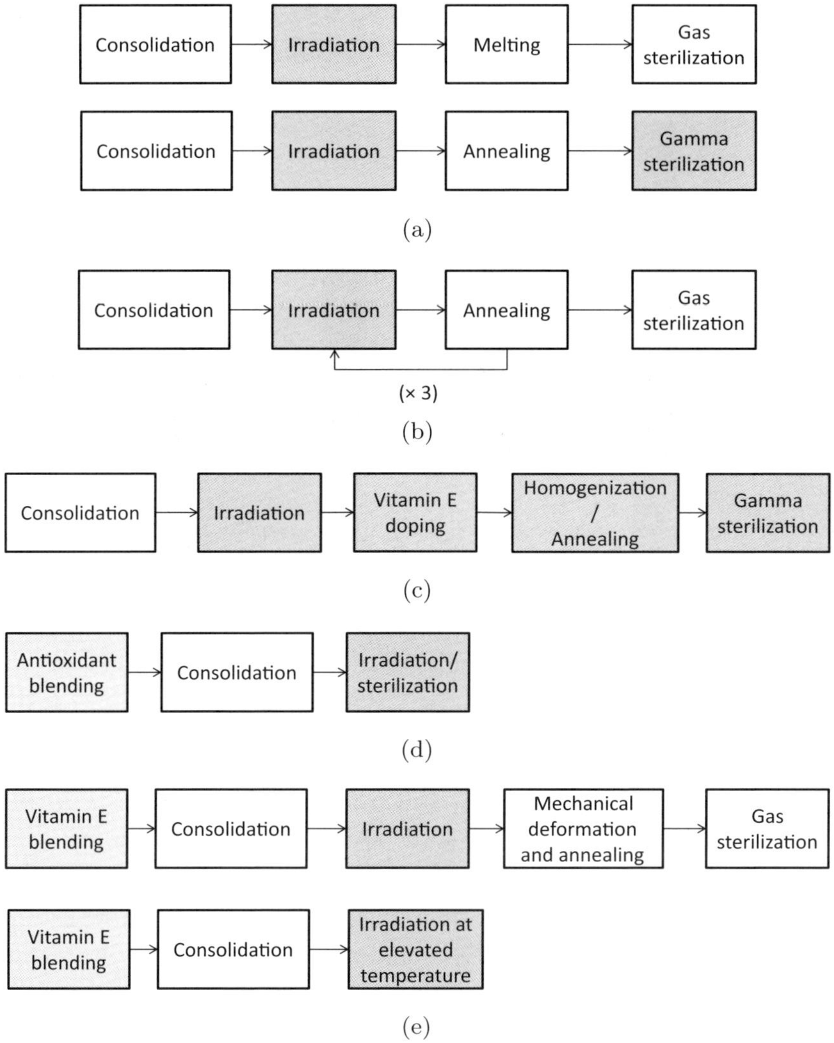

Figure 6-6. The production processes of different types of crosslinked UHMW-PEs. (a) First generation virgin crosslinked UHMWPEs with post-irradiation thermal treatment. Examples of irradiated and melted UHMWPEs are Longevity^{TM}, XLPE^{TM}, Marathon^{TM}, XLK^{TM}, while the sole example for irradiated and annealed UHMWPE was Crossfire^{TM}. (b) Second generation sequentially irradiated and annealed virgin UHMWPE (X3^{TM}). (c) Second generation vitamin E-diffused crosslinked UHMWPE (E1^{TM}). (d) Second generation antioxidant-blended crosslinked UHMWPEs. Examples are E-Plus^{TM}and AOX^{TM}. (e) Third generation vitamin E-blended crosslinked UHMWPEs with reduced residual free radicals. Examples are E-CiMa^{TM}and Vivacit-E^{TM}.

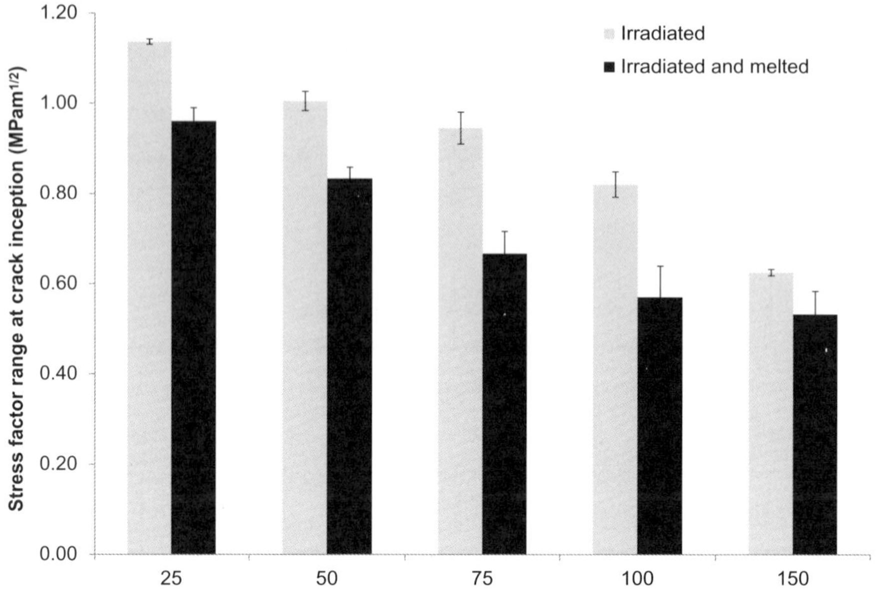

Figure 6-7. The effect of post-irradiation melting on the fatigue toughness of crosslinked UHMWPEs as a function of the radiation dose received.

of which can remain trapped in UHMWPE and cause embrittlement over time. The importance of these treatments to oxidation resistance will be discussed in the next section. The first method (post-irradiation melting) reduced residual free radicals to below detectable limits. However, re-crystallization of the polymer in the presence of crosslinks during this process caused a decrease in crystallinity, resulting in a decrease in fatigue toughness (Oral *et al.*, 2006) (Figure 6-7). The second method (post-irradiation annealing) exposed the crosslinked UHMWPE to temperatures close to but below the melting point. This resulted in a reduction of free radicals, thus preserved the fatigue toughness of the crosslinked UHMWPE (Medel *et al.*, 2007). However, this material still contained unstabilized free radicals and furthermore was terminally gamma sterilized, which introduced new free radicals and high oxidation potential. A second generation irradiated and annealed UHMWPE was further developed (Figure 6-6b; X3^{TM}, Stryker) with three sequential irradiation (30 kGy) and annealing steps and terminal gas plasma sterilization to effectively reduce the number of free radicals and prevent the introduction of new free radicals.

Hip and knee simulator studies of various designs with irradiated and melted UHMWPE all showed significantly improved wear resistance (60–90% decrease in wear) in comparison with conventional UHMWPE. Some studies used gamma in air-sterilized UHMWPE and others used ethylene oxide or gas plasma-sterilized UHMWPE as controls. Note that the gamma-sterilized controls would have some crosslinking and thus would also have a lower wear rate than the controls sterilized by non-ionizing methods. The hip simulator studies explored the influence of long-term use, artificial aging, presence of third-body particles, femoral head size, and, later, component placement on the wear of irradiated and melted UHMWPEs. Some studies were carried out to 30 million cycles, corresponding to 15–30 Yrs of *in vivo* service of an average total hip patient (Endo, 2002; McKellop, 1999b; Muratoglu, 2001a, 2001b, 2005b; Wang, 1998a). These studies showed that the marked reduction in wear was not affected by long-term testing and that there was no fatigue-induced wear. The addition of third-body particles, in the form of bone cement, increased the wear of both conventional and highly crosslinked UHMWPEs, yet the latter still exhibited better wear resistance. Standard artificial aging protocols did not oxidize the irradiated and melted UHMWPEs appreciably because of the improved oxidation resistance and as a result did not affect their wear rate.

While there are not many *in vitro* studies about the wear performance of first generation irradiated and annealed UHMWPE, it appeared to show similar wear rates to irradiated and melted UHMWPE irradiated to approximately the same dose in the available hip simulator studies (D'Lima *et al.*, 2003). Hip simulator wear testing for 5 million cycles of acetabular liners prepared from second generation sequentially irradiated and annealed UHMWPE (X3^{TM}) also showed that the wear rate was substantially reduced compared to gamma sterilized UHMWPE under normal gait (Essner *et al.*, 2005; Dumbleton *et al.*, 2006).

In hips, the femoral head size is an important factor, with larger heads increasing the wear rate of conventional UHMWPE

(Muratoglu, 2001b). Even though there is an increase in the contact area and hence a reduction in contact stress, wear is believed to increase with head size due to the dominant increase in the distance traveled at every gait cycle. Historically, smaller, 22 up to 28 mm diameter femoral heads had been used to minimize the wear of the liners. However, the disadvantage of smaller heads is the decrease in the stability and range of motion of the joint (Cuckler, 2004). Hip simulator studies also showed that there was not a significant increase in the wear rate of highly crosslinked UHMWPE when tested against larger femoral heads and the wear rate of an acetabular liner with an inner diameter of 46 mm and fabricated with irradiated and melted UHMWPE was lower than that of a 22 mm conventional UHMWPE acetabular liner (Muratoglu, 2001b). Similarly, there was no significant difference in the wear rate of sequentially irradiated and annealed UHMWPEs tested against femoral heads with inner diameters of 32–52 mm (Herrera *et al.*, 2007). Thus, it appeared to be feasible to use larger femoral heads (>32 mm) with highly crosslinked UHMWPEs without significant concern of increased wear rate and increased occurrence of osteolysis. It is estimated that about 50% of metal-on-polyethylene acetabular liners are used with femoral head sizes of 32 mm and about 10% with head sizes above 32 mm (personal communication with department surgeons).

3.1.3. *The development of crosslinked polyethylene (knees)*

The prevalence of adhesive/abrasive wear is thought to be less in total knees that in hips due to the more unidirectional articular motion in knees (Schwenke and Wimmer, 2013; Wang, 2001). In knees, in addition to adhesive wear caused by surface contact during articulation, delamination is a very common wear mechanism (Muratoglu *et al.*, 2003; Schmalzried and Callaghan, 1999). Delamination is caused by fatigue cracking initiated in the subsurface region of the implants, where the maximum stresses occur (D'Lima *et al.*, 2001). However, while infection and component loosening are the most common reasons for revision in total knees (Berger *et al.*, 2001; Berzins *et al.*, 2002; Bozic *et al.*, 2010; Colizza *et al.*, 1995; Diduch *et al.*, 1997), late failure is predominantly due to polyethylene wear and related

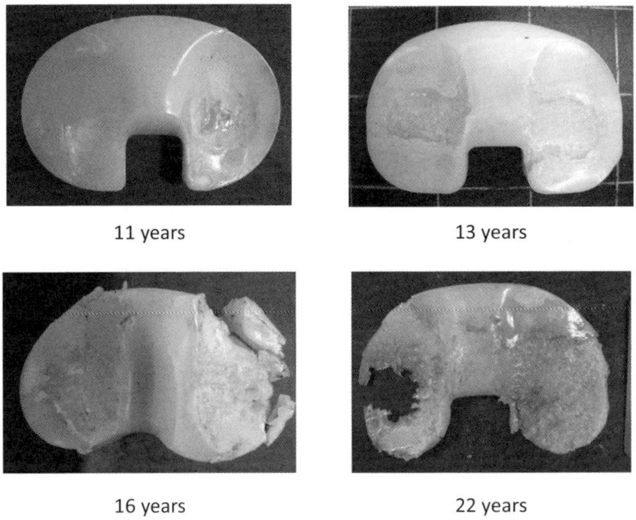

Figure 6-8. A selection of conventional, gamma-sterilized retrievals showing excessive wear and delamination with time.

loosening and instability (Sharkey *et al.*, 2002). While many failures may appear to be due solely to surgical factors (alignment, ligament balance), damage and failure mechanisms in total knees are often related to the performance of the bearing surface material (wear) and the forgiveness of the bearing surface to changes in factors such as implant design (conformity, modularity, polyethylene thickness) and articulation environment (third-body particulate) (Berend *et al.*, 2004; Wasiliewski *et al.*, 1994). Despite the poor long-term performance of conventional, gamma sterilized UHMWPEs in the knee (Figure 6-8), the benefits of using highly crosslinked UHMWPEs in total knees remains questionable (Jacofsky, 2008; Rodriguez, 2008) mainly due to the perceived increase in risk of fracture or fatigue damage with crosslinked UHMWPEs.

In vitro simulator studies have shown a reduction of 65–90% in knee wear compared to conventional, gamma-sterilized UHMWPEs (Hermida *et al.*, 2008; McEwen *et al.*, 2005; Muratoglu *et al.*, 2002, 2004; Wang *et al.*, 2008). In one wear resistance study, tibial inserts made of highly crosslinked, irradiated, and melted UHMWPE (95 kGy) showed 93% reduction in wear compared to that of conventional, gamma-sterilized (inert) UHMWPE after accelerated aging. In contrast to the aged conventional UHMWPE, which showed severe delamination and cracking, the highly crosslinked inserts did not delaminate or crack. Using sequentially irradiated and annealed UHMWPE with a cruciate-retaining design under normal gait, there was a 68% reduction in the volumetric wear rate of conventional UHMWPE. In the same study, using a posterior-stabilized design with stair climbing, there was also a 68% reduction in wear (Wang *et al.*, 2008). The wear rate of conventional UHMWPE increased significantly when the inserts were aged in an accelerated manner in addition to severe delamination and cracking. There was no change in the wear rate of the highly crosslinked UHMWPEs and no evidence of delamination.

In a fixed tibial bearing with modularity, posterior wear was quantified by measuring the protrusion of the material through the screw holes on the tibial plate for irradiated (65 kGy) and melted highly crosslinked UHMWPE and conventional, gamma-sterilized (inert) UHMWPE (Muratoglu *et al.*, 2007). A comparison of the wear volumes measured by a coordinate-measuring machine after melt recovery of plastic creep showed that the highly crosslinked UHMWPE had higher wear resistance than conventional UHMWPE. In another study which used both a fixed and a rotating platform design, there was also a clear reduction in wear and volume of wear particles using an irradiated (100 kGy) and melted highly crosslinked UHMWPE (Fisher *et al.*, 2004). Both in this study and others, the wear rates of both irradiated (100 kGy) and melted UHMWPE and conventional UHMWPEs increased when the counterface roughness increased. However, highly crosslinked UHMWPE still preserved its superior wear resistance compared to conventional UHMWPE (Muratoglu *et al.*, 2004).

In one simulator study (Hermida *et al.*, 2008), tibial inserts made of irradiated (65 kGy) and melted and sequentially irradiated (90 kGy) and annealed inserts were maligned in varus and tibial rotation at two standard deviations outside of average alignment. Gamma-sterilized (inert) and aged controls delaminated severely at 1 MC, especially on the medial side, leading the authors to stop their testing. In contrast, after accelerated aging and 5 MC testing under normal gait, there was no delamination or damage on the highly crosslinked inserts. In a similarly adverse fatigue model based on explanted components with cruciate-retaining design with ligamentous imbalance showing posterior damage, Muratoglu *et al.* (2002) combined stair climbing with a tight posterior cruciate ligament in a knee simulator. Irradiated (95 kGy) and melted UHMWPE as well as the unaged, conventional gamma-sterilized (inert) UHMWPE did not delaminate or crack after 0.5 MC, but accelerated aged conventional UHMWPE delaminated severely starting at 50,000 cycles, leading the authors to stop the study early for these inserts. In another knee simulator study investigating the effects of rotational malalignment on accelerated aged irradiated (95 kGy) and melted patellas, stair climbing load and kinematics were applied for 2 MC with and without the presence of a 4°femoral internal rotation (Burroughs *et al.*, 2006). In both the normal alignment and malalignment tests, the aged conventional controls developed extensive cracks whereas the highly crosslinked UHMWPE components did not crack or delaminate.

3.1.4. *Clinical methods and results*

It has already been mentioned in the previous sections that the calculation of a steady state linear penetration rate is done by separating the long-term wear rate of the material from the flow or creep of the material under stress. When measuring wear volumetrically in simulator components, creep deformation of UHMWPE has to be separated from wear. This can be done by melting the component after testing is completed, as UHMWPE has excellent shape memory and creep deformation can be eliminated by remelting the component (Muratoglu *et al.*, 2005). This is especially important in clinical studies, as gravimetric measurements cannot be made *in situ* and the wear rate is calculated by detecting changes in the location of the material. The location of the femoral head and the acetabular shell are calculated from two- or three-dimensional images taken of the implants *in vivo* at different time points (Charnley and Halley,

1975; Digas *et al.*, 2004; Hui *et al.*, 2003; Livermore, 1996). Currently, radiostereometric analysis (RSA) is considered the most accurate method in determining clinical wear rates in the hip (Bragdon *et al.*, 2004, 2006). This method utilizes embedded tantalum beads in the pelvis and the acetabular component at the time of implantation to accurately calculate the relative spatial orientation of the acetabular cup and the femoral head. Despite different proposals (Collier *et al.*, 2007; Price *et al.*, 2005; Teeter *et al.*, 2013; van Ijsseldijk *et al.*, 2013), there is currently no standard imaging technique to determine *in vivo* wear rates in the knee.

There are a number of clinical trials comparing the *in vivo* performance of highly crosslinked UHMWPEs to that of conventional UHMWPE acetabular liners (Digas, 2007a; Engh, 2006; Garcia-Rey, 2008). There is an 87% decrease in the risk of osteolysis in hips (there were not enough clinical studies to determine the risk for knees) after five years follow-up (Kurtz, 2011), representing a possible solution to one of the major problems limiting the life of joint implants.

A closely watched subset of acetabular liners is first generation irradiated and annealed Crossfire^{TM} implants (Stryker, Mahwah, NJ) due to their high oxidation potential (Currier *et al.*, 2007; Wannomae *et al.*, 2006). However, at about three years follow-up, liners manufactured from this material did not show increased wear rates (Kurtz *et al.*, 2010). A study comparing ceramic-on-ceramic articulation to ceramic-on-Crossfire^{TM} articulation found no significant differences in clinical performance in follow-ups up to five-years. In another study analyzing the reasons for revision of different highly crosslinked UHMWPE bearing surfaces, there was no significant differences between the linear penetration rates of irradiated and annealed, and of irradiated and melted first generation crosslinked UHMWPEs with up to three-year average implantation time (Kurtz *et al.*, 2010). At these early times, the clinical wear rates of highly crosslinked UHMWPEs appear to be following pre-clinical *in vitro* testing expectations.

Clinical outcome studies have been limited for knees. One retrospective series of 200 surgeries performed by a single surgeon (100 irradiated and melted highly crosslinked, 100 conventional) with a minimum follow up of 69 months (mean 75 months) showed reduction in radiolucency in the highly crosslinked (irradiated and melted) cohort when compared to conventional, gamma-sterilized UHMWPE (Hodrick *et al.*, 2008). Another study with a minimum follow-up of two years showed no revisions and no osteolysis for both irradiated/melted and conventional UHMWPEs (Minoda *et al.*, 2009).

3.1.5. *Surface coating*

One of the innate characteristics of articular cartilage is its superior lubricity. The dynamics between the osmotic pressure provided by the water in the cartilaginous network and the release of some of the free water from the network under load are partly responsible for the great wear and load-bearing properties of cartilage (Mankin *et al.*, 2000). In contrast, the wear of UHMWPE is governed by surface-on-surface contact with little load-sharing from a lubrication layer on the surface. Recently, a surface coating of UHMWPE comprising a phospholipid has been proposed to create a hydrophilic layer on the surface of UHMWPE, which can swell in water or synovial fluid and can create a fluid lubrication layer similar to cartilage under load (Moro *et al.*, 2004).

The incorporation and binding of the phospholipid 2-methacryloxyethyl phosphorylcholine (MPC) with the UHMWPE on the surface is enabled through a UV-mediated reaction (Ishihara *et al.*, 1990; Kyomoto *et al.*, 2008). In addition to the possible effects of wear reduction of the surface, MPC grafting was shown to reduce biological reactions *in vitro* (Ishihara *et al.*, 1990) and is proposed to also reduce the osteolytic potential of polyethylene wear particles. This method results in a roughly 100 nm-thick layer of the phospholipid on the surface (Moro *et al.*, 2004), which could be detected by a cross-sectional transmission electron microscope image. In addition, contact angle measurements showed that the resulting surface was predominantly hydrophilic (theta $<20°$) in contrast to the native UHMWPE surface, which is very hydrophobic (theta $\sim 70°$).

Despite the nanometer-level thickness of the surface layer, the coated surfaces were reported to have lower wear in a hip simulator study compared to the base material, which was 75 kGy irradiated virgin (no antioxidant) UHMWPE that had been annealed at 130°C, presumably to decrease the concentration of free radicals (Moro *et al.*, 2009).

The main concern with any coating in this load-bearing application is its shear and scratch-resistance due to the presence of high stresses and third-body particulate in the clinical environment. Despite the lack of testing in a third-body environment, the wear of coated acetabular liners did not change over 70 million cycles (MC) in a hip simulator test, nevertheless suggesting longevity of the bearing (Journal of Arthroplasty — In Press). Another drawback of this UHMWPE is the potential difficulty in incorporating an antioxidant in the UHMWPE before surface coating as free radical scavenging antioxidants can interfere with the UV-mediated reactions necessary for the binding of the coating.

The Japanese implant manufacturer Kyocera Medical introduced acetabular liners made out of this coated material for total hip arthroplasty applications in 2013 (Aquala™) in Japan.

3.2. *Oxidative Stability*

Our understanding of oxidative reactions in UHMWPE is based on the reactions of free radicals in the polymer that are caused by ionizing radiation. Free radicals are induced everywhere in this semicrystalline polymer as a result of irradiation used for sterilization or crosslinking and a large fraction of these free radicals are recombined in the amorphous regions of the polymer (Dole, 1972). However, some of these radicals are trapped in the rigid crystalline domains and are detectable in the polymer for long periods of time (Bhateja *et al.*, 1995). Since the interchain distance is too long for crosslinking to occur in the crystalline phase, these free radicals can only migrate along the chains and can react with diffused oxygen when they have reached the amorphous–crystalline interface. When these reactions occur, the primary alkyl and allyl radicals are transformed first into peroxy free radicals, after which these active free radicals attack nearby unreacted polymer chains to form hydroperoxides. During the eventual breakdown of these hydroperoxides, oxidation products are formed and the molecular weight of the polymer is degraded.

Also during the formation of each hydroperoxide, a new alkyl radical is formed, thereby furthering this cascade of degradation reactions (Al-Malaika, 1993).

Oxidation is detected in UHMWPE often using transmission Fourier transform infrared spectroscopy (FTIR). The carbonyl-containing species, which result from the slow degradation of hydroperoxides are measured and normalized against a standard crystalline polyethylene absorbance (Spiegelberg, 2009). The chain scissioning accompanying oxidation, also leads to the recrystallization of the shorter chains and can manifest as a gradual increase in crystallinity (Grood *et al.*, 1982; Keller and Ungar, 1983). While an increase in crystallinity without oxidation generally indicates increased strength in UHMWPE (Oral *et al.*, 2009), the increase in crystallinity with oxidation is a sign of decreased strength and elongation. In fact, there can be a white band visible in the highly oxidized regions of the oxidized polymer, often in the subsurface region and it is an indication of severe embrittlement (Figure 6-9).

The rate of oxidation of the historical gamma-sterilized UHMWPE, which was primarily a result of the oxidation mechanisms described above, causes significant oxidation within a decade of use (Premnath *et al.*, 1996). This oxidative degradation can manifest as increased adhesive/abrasive or delamination wear of the bearing surface (Bracco *et al.*, 2006; Walker *et al.*, 1998). In addition, the

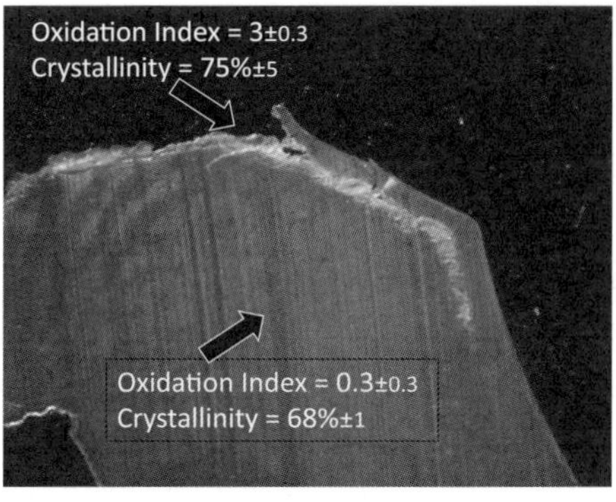

Figure 6-9. 'White banding' as a sign of oxidation and embrittlement in UHMWPE.

mechanical strength and toughness are both extremely sensitive to oxidation, increasing the risk of strain damage and fracture risk, especially under aggressive conditions.

The methods to stabilize UHMWPE bearing surfaces against oxidation were initially focused on the reduction or elimination of these so-called residual free radicals in a passive manner before implantation. Radiation sterilization in inert gas or vacuum and terminal sterilization methods other than radiation was introduced for UHMWPEs containing detectable free radicals at the time of implantation to limit the reintroduction of free radicals (Kurtz *et al.*, 1999).

3.2.1. *Post-irradiation thermal treatments*

Two methods were used in first generation crosslinked UHMWPEs to eliminate and reduce the concentration of free radicals after radiation crosslinking. The first was post-irradiation melting, which allowed the melting and disordering of the crystalline regions and the escape and recombination of the free radicals trapped within these regions. Then, implants fabricated from this type of material were sterilized using non-radiation methods such as gas plasma or ethylene oxide sterilization.

The second post-irradiation thermal method to address the residual free radicals was annealing below the melting point of the polymer. This method results in a decrease in the free radicals of the irradiated polymer with increasing annealing temperature. This is because the crystal melting range of the polydisperse polyethylene crystals is between 100°C and about 150°C, with the peak melting temperature at 137°C (Figure 6-2). Thus, about 10% of the free radicals remain after annealing at 130°C. A first generation irradiated and annealed UHMWPE was terminally sterilized using gamma irradiation, thus reintroducing a large number of free radicals into the polymer before implantation (Figure 6-6a).

The oxidative stability of these irradiated and melted UHMWPEs has been good in their first decade of use. Compared to conventional, gamma-sterilized UHMWPE and first generation irradiated annealed UHMWPE (Currier *et al.*, 2007), which showed significantly high levels of oxidation at five years implantation, the oxidation observed in irradiated and melted UHMWPEs in the same early follow-up period was low (Currier *et al.*, 2010). At the same time, there is an increasing trend with *in vivo* implantation time and the sporadic appearance of subsurface oxidation in these materials (Currier *et al.*, 2013) was without explanation based on our long-time understanding of oxidation and oxidative stabilization in UHMWPE.

The second generation irradiated and annealed UHMWPE was developed using a sequential scheme of three consecutive steps of 30 kGy irradiation and annealing below the melting point (Dumbleton *et al.*, 2006). It was hypothesized that the free radical reduction following a smaller radiation dose would be more effective, thus leaving a smaller amount of detectable free radicals at the end of the desired radiation crosslinking. In addition, this second generation material was sterilized without irradiation, preventing the introduction of new free radicals at the terminal step. Finally, the free radical concentration in this highly crosslinked UHMWPE was similar to conventional, gamma-sterilized UHMWPE (Wang *et al.*, 2006). There have been reports of low amounts of oxidation in these sequentially irradiated and annealed UHMWPE implants (Currier *et al.*, 2013), the rates being faster than in irradiated and melted UHMWPE and higher in total knee implants (Reinitz *et al.*, 2012), but the clinical effects of this oxidation, if any, are not clear.

3.2.2. *Antioxidant stabilization*

While the use of additives to stabilize against long-term oxidation is very common in industrial polymers, antioxidants were not used in medical grade UHMWPE until 2006. There were three separate hypotheses for the use of the antioxidant vitamin E in UHMWPE medical implants.

Vitamin E was investigated as an agent to prevent the formation of fatigue cracks especially in total knee implants (Tomita *et al.*, 1999), where subsurface fatigue crack formation and subsequent delamination are common (Muratoglu *et al.*, 2002). Thus, in Japan, vitamin E-stabilized UHMWPEs have been used clinically without radiation crosslinking (Nakashima Medical Ltd.), based also on one knee simulator study showing a wear reduction effect of vitamin E on UHMWPE (Teramura *et al.*, 2008), but this effect has not been confirmed.

Blending of vitamin E in UHMWPE resin powder before consolidation and radiation was introduced as a means of preventing the oxidation of conventional, gamma-sterilized UHMWPE (Bracco *et al.*, 2007). While this idea originated in the 1990s, there is still no clinical implant combining vitamin E stabilization and a sterilization dose of radiation (25–40 kGy). Because it became clear that highly crosslinked UHMWPEs performed very well clinically and decreased wear of implants, vitamin E-blended UHMWPEs were developed also to obtain high crosslink density. Since vitamin E is an antioxidant, which can also act as a powerful free radical scavenger, increasing vitamin E content decreases the crosslink density of irradiated UHMWPEs (Oral *et al.*, 2008). For this reason, to obtain a highly crosslinked UHMWPE, not only is the vitamin E concentration limited to 0.2 to 0.3 wt%, but also the radiation dose has to be increased compared to that used with virgin (no additive) UHMWPE (Table 6-2). Several clinical formulations of highly crosslinked, antioxidant-blended UHMWPEs, which have been developed following these guidelines, were introduced since 2011 (Table 6-3). While vitamin E remains the most common used in these implant materials, a different hindered phenol has also been introduced by DePuy.

Since the detrimental effects of radiation-induced free radicals on the oxidative stability of UHMWPE implants have been clearly

Table 6-2. The equivalent dose of radiation to obtain similar crosslink density in GUR1050 UHMWPE (260 mol/m^3) blended with different concentrations of vitamin E.

Vitamin E concentration (wt%)	Radiation dose (kGy)
0.02	111
0.05	118
0.1	123
0.2	150
0.3	189
0.5	245
1	540

Table 6-3. A compendium of vitamin E-stabilized joint implants in the US.

	E-Poly/E1™	Vivacit-E™	E+™	E-CiMa™	E-SYNTIAL™
Company	Biomet	Zimmer	DJO surgical	Corin	Mako/Stryker
Implant designs	Hip and knee	Hip and knee	Knee	Hip and knee	Knee
Available since	2008	2013	2011	2010	2013
Type of UHMWPE resin	GUR1020	GUR1020	Unknown	GUR1020	GUR1020
Consolidation method	Compression molding	Compression molding		Compression molding	Compression molding
Irradiation method	Gamma	E-beam (@elevated T)	Unknown	Gamma	Gamma
Irradiation dose	100 kGy	>100 kGy	Unknown	120 kGy	100 kGy
Oxidative stabilization method	Vitamin E diffusion	Vitamin E blending	Vitamin E blending	Vitamin E blending + mechanical annealing	Vitamin E blending + mechanical annealing
Sterilization method	Gamma irradiation	Ethylene oxide	Unknown	Ethylene oxide	Ethylene oxide

demonstrated, some formulations of antioxidant-blended UHMWPEs were developed with reduced or eliminated detectable free radicals from irradiation. One of these is a cold irradiated and mechanically annealed blend, in which the free radicals are reduced to below detectable levels by using mechanical deformation and thermal annealing after irradiation (Muratoglu *et al.*,; Oral *et al.*, 2014). The mobility induced in the crystalline regions by deformation results in the reduction of free radicals and thermal annealing uses the shape memory of UHMWPE to recover its original dimensions and obtain a more isotropic implant material. Another method to reduce the free radical content is irradiation close to the melting point of the polymer (Oral *et al.*, 2013), effectively crosslinking and reducing free radicals simultaneously. These vitamin E-blended UHMWPEs with reduced free radicals are expected to have high oxidative stability not only because they have vitamin E, but also because the vitamin E can be effective against oxidation for longer period of time *in vivo* with the reduced oxidative effect of radiation-induced free radicals.

Another method of incorporating vitamin E in highly crosslinked UHMWPE is by diffusion of the antioxidant in the already radiation-crosslinked material. Using this method, there is no limitation of the vitamin E content from the perspective of decreased crosslink density and vitamin E content can be as high as 0.7 wt% (estimated to be the solubility of vitamin E in crosslinked UHMWPE at body temperature (Rowell *et al.*, 2011)). Post-irradiation diffusion of vitamin E into irradiated UHMWPE is performed by a two-step process comprising doping with pure vitamin E at a temperature close to the peak melting point followed by annealing at a similarly high temperature to homogenize the high surface concentration obtained during doping throughout the implant (Oral *et al.*, 2007). A terminal gamma sterilization is used in implants fabricated using such a method. While this vitamin E-diffused implant has detectable free radicals (Oral *et al.*, 2006), it also contains a large amount of vitamin E, which is exposed to only a terminal sterilization dose of radiation. This type of implant has been used clinically in hips since 2007 and in knees since 2008. Its pre-clinical and clinical performance has been promising in terms of wear resistance (Greene *et al.*, 2013; Haider *et al.*,

2012; Oral *et al.*, 2006, 2008) and there are currently no reports of oxidation.

The incorporation of the antioxidant vitamin E has ushered in a new area in joint implant bearing surfaces and spurred the development of UHMWPEs with different formulations using vitamin E and also UHMWPEs using different antioxidants. Early clinical results with irradiated, vitamin E-diffused and gamma-sterilized highly crosslinked UHMWPE (E1^{TM}, Biomet, Warsaw, IN) corroborate the good wear resistance observed *in vitro* and the lack of oxidation or oxidative changes at mid-term follow-up (5–7 years) is promising for the large-scale adaptation of antioxidant technologies in UHMWPE bearing surfaces.

3.2.3. *Oxidation in the absence of radiation-induced free radicals*

Our understanding of oxidation and oxidative stability has been focused entirely on the effects of the free radicals residual from the radiation sterilization or crosslinking. While the oxidation reactions and oxidative effects of these radicals in UHMWPE are fairly well understood, the possible oxidation mechanisms *in vivo* in the absence of these reactions are not.

Implants made out of UHMWPEs without detectable free radicals have been used on a wide scale in the last decade in the form of irradiated and melted highly crosslinked UHMWPEs. While these materials have shown good oxidation resistance in their first decade of use, recently there have been reports of detectable subsurface oxidation in some retrievals that had been implanted for less than ten years (Currier *et al.*, 2010). In addition, there was evidence of oxidation in irradiated and melted implants after retrievals and shelf storage despite being exposed to the *in vivo* environment for as short a period of time as two months (Muratoglu *et al.*, 2010). These results suggested the possibility that there were oxidation initiation mechanisms *in vivo* other than those initiated by the trapped free radicals residual to the radiation crosslinking or sterilization processes.

Cyclic loading and lipid absorption from the synovial fluid were proposed as two possible environmental factors. It was shown that absorption of some synovial fluid lipids, which were previously

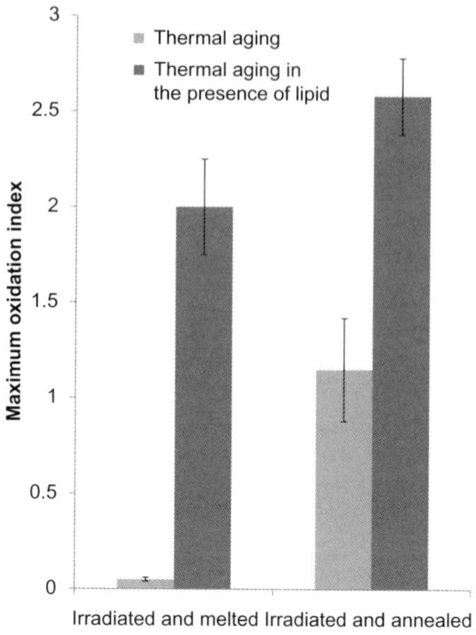

(a)

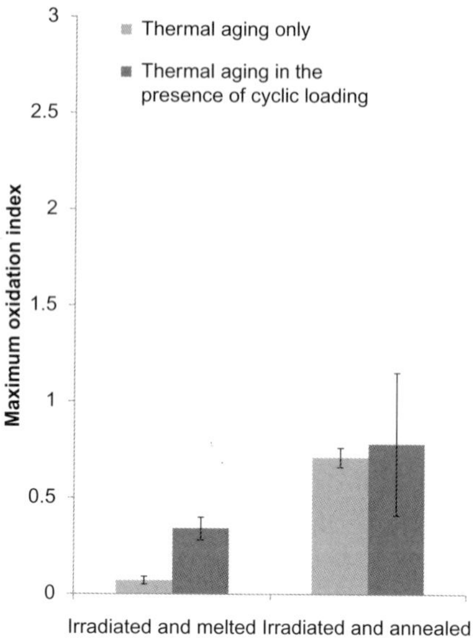

(b)

Figure 6-10. Oxidation of irradiated and melted UHMWPE in the presence of the synovial fluid lipid squalene (a) and cyclic loading (b).

detected in retrievals (Costa *et al.*, 2001), could initiate oxidation in highly crosslinked UHMWPE without detectable free radicals at implantation and could increase the rate of oxidative damage (Oral *et al.*, 2012) (Figure 6-10a).

It was possible for high-stress cyclic loading to cause chain scissioning through strain accumulation causing oxidative damage (Nabar *et al.*, 2008) (Figure 6-10b). This is hypothesized to occur through the production of new free radicals, which can then undergo oxidation reactions. In addition, chain scissioning can lead to direct deterioration of mechanical properties through molecular weight degradation.

These results suggested that there may be previously unknown oxidation mechanisms of oxidation initiation and propagation *in vivo*. Protecting against such mechanisms in an active manner may be another benefit of antioxidant stabilization of UHMWPE.

3.3. *Fatigue Toughness*

There are compressive and shear forces on UHMWPE during articulation, and there may be residual tensile stresses that arise from accumulated stress during repeated load cycles (Sathasivam and Walker, 1998). The reversal of stress direction causes fatigue cracks to initiate causing delamination (Bartel *et al.*, 1986, 1995). Therefore, fatigue resistance is a crucial material property of UHMWPEs developed for total joint replacements.

3.3.1. *In vitro testing*

Fatigue testing is performed *in vitro* in cyclic tension on a compact tension specimen (ASTM, 2008), which is designed to concentrate applied stress at a notch tip with an existing crack. A stress factor at crack inception (ΔKi) is calculated as a measure of fatigue crack propagation resistance. This is the stress factor range (dependent on the load ratio, sample geometry, and crack length), at which the crack growth rate exceeds 10^{-6} mm/cycle. The ΔKi of unirradiated UHMWPE is reported as 1.6–2.0 MPam$^{1/2}$ (Baker *et al.*, 2000; Oral *et al.*, 2009). Fatigue toughness of UHMWPE is often characterized by fatigue crack propagation resistance (ASTM, 2008). While this method is useful in ranking the toughness of different formulations of UHMWPE, the clinical relevance of this type of testing is not clear. Fatigue damage is common in all types of UHMWPEs under adverse stress conditions such as malaligned components. One fatigue-related damage mechanism of concern in total knee implants is delamination of the surface, which is a result of crack formation subsurface and the propagation of these cracks to the bearing surface. This mechanism is closely related to the oxidation level (Currier *et al.*, 2007; Wannomae *et al.*, 2010) of the material but a specific level of oxidation or fatigue toughness that leads to such damage has not been defined.

The fatigue strength of UHMWPE without subsequent radiation is the material with the highest among UHMWPE bearing surface formulations (Baker *et al.*, 2000; Oral *et al.*, 2006). However, the ductility of this material, which is the source of this high fatigue toughness, also leads to large-strain plastic deformation, a precursor to wear (Edidin *et al.*, 1999). Radiation crosslinking, which reduces plastic deformation and increases the wear resistance, thus also reduces the fatigue toughness (Baker *et al.*, 2003). In addition, oxidation severely degrades the ductility and the fatigue toughness of the material (Oral *et al.*, 2004) and the oxidative stability of the material as described above should be considered thoroughly for implantation.

The fatigue crack propagation resistance measurements, which are the most common indicator of fatigue toughness, can vary among laboratories for several reasons. The frequency of the test, the temperature and gas composition of the testing environment, the methodology of initiating and measuring crack propagation can all make a difference as well as the inherent variation in the prepared material (Baker *et al.*, 1999, 2003; Bradford *et al.*, 2004; Oral *et al.*, 2006; Pruitt *et al.*, 1994). Table 6-3 lists reported values for the fatigue crack propagation resistance of most clinically available UHMWPE formulations.

3.3.2. *Methods for improvement*

The fatigue strength of conventional gamma-sterilized UHMWPE in its freshly prepared and unoxidized state is considered a benchmark. While there is no clear guideline for surgeons on how thin/thick an implant bearing surface they can use, the 6 mm thickness that Bartel *et al.* (1996) defined based on this conventional UHMWPE is still considered the minimum thickness. In addition, although the discussion of how thin/or thick the bearing surface can be is based on the thickness at the articulating surface, the thickness of the thinnest parts of the component such as the locking mechanisms or rims are usually unknown. So, there is concern about increased risk of fatigue damage or even fracture for new formulations of UHMWPE with low/lower fatigue toughness than unoxidized conventional UHMWPE at implantation.

For highly crosslinked UHMWPEs with high dose irradiation, the concern of fatigue damage has been heightened due to their much lower fatigue toughness compared to unoxidized conventional UHMWPE at the time of implantation (Table 6-4). In addition, in those materials that were melted post-irradiation, the fatigue

Table 6-4. The stress factor range at crack inception as an indicator of fatigue toughness of different formulations of GUR1050 UHMWPE.

Material	$\Delta K_i (MPam^{1/2})$
Conventional (~25–40 kGy)[1]	0.93 ± 0.03
Conventional (aged)[2]	0.18 ± 0.06
0.1 wt% vitamin E + 150 kGy	0.73 ± 0.04
100 kGy[2]	0.74 ± 0.01
100 kGy + melting[2]	0.56 ± 0.02
85 kGy + vitamin E diffusion + gamma sterilization[3]	0.77 ± 0.02

Note: [1]Oral (2010), [2]Oral (2004), [3]Oral (2006).

toughness was decreased even further due to a loss of crystallinity after melting and recrystallization in the presence of crosslinks (Oral *et al.*, 2006). These materials have shown excellent clinical performance in the hip over the last ten years, but there have been reports of adverse events such as rim fracture in vertically placed cups (Tower *et al.*, 2007). In knees, where the concern for fatigue damage is highest due to the high stresses and the historically high incidence of delamination, there have been no reports of fracture or delamination in any type of highly crosslinked UHMWPEs. However, there is a great need for increasingly detailed reports of the clinical performance of highly croslinked UHMWPEs in knees.

In order to alleviate concerns over the performance of highly crosslinked UHMWPEs, whose wear resistance has been excellent, one approach is to improve the fatigue toughness without sacrificing wear and oxidative stability. This can be done either by improving the fatigue toughness of the UHMWPE before radiation crosslinking (to compensate for losses in ductility due to crosslinking) or by improving the toughness of radiation crosslinked UHMWPE.

One approach in improving the fatigue toughness of UHMWPE was increasing its crystalline content. This can be done by high pressure crystallization (or HPC), where the material is crystallized at high pressure (>210 MPa) and allowed to crystallize in its hexagonal phase. In this phase, the crystals have enough mobility to slide past each other and crystallization is less hindered, enabling the formation of the so-called extended chain crystals. Crystallization in this manner increases the crystallinity and the crystal size of UHMWPE, thus improving its fatigue toughness. Interestingly, the inclusion of vitamin E was shown to amplify this effect and result in higher crystallinity and higher fatigue toughness under the same conditions (Oral *et al.*, 2009). The radiation crosslinking of such a highly crystalline UHMWPE can be done to improve the toughness of highly crosslinked UHMWPE.

Another approach to improve the toughness of UHMWPE is high temperature melting (HTM), which is defined as the exposure of UHMWPE to temperatures high above its melting point (>200°C). Due to the very high molecular weight of UHMWPE, the time for UHMWPE chains to diffuse past each other and find an equilibrium state is extremely long (calculated to be around 15 hours at 180°C). But, the consolidation of UHMWPE in the manufacturing of medical implants relies on a relatively short high temperature/pressure dwell period. Thus, by HTM of consolidated UHMWPE, the diffusion of chains in the inter-particle regions can be improved and fusion defects can be healed, resulting in a UHMWPE with improved toughness (Fu *et al.*, 2010). In addition, when the temperature is close to 300°C, chain scissioning starts occurring to a significant degree, resulting in a large amount of terminal vinyl groups forming and an increase in the elongation of the material. When this material is radiation crosslinked, the result is a highly wear resistant UHMWPE with improved toughness (Fu *et al.*, 2011, 2013).

Another approach to improve the fatigue toughness of crosslinked UHMWPE is limiting the crosslinking of the bearing material to the surface or surfaces where it is needed. *In vivo* measurements of UHMWPE wear in the hip have estimated the wear of highly crosslinked UHMWPEs to be in the worst case 0.05 mm/yr (Kurtz *et al.*, 2011), which would result in a total loss of material of 2 mm in 40 years. Therefore, by limiting the crosslinking to the surface 2 mm of the implant, the wear resistance requirements can be satisfied while protecting the fatigue toughness of the implant by protecting the rest of the implant from crosslinking. This can be achieved by spatially controlling the vitamin E content throughout the implant material during radiation exposure (Oral *et al.*, 2010, 2013). Since vitamin E can act as a free radical scavenger, the surface of the implant with low vitamin E concentration can have a higher crosslink density than the bulk, where the vitamin E concentration is higher. Alternatively, the penetration of the radiation energy can be controlled to limit crosslinking at the surface (Neils *et al.*, 2013). In each case, the result is improved toughness compared to uniformly crosslinked implant material. In fact, since the fatigue toughness improvement is linearly affected by the fraction of the implant that is crosslinked (Oral *et al.*, 2011), the fatigue strength improvement would be higher for thicker implant components.

4. Conclusions

Overall, total joint arthroplasty is a very successful operation, restoring function to the joints of millions of patients with debilitating diseases and improving their lives. The knowledge gained about the design of the implants and the reaction of the body to these implants has enabled the development of better products. While the manufacturing of UHMWPE (in sterilized form) originally enabled hard-on-soft articulations and the use of most total joint implants as we know them today, the development of highly crosslinked UHMWPEs in the last decade has to a large extent eliminated the incidence of osteolysis in the first decade, making great strides in the quest to solve one of the major problems threatening the longevity of joint implants.

Another major problem in hip replacements is dislocation, comprising approximately 19% of all revisions in the US (Bozic *et al.*, 2009). This early complication can threaten the early stability and fixation of a joint. The use of larger femoral heads was shown to decrease the incidence of dislocation and hard-on-hard bearing couples were preferred to prevent dislocation, especially in younger patients. However, the unexpected catastrophic periprosthetic tissue reactions caused by metal debris and metal ions have almost eliminated the use of metal-on-metal implants, the most commonly used hard-on-hard bearing surface in the US. Thus, better strength and wear performance is now expected of metal-on-UHMWPE or ceramic-on-UHMWPE bearings to address not only the problem of dislocation but also for the continued use in young and active patients. It is therefore necessary to continue improving the fatigue toughness of crosslinked UHMWPEs to increase their safety for use with larger femoral heads as well as under adverse conditions such as the vertical alignment of the cup.

References

Al-Malaika, S. (1993). *Autoxidation. Atmospheric Oxidation and Antioxidants.* G. Scott, Elsevier, Amsterdam, 45–82.

ASTM. (2008). E647-08 Standard test method for measurement of fatigue crack growth rates.

Baker, D.A., Bellare, A. and Pruitt, L. (2003). The effect of degree of crosslinking on the fatigue crack initiation and propagation resistance of orthopedic-grade polyethylene, *J Biomed Mater Res A*, **66**, 146–154.

Baker, D.A., Hastings, R.S. and Pruitt, L. (1999). Study of fatigue resistance of chemical and radiation crosslinked medical grade ultrahigh molecular weight polyethylene, *J Biomed Mater Res*, **46**(4), 573–581.

Baker, D.A., Hastings, R.S. and Pruitt, L. (2000). Compression and tension fatigue resistance of medical grade ultra high molecular weight polyethylene: The effect of morphology, sterilization, aging and temperature, *Polymer*, **41**(2), 795–808.

Bartel, D.I., Bicknell, I. and Wright, T.M. (1986). The effect of conformity, thickness, and material on stresses in ultra-high molecular weight components for total joint replacement. *J Bone Joint Surg Am*, **68**(7), 1041–1051.

Bartel, D.I., Bicknell, I., Wright, T.M. (1996). The effect of conformity, thickness, and material on stresses in ultra-high molecular weight components for total joint replacement, *J Bone Joint Surg Am*, **68**(7), 1041–1048.

Bartel, D.L., Rawlinson, J.J., Burstein, A.H., Ranawat, C.S. and Flynn Jr., W.F. (1995). Stresses in polyethylene components of contemporary total knee replacements, *Clin Orthop Relat R*, **317**, 76–82.

Bassett, D.C., Block, S. and Piermarini, G.J. (1974). A high-pressure phase of polyethylene and chain-extended growth, *J Appl Phys*, **45**, 4146–4150.

Beaule, P., Schmalzried, T., Udomkiat, P. and Amstutz, H.C. (2002). Jumbo femoral head for the treatment of recurrent dislocation following total hip replacement, *J Bone and Joint Surg Am*, **84**, 256–263.

Berend, M., Ritter, M., Meding, J.B., Faris, P.M., Keating, E.M., Redelman, R. *et al.* (2004). Tibial component failure mechanisms in total knee arthroplasty, *Clin Orthop Relat R*, **428**, 26–34.

Berger, R.A., Rosenberg, A.G., Barden, R.M., Sheinkop, M.B., Jacobs, J.J. and Galante, J.O. (2001). Long-term followup of the Miller–Galante total knee replacement, *Clin Orthop Relat R*, **388**, 58–67.

Bergmann, G., Graichen, F. and Rohlmann, A. (1993). Hip joint loading during walking and running, measured in two patients, *J Biomech*, **26**(8), 969–990.

Berzins, A., Jacobs, J.J., Berger, R., Ed, C., Natarajan, R., Andriacchi, T. *et al.* (2002). Surface damage in machined ram-extruded and net-shape molded retrieved polyethylene tibial inserts of total knee replacements, *J Bone Joint Surg Am*, **84**(9), 1534–1540.

Bhateja, S., Duerst, R., Aus, E.B. and Andrews, E.H. (1995). Free radicals trapped in polyethylene crystals, *J Macromol Sci B*, **34**(3), 263–272.

Bozic, K., Kurtz, S., Lau, E., Ong, K., Chiu, V., Vail, T.P. *et al.* (2010). The epidemiology of revision total knee arthroplasty in the United States, *Clin Orthop Relat R*, **468**(1), 45–51.

Bozic, K., Kurtz, S., Lau, E., Ong, K., Vail, T.P. and Berry, D.J. (2009). The epidemiology of revision total hip arthroplasty in the United States, *J Bone Joint Surg Am*, **91**, 128–133.

Bracco, P., Brach del Prever, E.M., Cannas, M., Luda, M.P. and Costa, L. (2006). Oxidation behaviour in prosthetic UHMWPE components sterilized with high energy radiation in a low-oxygen environment, *Polym Degrad Stabil*, **91**, 2030–2038.

Bracco, P., Brunella, V., Zanetti, M., Luda, M.P. and Costa, L. (2007). Stabilisation of ultra-high molecular weight polyethylene with vitamin E, *Polym Degrad Stabil*, **92**, 2155–2162.

Bracco, P. and Oral E. (2011). Vitamin E-stabilized UHMWPE for total joint implants, *Clin Orthop Relat R*, **469**, 2286–2293.

Bradford, L., Baker, D., Ries, M.D. and Pruitt, L.A. (2004). Fatigue crack propagation resistance of highly crosslinked polyethylene, *Clin Orthop Relat R*, **429**, 68–72.

Bragdon, C., Estok, D., Malchau, H., Kärrholm, J., Yuan, X., Bourne, R. *et al.* (2004). Comparison of two digital radiostereometric analysis (RSA) methods in the determination of femoral head penetration in a total hip replacement phantom, *J Orthop Res*, **22**(3), 659–664.

Bragdon, C., Martell, J., Greene, M.E., Estok, D.M., Thanner, J., Kärrholm, J. *et al.* (2006). Comparison of femoral head penetration using RSA and the Martell method, *Clin Orthop Relat R*, **448**, 52–57.

Bragdon, C.R., O'Connor, D.O., Lowenstein, J.D., Jasty, M., Biggs, S.A. and Harris, W.H. (2001). A new pin-on-disk wear testing method for simulating wear of polyethylene on cobalt–chrome alloy in total hip arthroplasty, *J Arthroplasty*, **16**(5), 658–665.

Bragdon, C.R., O'Connor, D.O., Lowenstein, J.D., Jasty, M. and Syniuta, W.D. (1995). The importance of multidirectional motion on the wear of polyethylene, *Proc Inst Mech Eng H*, **210**, 157–165.

Burgess, I.C., Kolar, M., Cunningham, J.L. and Unsworth, A. (1997). Development of a six station knee wear simulator and preliminary wear results, *Proc Inst Mech Eng H*, **211**(1), 37–47.

Burroughs, B., Rubash, H., Estok, D., Jasty, M., Krevolin, J. and Muratoglu, O.K. (2006). Comparison of conventional and highly crosslinked UHMWPE patellae evaluated by a new *in vitro* patellofemoral joint simulator, *J Biomed Mater Res B Appl Biomater*, **79**, 268–274.

Campbell, P., Shen, F.W. and McKellop, H. (2004). Biologic and tribologic considerations of alternative bearing surfaces, *Clin Orthop Relat R*, **418**, 98–111.

Charnley, J. (1961). Arthroplasty of the Hip: A new operation, *Lancet*, **1**(7187), 1129–1132.

Charnley, J. (1970). Total hip replacement by low-friction arthroplasty, *Clin Orthop Relat R*, **72**, 7–21.

Charnley, J. and Halley D. (1975). Rate of wear in total hip replacement, *Clin Orthop Relat R*, **112**, 170–180.

Colizza, W.A., Insall, J.N. and Scuderi, G.R. (1995). The posterior stabilized total knee prosthesis. Assessment of polyethylene damage and osteolysis after a ten-year-minimum follow-up, *J Bone Joint Surg Am*, **77**(11), 1713–1720.

Collier, M., Engh Jr., C., McAuley, J.P. and Engh, G.A. (2007). Factors associated with the loss of thickness of polyethylene tibial bearings after knee arthroplasty, *J Bone Joint Surg Am*, **89**, 1306–1314.

Cooper, J., Dowson, D. and Fisher, J. (1993). Macroscopic and microscopic wear mechanisms in UHMWPE, *Wear*, **162–164**, 378–384.

Costa, L., Bracco, P., del Prever, E.B., Luda, M.P. and Trossarelli, L. (2001). Analysis of products diffused into UHMWPE prosthetic components *in vivo*, *Biomaterials*, **22**(4), 307–315.

Counsell, A., Heasley, R., Arumilli, B. and Paul, A. (2008). A groin mass caused by metal particle debris after hip resurfacing, *Acta Orthop Belg*, **74**(6), 870–874.

Cuckler, J., Moore, K., Lombardi, A.V., McPherson, E. and Emerson, R. (2004). Large versus small femoral heads in metal-on-metal total hip arthroplasty, *J Arthroplasty*, **19**(8 Suppl. 3), 41–44.

Currier, B., Van Citters, D., Currier, J.H. and Collier, J.P. (2010). *In vivo* oxidation in remelted highly crosslinked retrievals, *J Bone Joint Surg Am*, **92**, 2409–2418.

Currier, B., Van Citters, D., Currier, J.H., Carlson, E.M., Tibbo, M.E. and Collier, J.P. (2013). *In vivo* oxidation in retrieved highly crosslinked tibial inserts, *J Biomed Mater Res B Appl Biomater*, **101**, 441–448.

Currier, B.H., Currier, J.H., Collier, J.P. and Mayor, M.B. (2000). Effect of fabrication method and resin type on performance of tibial bearings, *J Biomed Mater Res*, **53**(2), 143–151.

Currier, B.H., Currier, J.H., Mayor, M.B., Lyford, K.A., Collier, J.P. and Van Citters, D.W. (2007). Evaluation of oxidation and fatigue damage of retrieved Crossfire polyethylene acetabular cups, *J Bone Joint Surg Am*, **89**, 2023–2029.

Currier, B.H., Currier, J.H., Mayor, M.B., Lyford, K.A., Van Citters, D.W. and Collier, J.P. (2007). *In Vivo* oxidation of y- barrier- sterilized ultra-high-molecular-weight polyethylene bearing, *J Arthroplasty*, **22**, 721–731.

D'Lima, D., Chen, P. and Colwell, C.W. (2001). Polyethylene contact stresses, articular congruity and knee alignment, *Clin Orthop Relat R*, **392**, 232–238.

D'Lima, D., Hermida, J., Chen, P.C. and Colwell, C.W. (2003). Polyethylene cross-linking by two different methods reduces acetabular liner wear in a hip joint wear simulator, *J Orthop Res*, **21**, 761–766.

Dahl, J., Snorrason, F., Nordsletten, L. and Röhrl, S.M. (2013). More than 50% reduction of wear in polyethylene liners with alumina heads compared to cobalt-chrome heads in hip replacements, *Acta Orthop*, **84**(4), 360–364.

Diduch, D.R., Insall, J.N., Scott, W.N., Scuderi, G.R. and Font-Rodriguez, D. (1997). Total knee replacement in young, active patients. Long-term follow-up and functional outcome, *J Bone Joint Surg Am*, **79**(4), 575–582.

Digas, G., Karrholm, J., Thanner, J., Malchau, H. and Herberts, P. (2004). Highly cross-linked polyethylene in total hip arthroplasty: Randomized evaluation of penetration rate in cemented and uncemented sockets using radiostereometric analysis, *Clin Orthop Relat R*, **429**, 6–16.

Dole, M. (1972). Free radicals in irradiated polyethylene, in Dole, M. (ed), *The Radiation Chemistry of Macromolecules*, Academic Press, New York, 335–348.

Dumbleton, J., Miller, D.A. and Miller, E.H. (1972). A simulator for load bearing joints, *Wear*, **20**, 165.

Dumbleton, J., D'Antonio, J., Manley, M.T., Capello, W.N. and Wang, A. (2006). The basis for a second-generation highly cross-linked UHMWPE, *Clin Orthop Relat R*, **453**, 265–271.

Du Plessis, T., Grobbelaar, C. and Marais, F. (1977). The improvement of polyethylene prostheses through radiation crosslinking, *Radiat Phys Chem*, **9**, 647–652.

Edidin, A.A., Pruitt, L., Jewett, C.W., Crane, D.J., Roberts, D. and Kurtz, S.M. (1999). Plasticity-induced damage layer is a precursor to wear in radiation-cross-linked UHMWPE acetabular components for total hip replacement. Ultra-high-molecular-weight polyethylene, *J Arthroplasty*, **14**(5), 616–627.

Essner, A., Schmidig, G., Herrera, L., Yau, S.S., Wang, A., Dumbleton, J.H. *et al.* (2005). Hip wear performance of a nest generation cross-linked and annealed polyethylene. *Trans Ann Meet Orthop Res Soc 2005*, Washington D.C.

Fisher, J., McEwen, H., Tipper, J.L., Galvin, A.L., Ingram, J., Kamali, A. *et al.* (2004). Wear, debris, and biological activity of crosslinked polyethylene in the knee: Benefits and potential concerns, *Clin Orthop Relat R*, **428**, 114–119.

Fu, J., Doshi, B., Oral, E. and Muratoglu O.K. (2013). High temeprature melted, radiation cross-linked, vitamin E stabilized oxidation resistance UHMWPE with low wear and high impact strength, *Polymer*, **54**, 199–209.

Fu, J., Ghali, B., Lozynsky, A.J., Oral, E. and Muratoglu, O.K. (2010). Ultrahigh molecular weight polyethylene with improved plasticity and toughness by high temperature melting, *Polymer*, **51**(12), 2721–2731.

Fu, J., Ghali, B., Lozynsky, A.J., Oral, E. and Muratoglu, O.K. (2011). Wear resistant UHMWPE with high toughness by high temperature melting and subsequent radiation cross-linking, *Polymer*, **52**, 1155–1162.

Green, J., Hallab, N., Liao, Y.S., Narayan, V., Schwarz, E.M. and Xie, C. (2013). Antioxidant treatment of UHMWPE components to decrease periprosthetic osteolysis-evaluation of osteolytic and osteogenic properties of wear debris particles in a murine calvaria model, *Curr Rheumatol Rep*, **15**(325), 1–5.

Greene, M., Bragdon, C., Kwon, Y.M., Rubash, Y.M. and Malchau, H. (2012). Three year evaluation of the wear of vitamin E stabilized highly crosslinked polyethylene, the stability of Regenerex acetabular shells and femoral components with 32 mm heads. *Trans Ann Meet Orthop Res Soc 2012*, San Francisco.

Greene, M., Sillesen, N., Nebergall, A. *et al.* (2013). RSA Evaluation of vitamin E diffused highly crosslinked polyethylene and acetabular and femoral component stability. *Ann Meet Am Acad Orthop Surg 2013*, Chicago.

Grobbelaar, C.J., Weber, F.A., Spirakis, A., Du Plessis, T.A., Cappaeri, G. and Cakic, J.N. (1999). Clinical experience with gamma irradiation-crosslinked polyethylene: A 14 to 20 year follow-up report, *South Afr Bone Joint Surg*, **11**(3), 140–147.

Grood, E.S., Shastri, L. and Hopson, C.N. (1982). Analysis of retrieved implants: Crystallinity changes in ultrahigh molecular weight polyethylene, *J Biomed Mater Res*, **16**, 399–405.

Gul, R., McGarry, F., Bragdon, C.R., Muratoglu, O.K. and Harris, W.H. (2003). Effect of consolidation on adhesive and abrasive wear of UHMWPE, *Biomaterials*, **24**(19), 3193–3199.

Haider, H. (2009). Tribological assessment of UHMWPE in the knee, in Kurtz, S. (ed), *UHMWPE Biomaterials Handbook*, Elsevier, New York, pp. 381–408.

Haider, H., Weisenburger, J., Kurtz, S.M., Rimnac, C.M., Freedman, J., Schroeder, D.W. *et al.* (2012). Does vitamin E-stabilized UHMWPE address concerns of cross-linked polyethylene in total knee arthroplasty?, *J Arthroplasty*, **27**(3), 461–469.

Han, K., Wallace, J., Truss, R.W. and Geil, P.H. (1981). Powder compaction, sintering and rolling of UHMWPE and its composites, *J Macromol Sci Phys*, **B19**, 313–349.

Harris, W. (1994). Osteolysis and particle disease in hip replacement: A review, *Acta Orthop Scand*, **65**, 113–123.

Hermida, J., Fischler, A., Colwell, C.W. and D'Lima, D.D. (2008). The effect of oxidative aging on the wear performance of highly crosslinked polyethylene knee inserts under conditions of severe malalignment, *J Orthop Res*, **26**(12), 1585–1590.

Herrera, L., Lee, R., Longaray, J., Essner, A. and Wang, A. (2007). Hip simulator evaluation of the effect of femoral head size on sequentially cross-linked acetabular liners, *Wear*, **263**, 1034–1037.

Hodrick, J.T., Severson, E.P., McAlister, D.S., Dahl, B. and Hofmann, A.A. (2008). Highly crosslinked polyethylene is safe for use in total knee arthroplasty, *Clin Orthop Relat R*, **466**, 2806–2812.

Hui, A., McCalden, Martell, J.M., MacDonald, S.J., Bourne, R.B. and Rorabeck, C.H. (2003). Validation of two and three-dimensional radiographic techniques for measuring polyethylene wear after total hip arthroplasty, *J Bone Joint Surg Am*, **85**(3), 505–511.

Hunziker, E.B. (2002). Articular cartilage repair: Basic science and clinical progress. A review of the current status and prospects, *Osteoarthr Cartilage*, **10**(6), 432–463.

Canadian Institute for Health Information. (2013). *Hip and Knee Replacements in Canada: Canadian Joint Replacement Registry 2013 Annual Report.* Ottawa, ON.

Ishihara, K., Aragaki, R., Ueda, T., Watenabe, A. and Nakabayashi, N. (1990). Reduced thrombogenicity of polymers having phospholipid polar groups, *J Biomed Mater Res*, **24**, 1069–1077.

Jacofsky, D.J. (2008). Highly crosslinked polyethylene in total knee arthroplasty, *J Arthroplasty*, **23**(7 Suppl 1), 28–30.

Jarrett, B., Cofske, J., Rosenberg, A.E., Oral, E., Muratoglu, O. and Malchau, H. (2010). *In vivo* biological response to vitamin E and vitamin E-doped polyethylene, *J Bone Joint Surg Am*, **92**(13), 2672–2681.

Jasty, M.J., Goetz, D.D., Bragdon, C.R., Lee, K.R., Hanson, A.E., Elder, J.R. *et al.* (1997). Wear of polyethylene acetabular components in total hip arthroplasty. An analysis of 128 components retrieved at autopsy or revision operation, *J Bone Joint Surg Am*, **79**, 349–358.

Johnston, R. and Smidt, G. (1969). Measurement of hip-joint motion during walking. Evaluation of an electrogoniometric method, *J Bone Joint Surg Am*, **51**, 1082–1094.

Keller, A. and Ungar, G. (1983). Radiation effects and crystallinity in polyethylene, *Radiat Phys Chem*, **22**(1-2), 155–181.

Keurentjes, J., Kuipers, R., Wever, D.J. and Schreurs, B.W. (2008). High incidence of squeaking in THAs with alumina ceramic-on-ceramic bearings, *Clin Orthop Relat R*, **466**(6), 1438–1443.

King, R., Narayan, V.S., Ernsberger, C. and Hanes, M. (2009). Characterization of gamma-irradiated UHMWPE stabilized with a hindered-phenol antioxidant. *Trans Ann Meet Orthop Res Soc 2009*, Las Vegas.

Kurtz, S. (2009). Compendium of highly crosslinked UHMWPEs, in Kurtz, S. (ed), *UHMWPE Biomaterials Handbook*, Elsevier, New York, 291–308.

Kurtz, S. (2009). From ethylene gas to UHMWPE component: The process of producing orthopaedic implants', in Kurtz, S. (ed), *UHMWPE Biomaterials Handbook*, Elsevier, New York, 7–19.

Kurtz, S. (2009). A Primer on UHMWPE, in Kurtz, S. (ed), *UHMWPE Biomaterials Handbook*, Elsevier, New York, 1–6.

Kurtz, S., Gawel, H. and Patel, J.D. (2011). History and systematic review of wear and osteolysis outcomes for first-generation highly crosslinked polyethylene, *Clin Orthop Relat R*, **469**, 2262–2277.

Kurtz, S.M., Muratoglu, O.K., Evans, M. and Edidin, A.A. (1999). Advances in the processing, sterilization, and crosslinking of ultra-high molecular weight polyethylene for total joint arthroplasty, *Biomaterials*, **20**(18), 1659–1688.

Kurtz, S.M., Ong, K., Lau, E., Mowat, F. and Halpern, M. (2007). Projections of primary and revision hip and knee arthroplasty in the united states from 2005 to 2030, *J Bone Joint Surg Am*, **89**, 780–785.

Kurtz, S., Medel, F., MacDonald, D.W., Parvizi, J., Kraay, M.J. and Rimnac, C.M. (2010). Reasons for revision of first generation highly crosslinked polyethylenes, *J Arthroplasty*, **25**(6), 67–74.

Kurtz, S., Austin, M., Azzam, K., Sharkey, P.F., MacDonald, D.W., Medel, F.J. *et al.* (2010). Mechanical properties, oxidation and clinical performance of retrieved highly crosslinked Crossfire liners after intermediate-term implantation, *J Arthroplasty*, **25**(4), 614–625.

Kyomoto, M., Moro, T., Miyaji, F., Hashimoto, M., Kawaguchi, H., Takatori, Y. *et al.* (2008). Effect of 2-methacryloyloxyethyl phosphorylcholine concentration on photo-induced graft polymerization of polyethylene in reducing the wear of orthopaedic bearing surface, *J Biomed Mater Res A*, **86**, 439–447.

Leung, S.B., Egawa, H., Stepniewski, A., Beykirch, S., Engh Jr., C.A. and Engh Sr., C.A. (2007). Incidence and volume of pelvic osteolysis at early follow-up with highly cross-linked and noncross-linked polyethylene, *J Arthroplasty*, **22**(6 Suppl 2), 134–139.

Liao, Y.S., Benya, P. and McKellop, H.A. (1999). Effect of protein lubrication on the wear properties of materials for prosthetic joints, *J Biomed Mater Res*, **48**(4), 465–473.

Livermore, J.T. (1996). Polyethylene wear in total hip arthroplasty, *Semin Arthroplasty*, **7**(1), 40–46.

Maibauer, A. and Myers, C. (1946). Polyethylenes, *J Electrochem Soc*, **90**(1), 341–360.

Mankin, H., Mow, V. and Buckwalter, J.A. (2000). Articular cartilage structure, composition and function, in Buckwalter, J., Einhorn, T. and Simon, S. (eds), *Orthopaedic Basic Science: Biology and Biomechanics of the Musculoskeletal System*, American Academy of Orthopedic Surgeons, Rosemont, 443–470.

Matthies, A., Skinner, J., Osmani, H., Henckel, J. and Hart, A.J. (2012). Pseudotumors are common in well-positioned, low-wearing metal-on-metal hips, *Clin Orthop Relat R*, **470**(7), 1895–1906.

McEwen, H., Barnett, P., Bell, C.J., Farrar, R., Auger, D.D., Stone, M.H. *et al.* (2005). The influence of design, materials and kinematics on the *in vitro* wear of total knee replacements, *J Biomech*, **38**, 357–365.

McKellop, H., Shen, F.W., Lu, B., Campbell, P. and Salovey, R. (1999). Development of an extremely wear resistant ultra-high molecular weight polyethylene for total hip replacements, *J Orthop Res*, **17**(2), 157–167.

Medel, F.J., Pena, P., Cegonino, J., Gomez-Barrena, E. and Puertolas, J.A. (2007). Comparative fatigue behavior and toughness of remelted and annealed highly crosslinked polyethylenes, *J Biomed Mater Res B Appl Biomater*, **83**(2), 380–390.

Minoda, Y., Aihara, M., Sakawa, A., Fukuoka, S., Hayakawa, K., Tomita, M. *et al.* (2009). Comparison between highly crosslinked and conventional polyethylene in total knee arthroplasty, *Knee*, **16**(5), 348–351.

Moro, T., Kawaguchi, H., Ishihara, K., Kyomoto, M., Karita, T., Ito, H. *et al.* (2009). Wear resistance of artificial hip joints with poly(2-methacryloyloxyethyl phosphorylcholine) grafted polyethylene: Comparisons with the effect of polyethylene cross-linking and ceramic femoral heads, *Biomaterials*, **30**, 2995–3001.

Moro, T., Takatori, Y., Ishihara, K., Konno, T., Takigawa, Y., Matsushita, T. *et al.* (2004). Surface grafting of artificial joints with a biocompatible polymer for preventing periprosthetic osteolysis, *Nat Mater*, **3**(11), 829–836.

Muratoglu, O., Mark, A., Vittetoe, D.A., Harris, W.H. and Rubash, H.E. (2003). Polyethylene damage in total knees and use of highly crosslinked polyethylene, *J Bone Joint Surg Am*, **85**(Suppl 1), 7–13.

Muratoglu, O., Wannomae, K., Rowell, S.L., Micheli, B.R. and Malchau, H. (2010). Ex vivo stability loss of irradiated and melted UHMWPE, *J Bone Joint Surg Am*, **92**, 2809–2816.

Muratoglu, O., Burrough, B.R., Malhi, A., Christensen, S., Wannomae, K., Oral, E. *et al.* (2005). Two second generation crosslinked UHMWPEs show improved mechanical properties and fatigue strength. *Trans Ann Meet Orthop Res Soc 2005*, Washington, D.C.

Muratoglu, O.K., Vittetoe, D. and Rubash, H.E. (2002). Damage of implant surfaces in total knee arthroplasty, in Callaghan, J., Rosenberg, A., Rubash, H., Simonian, P. and Wickiewicz, T. (eds), *The Adult Knee*, Lippincott Williams and Wilkins, Philadelphia.

Muratoglu, O.K., Wannomae, K., Christensen, S., Rubash, H.E. and Harris, W.H. (2005). Ex vivo wear of conventional and cross-linked polyethylene acetabular liners, *Clin Orthop Relat R*, **438**, 158–164.

Muratoglu, O.K., Bragdon, C.R., Jasty, M., O'Connor, D.O., Von Knoch, R.S. and Harris, W.H. (2004). Knee simulator testing of conventional and crosslinked polyethylene tibial inserts, *J Arthroplasty*, **19**(7), 887–897.

Muratoglu, O.K., Bragdon, C.R., O'Connor, D.O., Perinchief, R.S., Jasty, M. and Harris, W.H. (2002). Aggressive wear testing of a cross-linked polyethylene in total knee arthroplasty, *Clin Orthop Relat R*, **404**, 89–95.

Muratoglu, O.K., Burroughs, B.R., Bragdon, C.R., Christensen, S., Lozynsky, A. and Harris, W.H. (2004). Knee simulator wear of polyethylene tibias articulating against explanted rough femoral components, *Clin Orthop Relat R*, **428**, 108–113.

Muratoglu, O.K., Rubash, H.E., Bragdon, C.R., Burroughs, B.R., Huang, A. and Harris, W.H. (2007). Simulated normal gait wear testing of a highly crosslinked polyethylene tibial insert, *J Arthroplasty*, **22**(3), 435–444.

Muratoglu, O.K., Bragdon, C.R., O'Connor, D.O., Jasty, M., Harris, W.H., Gul, R. *et al.* (1999). Unified Wear model for highly crosslinked ultra-high molecular weight polyethylenes (UHMWPE), *Biomaterials*, **20**(16), 1463–1470.

Nabar, S., Wannomae, K. and Muratoglu, O. (2008). Environmental stress cracking of contemporary and alpha-tocopherol doped UHMWPEs. *Trans Ann Meet Orthop Res Soc 2008*, San Francisco.

Narayan, V., Ernsberger, C. and King, R. (2009). Pin-on-disk wear studies of antioxidant stabilized UHMWPE materials. *Trans Ann Meet Orthop Res Soc 2009*, Las Vegas.

Neils, A., Ward, J., Doshi, B., Oral, E. and Muratoglu, O.K. (2013). Surface cross-linking of vitamin E-blended UHMWPE by low energy irradiation. *Trans Ann Meet Orthop Res Soc 2013*, San Antonio.

Oonishi, H., Kim, S.C., Takao, Y., Kyomoto, M., Iwamoto, M. and Ueno, M. (2006). Wear of highly crosslinked polyethylene acetabular cup in Japan, *J Arthroplasty*, **21**(7), 944–949.

Oral, E., Ghali, B. and Muratoglu, O.K. (2010). A surface cross-linked UHMWPE stabilized by vitamin E with low wear and high fatigue strength, *Biomaterials*, **31**, 7051–7060.

Oral, E., Malhi, A. and Muratoglu, O.K. (2006). Mechanisms of decrease in fatigue crack propagation resistance in irradiated and melted UHMWPE, *Biomaterials*, **27**, 917–925.

Oral, E., Rowell, S.L. and Muratoglu, O.K. (2006). The effect of alpha-tocopherol on the oxidation and free radical decay in irradiated UHMWPE, *Biomaterials*, **27**, 5580–5587.

Oral, E., Ghali, B., Neils, A. and Muratoglu, O.K. (2012). A new mechanism of oxidation in UHMWPE caused by squalene absorption, *J Biomed Mater Res B Appl Biomater*, **100**, 742–751.

Oral, E., Godleski Beckos, C., Malhi, A.S. and Muratoglu, O.K. (2008). The effects of high dose irradiation on the cross-linking of vitamin E-blended UHMWPE, *Biomaterials*, **29**, 3557–3560.

Oral, E., Malhi, A. Wannomae, K.K. and Muratoglu, O.K. (2008). Highly cross-linked UHMWPE with improved fatigue resistance for total joint arthroplasty, *J Arthroplasty*, **23**(7), 1037–1044.

Oral, E., Neils, A., Lozynsky, A.J. and Muratoglu, O.K. (2011). The modulation of impact strength of surface crosslinked UHMWPE by surface thickness. *Trans Ann Meet Orthop Res Soc 2011*, Long Beach.

Oral, E., Neils, A., Wannamae, K.K. and Muratoglu, O.K. (2014). Novel active stabilization technology in highly crosslinked UHMWPEs for superior stability. *Radiat Phys Chem*, **105**, 6–11.

Oral, E., Wannomae, K.K., Rowell, S.L. and Muratoglu, O.K. (2007). Diffusion of vitamin E in ultra-high molecular weight polyethylene, *Biomaterials*, **28**(35), 5225–5237.

Oral, E., Christensen, S. Malhi, A.S., Wannomae, K.K. and Muratoglu, O.K. (2006). Wear resistance and mechanical properties of highly crosslinked UHMWPE doped with vitamin E, *J Arthroplasty*, **21**(4), 580–591.

Oral, E., Godleski Beckos, C., Lozynsky, A.J., Malhi, A.S. and Muratoglu, O.K. (2009). Improved resistance to wear and fatigue fracture in high pressure crystallized vitamin E-containing ultrahigh molecular weight polyethylene, *Biomaterials*, **30**, 1870–1880.

Oral, E., Neils, A., Rowell, S.L., Lozynsky, A.J. and Muratoglu, O.K. (2013). Increasing irradiation temperature maximizes vitamin E grafting and wear resistance of UHMWPE, *J Biomed Mater Res B Appl Biomater*, **101**(3), 436–440.

Oral, E., Wannomae, K.K., Hawkins, N., Harris, W.H. and Muratoglu, O.K. (2004). Alpha-Tocopherol doped irradiated UHMWPE for high fatigue resistance and low wear, *Biomaterials*, **25**(24), 5515–5522.

Oral, E., Neils, A., Lyons, C., Fung, M., Doshi, B. and Muratoglu, O.K. (2013). Surface cross-linked UHMWPE can enable the use of larger femoral heads in total joints, *J Orthop Res*, **31**(1), 59–66.

Pandit, H., Glyn-Jones, S., McLardy-Smith, P., Gundle, R., Whitwell, D., Gibbons, C.L. *et al.* (2008). Pseudotumours associated with metal-on-metal hip resurfacings, *J Bone Joint Surg Br*, **90**(7), 847–851.

Parth, M., Aust, N. and Lederer, K. (2002). Studies on the effect of electron beam radiation on the molecular structure of ultra-high molecular weight polyethylene under the influence of alpha-tocopherol with respect to its application in medical implants, *J Mater Sci Mater Med*, **13**(10), 917–921.

Paul, J. (1966). Biomechanics. The biomechanics of the hip-joint and its clinical relevance, *P Roy Soc Med*, **59**, 943–948.

Peacock, A.J. (2000). *Handbook of Polyethylene*. CRC Press, New York.

Premnath, V., Harris, W., Jasty, M. and Merrill, E.W. (1996). Gamma sterilization of UHMWPE articular implants: An analysis of the oxidation problem. Ultra high molecular weight poly ethylene, *Biomaterials*, **17**, 1741–1753.

Price, A., Short, A., Kellett, C., Beard, D., Gill, H., Pandit, H. *et al.* (2005). Ten-year *in vivo* wear measurement of a fully congruent mobile bearing unicompartmental knee arthroplasty, *J Bone Joint Surg Br*, **87**(11), 1493–1497.

Pruitt, L., Koo, J., Rimnac, C.M., Suresh, S. and Wright, T.M. (1994). Cyclic compressive loading results in fatigue cracks in ultra high molecular weight polyethylene, *J Orthop Res*, **13**(1), 143–146.

Rahaman, M., Yao, A., Bal, S., Garino, J.P. and Ries, M.D. (2007). Ceramics for prosthetic hip and knee replacement, *J Am Ceram Soc*, **90**(7), 1965–1988.

Ramamurti, B., Muratoglu, O., Bragdon, C. and O'Connor, D. (1996). How realistically do contemporary hip joint simulators reproduce physiologic gait motion. *Trans Ann Meet Orthop Res Soc 1996*, Atlanta.

Ramamurti, B.S., Estok, D.M., Jasty, M. and Harris W.H. (1998). Analysis of the kinematics of different hip simulators used to study wear of candidate materials for the articulation of total hip arthroplasties, *J Orthop Res*, **16**(3), 365–369.

Reinitz, S., Franklin, K.J., Gray L.T., Dansu, H.S., Currier, B.H. and Van Citters, D.W. (2012). Comparison of the *In Vivo* Perfomance of Two Highly Crosslinked UHMWPE Materials in the Hip and Knee. *Trans Ann Meet Orthop Res Soc 2012*, San Francisco.

Rodriguez, J. (2008). Crosslinked polyethylene in total knee arthroplasty. In opposition, *J Arthroplasty*, **23**(7 Suppl 1), 31–34.

Rowell, S., Oral, E. and Muratoglu, O.K. (2011). Comparative oxidative stability of a-tocopherol blended and diffused UHMWPEs at 3 years of real-time aging, *J Orthop Res*, **29**, 773–780.

Saikko, V., Paavolainen, P., Kleimola, M. and Stätis, P. (1992). A five-station hip joint simulator for wear rate studies, *Proc Inst Mech Eng H*, **206**, 195–200.

Sathasivam, S. and Walker, P. (1998). Computer model to predict subsurface damage in tibial inserts of total knees, *J Orthop Res*, **16**, 564–571.

Scales, J., Kelly, P. and Goddard, D. (1969). Friction torque studies of total joint replacements. The use of a simulator, *Ann Rheum Dis*, **28**(5), 30–35.

Schmalzried, T. and Callaghan, J. (1999). Wear in total hip and knee replacements. *J Bone Joint Surg Am*, **81**(1), 115–136.

Schwenke, T. and Wimmer, M. (2013). Cross-shear in metal-on-polyethylene articulation of orthopaedic implants and its relationship to wear, *Wear*, **301**(1–2), 727–734.

Sharkey, P., Hozack, W., Rothman, R.H., Shastri, S. and Jacoby, S.M. (2002). Why are total knee arthroplasties failing today?, *Clin Orthop Relat R*, **404**, 7–13.

Shaw, J.A. and Murray, D.G. (1973). Knee joint simulator, *Clin Orthop Relat R*, **94**, 15–23.

Shikata, T., Oonishi, H. and Hashimato, Y. (1977). Wear resistance of irradiated UHMW polyethylenes to Al2O3 ceramics in total hip prostheses, *Trans Ann Meet Soc Biomater 1977*.

Spiegelberg, S. (2009). Characterization of physical, chemical, and mechanical properties of UHMWPE, in Kurtz, S. (ed), *UHMWPE Biomaterials Handbook*, Elsevier, New York, 355–368.

Stallforth, H. and Ungethum, M. (1977). Development of a knee-joint simulator, *Arch Orthop Unfallchir*, **90**(3), 343–353.

Teeter, M., Seslija, P., Milner, J.S., Nikolov, H.N., Yuan, X., Naudie, D.D. *et al.* (2013). Quantification of *in vivo* implant wear in total knee replacement from dynamic single plance radiography, *Phys Med Biol*, **58**, 2751–2767.

Teramura, S., Sakoda, H., Terao, T., Endo, M.M., Fujiwara, K. and Tomita, N. (2008). Reduction of wear volume from ultrahigh molecular weight polyethylene knee components by the addition of vitamin E, *J Orthop Res*, **26**(4), 460–464.

Tomita, N., Kitakura, T., Onmori, N., Ikada, Y. and Aoyama, E. (1999). Prevention of fatigue cracks in ultrahigh molecular weight polyethylene joint components by the addition of vitamin E, *J Biomed Mater Res*, **48**(4), 474–478.

Tower, S.S., Currier, J.H., Currier, B.H., Lyford, K.A., Van Citters, D.W. and Mayor, M.B. (2007). Rim cracking of the cross-linked longevity polyethylene acetabular liner after total hip arthroplasty, *J Bone Joint Surg Am*, **89**(10), 2212–2217.

Truss, R., Han, K.S., Wallace, J.F. and Geil, P.H. (1981). Cold compaction molding and sintering of UHMWPE, *J Appl Polymer Sci*, **26**, 79–88.

Tung, L. (1957). Molecular weight-intrinsic viscosity relationship and molecular weight distribution of low pressure polyethylenes, *J Appl Polymer Sci*, **24A**(107), 333—348.

van Ijsseldijk, E., Lebel, B., Stoel, B.C., Valstar, E.R., Gouzy, S., Vielpeau, C. *et al.* (2013). Validation of the *in vivo* volumetric wear measurement for total knee prostheses in model-based RSA, *J Biomech*, **46**(7), 1387–1391.

Walker, P., Bell, C. Abeysundera, M.R., Simmons, J.M., King, P.M. and Blunn, G.W. (1998). Effect of oxidation on delamination of ultrahigh-molecular-weight polyethylene tibial components, *J Arthroplasty*, **13**(3), 280–290.

Walker, P., Blunn, G., Broome, D.R., Perry, J., Watkins, A., Sathasivam, S. *et al.* (1997). A knee simulating machine for performance evaluation of total knee replacements, *J Biomech*, **30**(1), 83–89.

Wang, A. (2001). A unified theory of wear for ultra-high molecular weight polyethylene in multi-directional sliding, *Wear*, **248**, 38–47.

Wang, A., Essner, A., Stark, C. and Dumbleton, J.H. (1996). Comparison of the size and morphology of UHMWPE wear debris produced by a hip joint simulator under serum and water lubricated conditions, *Biomaterials*, **17**(9), 865–871.

Wang, A., Essner, A., Polineni, V.K., Stark, C. and Dumbleton, J.H. (1998). Lubrication and wear of uhmwpe in total joint replacements, *Tribol Int*, **31**, 17–33.

Wang, A., Yau, S.S., Essner, A., Herrera, L., Manley, M. and Dumbleton, J. (2008). A highly crosslinked UHMWPE for CR and PS total knee arthroplasties, *J Arthroplasty*, **23**(4), 559–566.

Wang, A., Zeng, H., Yau, S.S., Essner, A., Manely, M. and Dumbleton, J. (2006). Wear, oxidation and mechanical properties of a sequentially irradiated and annealed UHMWPE in total joint replacement, *J Phys Appl Phys*, **39**, 3213–3219.

Wannomae, K., Bhattacharyya, S., Freiberg, A., Estok, D., Harris, W.H. and Muratoglu, O. (2006). *In vivo* oxidation of retrieved crosslinked UHMWPE acetabular components with residual free radicals, *J Arthroplasty*, **21**(7), 1005–1011.

Wannomae, K., Christensen, C., Micheli, B.R., Rowell, S.L., Schroeder, D.W. and Muratoglu, O.K. (2010). Delamination and adhesive wear behavior of alpha-tocopherol-stabilized irradiated UHMWPE, *J Arthroplasty*, **25**(4), 635–643.

Wasiliewski, R., Galante, J., Leighty, R.M., Natarajan, R.N. and Rosenberg, A.G. (1994). Wear patterns on retrieved polyethylene tibial inserts and their relationship to technical considerations in total knee arthroplasty, *Clin Orthop Relat R*, **299**, 31–43.

Willert, H.G., Bertram, H. and Buchhorn, G.H. (1990). Osteolysis in alloarthroplasty of the hip: The role of ultra-high molecular weight polyethylene wear particles, *Clin Orthop Relat R*, **258**, 95–107.

Wright, T.M., Astion, D.J., Bansal, M., Rimnac, C.M., Green, T., Insall, J.N. *et al.* (1988). Failure of carbon fiber-reinforced polyethylene total knee-replacement components. A report of two cases, *J Bone Joint Surg Am*, **70**, 926–932.

Wunderlich, B. and Davidson, T. (1969). Extended-chain crystals. I. General crystallization conditions and review of pressure crystallization of polyethylene, *J Polymer Sci 2 Polymer Phys*, **7**(12), 2043–2050.

Zhang, W., Moskowitz, R., Nuki, G., Abramson, S., Altman, R.D., Arden, N. *et al.* (2008). OARSI recommendations for the management of hip and knee osteoarthritis, Part II: OARSI evidence-based, expert consensus guidelines, *Osteoarthr Cartilage*, **16**(2), 137–162.

Chapter 7

Non-Oxide Ceramics

Valentina Medri, Elena Landi and Alida Bellosi
CNR-ISTEC, National Research Council of Italy —
Institute of Science and Technology for Ceramics, Faenza, Italy

1. Introduction

Rapid technological advancements in the prosthesis market are contributing to the development of improved implant materials and devices, featuring better design and offering longer life. The need for high performance materials (Sonntag *et al.*, 2012) has pushed research in the direction of advanced materials normally used in industrial engineering applications.

Advanced ceramics (also named 'fine ceramics' or 'technical ceramics') are defined by ISO/TC 206 (International Organization for Standardization, 1992) as "...highly engineered, high performance, predominantly non-metallic, inorganic material having specific functional attributes". This definition underlines the complexity of ceramics, now moving away from traditional 'clayey' ceramics due to the raw materials, which are the product of chemical syntheses and not naturally occurring, the complexity of the production technologies, and the final functional or thermo-mechanical properties.

Advanced ceramics can be classified in three main categories:

— oxide ceramics (alumina, zirconia, ceria, magnesia etc.);
— non-oxide ceramics (carbides, borides, nitrides, and silicides);
— composite ceramics (particulate- or fiber-reinforced composites, which can be a combination of oxides and/or non-oxide phases).

Focusing on the specific application in arthroplasty, high strength and low wear oxide ceramics (alumina- and zirconia-based) are widely used as bearing materials for orthopedic implants and prostheses (Rahaman *et al.*, 2007). Other biomaterials, such as titanium (Ti) alloys, cobalt–chromium (CoCr), and high-density polyethylene (PE), greatly reduce the risk of inflammatory disease due to the adverse host biological response to accumulated microscopic wear debris in the periprosthetic joint space (Rahaman *et al.*, 2007).

The major concern regarding the use of oxide ceramics components is the possibility of brittle fracture, i.e. fracture spontaneously occurring within a post-surgical follow-up period ranging from a few months to several years (Bal and Rahaman, 2012). In this regard, oxide ceramics generally exhibit relatively low fracture toughness and are thus prone to brittle fracture both after short (fast fracture) or prolonged time (following sub-critical crack growth (Rahaman *et al.*, 2007). Their mechanical properties are the reason that thin-walled resurfacing implant components for bone conserving application, for example, are not made of oxide ceramics (Back *et al.*, 2005; McMinn *et al.*, 1996).

Until 1970, non-oxide ceramics were primarily used in the iron/steel industry or in the chemical industry (Goursat and Foucaud, 2007) because of their high melting points and high chemical inertia. During the last decades, the development of new processes of powder synthesis, shaping and sintering, and a better understanding of the correlation between process, microstructure, and functional properties have opened the way to the proper design of non-oxide ceramics in view of novel applications (Hampshire, 2007; Petzow and Herrmann, 2002; Riley, 2000). Nowadays, non-oxide ceramics as bulk materials, composites, or coatings cover many application areas, including mechanics, automotive, aerospace, electronics, telecommunications, chemistry, energetics, and medicine (Goursat and Foucaud, 2007; Riley, 2000).

Highly engineered non-oxide ceramics such as silicon carbide (SiC) or silicon nitride (Si_3N_4) (Cappi *et al.*, 2009; Chevalier and Gremillard, 2009); are a possible solution to overcome the aforementioned problems related to the use of oxide ceramics in arthroplasty. In fact, they possess outstanding mechanical properties (wear resistance, strength, toughness) thanks to a microstructure containing elongated grains able to bridge a propagating crack. Moreover, they show a better reliability than oxide ceramics because they are less sensitive to slow crack growth with a consequent lower risk of delayed failure (Bal and Rahaman, 2012).

Silicon carbide is employed in clinical use as a coating for stents (Kalnins *et al.*, 2002; Monnink *et al.*, 1999), while biomorphic wood-based SiC (Ramirez-Rico *et al.*, 2010; Varela-Feria *et al.*, 2002) is very promising as a load-bearing light implant material.

Silicon nitride has already become an established biomaterial, and is manufactured by Amedica Corp. (Salt Lake City, UT) who have put Si_3N_4 spinal spacers on the market (Khandkar *et al.*, 2008) and have already developed innovative total hip Si_3N_4 femoral head technology and knee prostheses under the trade name MC^2 (Bal *et al.*, 2008, 2009; Bal and Rahaman, 2012; Bernero *et al.*, 2006; Ely *et al.*, 2005; Khandkar, 2010; Rahaman *et al.*, 2007). In particular, Si_3N_4 is characterized by biocompatibility, good cell/material interaction, low specific weight, hydrophilic behavior, chemical stability, and low friction coefficient. An overview on the state of the art concerning structure and fabrication of Si_3N_4- and SiC-based ceramics with improved performances is presented in the following sections. This chapter presents mechanical and biotribological properties and *in vivo*/ *in vitro* applications of these non-oxide materials, focusing mainly on silicon nitride as it is the most mature product for the market and an extensive use in arthroplasty is expected within the near future.

2. Silicon Nitride

2.1. *Si_3N_4-Based Ceramics*

2.1.1. *Structure and synthesis of Si_3N_4*

Silicon nitride does not exist in nature and thus it must be produced synthetically. Moreover, it does not possess a true melting point, rather it decomposes at 0.1 MPa of N_2 and 1,775°C (Ray, 1993):

$$Si_3N_{4(s)} = 3Si_{(l)} + 2N_{2(g)}. \qquad (7.1)$$

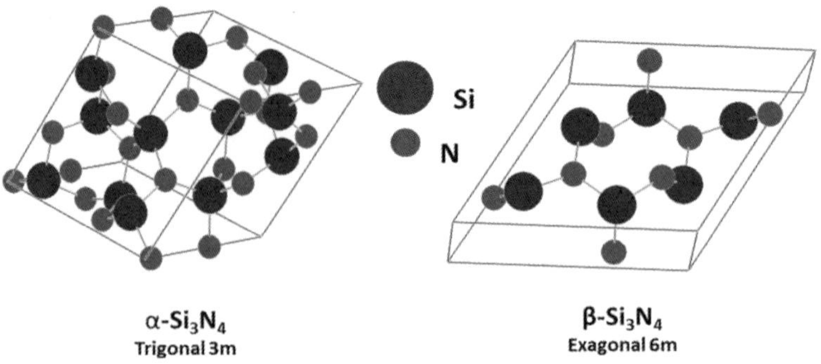

Figure 7-1. Crystallographic structures of α-Si_3N_4 and β-Si_3N_4.

The synthesized silicon nitride occurs primarily as a metastable α-phase, that converts into more stable β-phase with increasing temperature: The energy of activation for this $\alpha \rightarrow \beta$ transformation in the liquid phase during sintering is 435 ± 38 kJ/mol, corresponding to the energy of the Si–N bond. Figure 7-1 reports the crystallographic aspect of Si_3N_4. The hexagonal modifications α and β are both constituted by tetrahedral units SiN_4 and trigonal planar NSi_3: The tetrahedra share a nitrogen atom (Wild *et al.*, 1972).

In addition to the α- and β-phases, silicon nitride forms solid solutions with aluminum and beryllium by substitution of Si^{4+} and N^{3+} with Al^{3+}, Be^{2+}, and O^{2-} without varying the ratio cation/anion of 3/4 (Cao and Metselaar, 1991). For example, aluminum and β-phase constitute $Si_{6-x}Al_xO_xN_{8-x}$ with $x < 4.2$. These phases are named 'Sialon' and 'Sibeon' with aluminum and beryllium substitution, respectively.

The industrial production of silicon nitride powders is fundamentally based on three processes (van Dijen *et al.*, 1994) as follows:

— **Direct nitridation:** This process was first developed in 1910 and it is still the most widespread methodology in the temperature range 1,100–1,400°C.

$$3Si_{(s)} + 2N_{2(g)} \rightleftarrows Si_3N_{4(s)}. \tag{7.2}$$

The resulting powder consists mainly of α-phase. Usually, the powder is ground after synthesis, resulting in an elongated particle morphology. The powder produced by this method has a high content of impurities.

— **Carbothermic reduction:** This synthesis starts from a mixture of SiO_2 and carbon in excess which is treated under N_2 at 1500°C:

$$3SiO_{2(s)} + 6C_{(s)} + 2N_{2(g)} \rightleftarrows Si_3N_{4(s)} + 6CO_{(g)}. \quad (7.3)$$

Very pure powders are obtained using synthetic starting materials deriving from pyrolysis reactions.

— **Reaction in the liquid phase (imide decomposition):** This method consists of the reaction of ammonolysis of clorosilane in the liquid phase at 0–25°C which liberates a polymeric diimide:

$$nSiCl_{4(l)} + 6nNH_{3(l)} \leftrightarrows 4nNH_4Cl_{(l)} + [Si(NH)_2]_{n(s)}$$
$$\text{diimide polymer.} \quad (7.4)$$

This product is then calcined (5) with evolution of hydrogen and nitrogen. At 1200–1500°C amorphous silicon nitride crystallizes in α-phase:

$$3/n[Si(NH)_2]_{n(s)} \leftrightarrows \alpha - Si_3N_{4(s)} + N_{2\uparrow} + 3H_{2\uparrow}. \quad (7.5)$$

The gas phase synthesis helps to get the most pure and fine powders, ideal for more advanced applications. For example, in a laser-heated gas phase reaction, a gaseous mixture of silane and ammonia is exposed to the coherent light of a CO_2 laser. The silane has a high absorption power of the wavelength involved for which an increase in temperature is necessary to the reaction.

$$3SiH_4(g) + 4NH_3(g) = Si_3N_4 \text{ amorph} + 12H_2(g). \quad (7.6)$$

Particle sizes of the amorphous product are typically 10–25 nm, from which equiaxed α-Si_3N_4 is produced by crystallization at 1400°C (Cannon *et al.*, 1982).

2.1.2. *Sintering and microstructure of Si_3N_4*

Silicon nitride is a compound characterized by a remarkable covalent character, greater than 70% (Thompson and Pratt, 1966), which implies great bond strength and low coefficients of auto-diffusion. Consequently, Si_3N_4 has a low sinterability (Riley, 2000). However, structural applications of silicon nitride require dense materials. It is therefore necessary to provide an adequate temperature gradient along with a considerable pressure to activate a mass transport mechanism supported then by energy gradients. For this reason, Si_3N_4 powder is usually admixed with sintering aids, typically oxides of metals, especially rare earths, such as MgO, Y_2O_3, Al_2O_3, La_2O_3, Lu_2O_3 etc., or a combination of these, to obtain a liquid-phase sintering (LPS) generally by pressure assisted method such as:

— hot pressing (HP) (Bowen *et al.*, 1978);
— hot isostatic pressing (HIPping) (Iturriza *et al.*, 1989);
— a combination of pressureless sintering and post-HIPping to obtain complex shapes, as in the case of femoral heads and acetabular cups (Bal *et al.*, 2009);
— spark plasma sintering (SPS) (Belmonte *et al.*, 2010), which allows a shortening of the sintering time from hours to minutes, getting total densification with negligible grain growth and/or phase transformation.

Since silicon nitride is prone to oxidize due to its instability in air and in the function of hydrolysis (even at room temperature), the surface of the grains is naturally covered with a layer of intermediate composition between SiO_2 and oxynitride Si_2N_2O. At high temperatures, the sintering additives react with the silica present on the surface of the nitride particles to give a liquid secondary phase of silicate/oxynitride composition, according to the reaction:

$$\alpha - \mathrm{Si_3N_4} + \mathrm{SiO_2} + \mathrm{M_xO_y} \leftrightarrows \beta - \mathrm{Si_3N_4} + \mathrm{M_zSi_zO_zN_z}. \qquad (7.7)$$

This liquid phase promotes a range of matter transport mechanisms and a series of chemical and physical phenomena that make possible the full densification.

If the liquid phase reaches a sufficient volume concentration and a not too high viscosity, the capillary forces initially give rise to a process of rearrangement whose speed is strongly influenced by the size and shape of the α-Si_3N_4 particles.

With increasing temperature, the smaller particles begin to dissolve due to the difference in chemical potential between small and large particles and the capillary forces that increase the solubility of the silicon nitride at the contact points. This is known as the phenomenon of Ostwald ripening (Wagner, 1961). The particles spread and reprecipitate as β-phase. The external pressure increases the speed of this process of solution–diffusion–reprecipitation. During cooling, the liquid system glazes, forming a partially crystalline phase at the grain boundaries. The LPS process then implies a profound transformation phase of spheroidal particles α-Si_3N_4 to give a final system of elongated grains of β-Si_3N_4, immersed in a partially crystalline secondary phase (Figure 7-2a).

Raw powders normally contain an initial α-phase amount up to 95%, which decreases during sintering because the kinetically favored

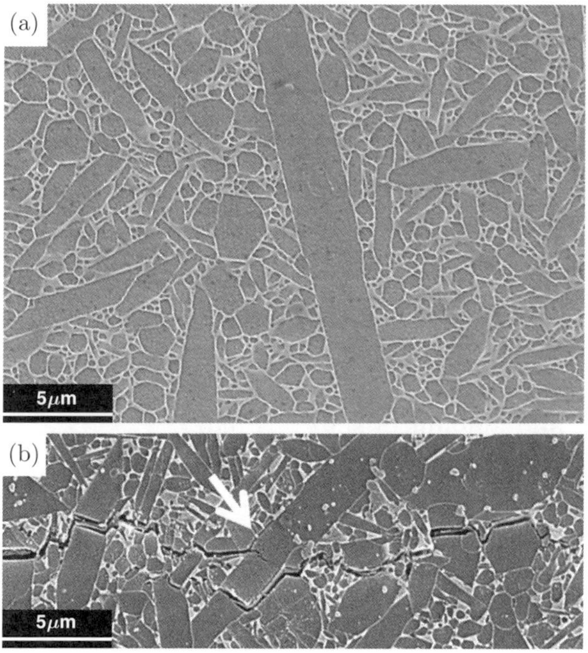

Figure 7-2. SEM micrographs showing a dense Si_3N_4 in which LPS process induced the phase transformation of spheroidal α-Si_3N_4 grains. The final microstructure is mainly composed of elongated β-Si_3N_4 grains immersed in a partially crystalline secondary phase (a). The elongated grains form an interconnected matrix which promotes crack bridging as indicated by the arrow (b). *Courtesy of Dr. Frederic Monteverde.*

α-phase over 1400°C spontaneously converts into β-phase, which is thermodynamically more stable (Lange, 1979).

The amount of additives is closely related to the sintering technique. In the case of HP, the amount of additive is usually between 2% and 10% by weight. By means of HIPping, Themelin *et al.* (1993) sintered Si_3N_4 powder in the presence of 0.5 wt% Y_2O_3 and 0.025 wt% of Al_2O_3 with a relative final density of 99%. By combining pressureless sintering and post HIPping, Bal *et al.* (2008; 2009) proposed a Si_3N_4 with 6 wt% Y_2O_3 and 4 wt% Al_2O_3. Using SPS and 2 wt% of Al_2O_3 and 5 wt% of Y_2O_3, a relative density >95%, a limited phase transformation (76% α-phase), and negligible grain growth (190 nm) at temperatures as low as 1500°C was achieved (Belmonte *et al.*, 2010). At 1600°C, fully dense materials retaining an α-phase content (41%) were produced.

2.1.3. *Properties — microstructure correlation*

The functional and mechanical properties (fracture toughness, strengths etc.) of densified Si_3N_4 ceramics are strongly correlated to the microstructure (Hampshire, 2007; Lange, 1979; Riley, 2000).

The microstructure of Si_3N_4-based ceramics can be tailored by:

— the amount of α silicon nitride in the starting raw powders (Lange, 1979);
— sintering procedure;
— the type and amount of sintering aids;
— addition of secondary phases (composite material).

High fracture toughness (>10 MPa·m$^{1/2}$) combined with a high bending strength (>1 GPa) can be developed by careful control of the size and amount of well-dispersed large elongated grains in a fine-grained matrix (Becher *et al.*, 1998). High toughness values are also associated with resistance to machining damage and improved fatigue behavior (Hampshire, 2007).

The microstructural evolution of α silicon nitride by LPS leads to a morphology in elongated grains as explained in the previous section (Figure 7-2). The elongated grains form an interconnected matrix which can promote crack bridging (Figure 7-2b), resulting in a significant toughening effect (Lange, 1979). Fracture toughness increases as the square root of the elongated grain diameter (Kawashima *et al.*, 1991), in much the same way as a reinforcing fibrous phase in a composite material.

In the applications of silicon nitride as biomaterial, a key aspect is the presence in this ceramic of a grain boundary phase, deriving from the necessary use of sintering aids. In particular, the silicon nitride microstructure could be tailored by the proper selection and addition of sintering aids. This has a strong influence on the mechanical properties: The fracture toughness, for example, is increased by increasing the Y:Al ratio in the sintering aid composition (Sun *et al.*, 1998). Moreover, the thermal expansion coefficient (CTE) of the secondary phases, up to three times higher than that of Si_3N_4 ($\sim 3 \cdot 10^{-6\circ}C^{-1}$), produces after sintering a mean compression stress in the matrix, which improves the mechanical properties with a toughening and strengthening effect (Gogotsi, 1994). Therefore, silicon nitride-based ceramics can be regarded as ceramic-glass composites. The β-Si_3N_4 grain morphology is known to be very sensitive to the particular additive used, especially in the case of the oxides of the rare earths (RE). The aspect ratio of β-Si_3N_4 grain increases with the increasing preference of the additive element to segregate to the Si_3N_4 grain surface, following the sequence Lu<Yb<Sc<Y<La (Becher *et al.*, 2006). Moreover, toughness increases with increasing ion size of the RE^{3+}, as a consequence of an increasingly intergranular crack path (Satet *et al.*, 2006).

The design of advanced ceramic devices requires a probabilistic approach based on the concept of a fracture probability as a function of the applied load and the volume of the material under load. Ceramics are brittle materials and they do not allow any relaxation by plastic deformation of the stresses that build up at the apex of microstructural defects which act as the fracture origin. Typical microstructural defects of ceramics are microcracks, inclusions, inhomogeneities, or pores, and the fracture strength is related to the size of these defects and the fracture toughness (Petzow *et al.*, 1991). For a material with a flat toughness (no R-curve), the size, orientation, and shape of the defects present in the material determine the variability of the failure stress.

The function that describes the cumulative statistical probability of fracture of a given volume is the Weibull distribution function (Weibull, 1939). The Weibull modulus (m) is a dimensionless parameter of the Weibull distribution function which is used to describe the variability of measured material strengths (Bergman, 1984). Materials with low Weibull modulus exhibit low reliability and their strength values will be broadly distributed. The value of m generally ranges from 10 to 12 for dense technical ceramics. Higher Weibull moduli (from 20 to 50) can be reached by a proper design of the microstructure as in the case of toughened Si_3N_4 ceramics (Bal *et al.* 2008; Hirosaki *et al.*, 1993; Li *et al.*, 1995).

Finally, to induce functional properties such as electrical conductivity, since the 1980s attention has been devoted to composite ceramics with a second phase, mainly in the form of particles (Kamijo *et al.*, 1985). The use of electrically conductive phases such as TiN, TiB_2, TaN, TiCN, TiC, ZrN, and $MoSi_2$, in amount over 20 vol% (generally 30 vol%) allows the manufacture of components of complex shape by electro-discharge machining (EDM) (König *et al.*, 1988; Martin *et al.*, 1989). The EDM technique is highly cost-effective and opens the possibility of customizing the large bearing surfaces with complex topographies and shapes through CAD–CAM rendering.

A Si_3N_4-TiN composite has been proposed (Bucciotti *et al.*, 2010; Mazzocchi and Bellosi, 2008; Mazzocchi *et al.*, 2008; for the production of complex-shaped implantable devices. Some key properties are: Hardness 15 GPa; Young's modulus 343 GPa; flexural strength 900 MPa; fracture toughness 5.7 $MPa{\cdot}m^{1/2}$; electro-conductivity $6{\cdot}10^{-4}$ $\Omega{\cdot}cm$ (Bracisiewicz *et al.*, 2002; Guicciardi *et al.*, 2003). Figure 7-3 reports the microstructure of the surface of a Si_3N_4-35 vol% TiN before and after EDM treatment. The material removing mechanisms (melting and evaporation) operating during EDM form a surface layer of 10–20 μm in thickness (Mazzocchi and Bellosi, 2008) that evidences the presence of craters and droplets (Figure 7-3b). For clinical applications, the final polishing with tribochemical methods or mechanical routes should be performed to restore the bulk properties in the exposed surface (Mazzocchi and Bellosi, 2008).

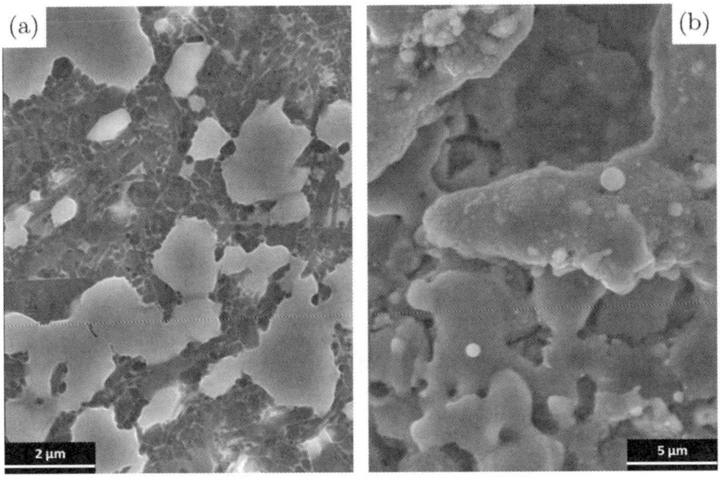

Figure 7-3. SEM micrographs of a Si_3N_4-35 vol% TiN composite showing the mirror polished surface (a) with the dispersion of TiN particles (light gray phase) in the Si_3N_4 matrix and (b) the surface degradation after EDM.

3. Silicon Carbide

3.1. *SiC-Based Ceramics*

3.1.1. *Structure and synthesis of SiC*

Silicon carbide was synthesized for the first time at the beginning of the 19th century by Berzelius (1824). The technological importance of silicon carbide only began to be appreciated after the invention of the electric arc furnace, which allowed Acheson (1893) to apply to carbonaceous compounds for the production of silicon carbide. In nature, silicon carbide in its α form has occasionally been found in association with diamond or iron meteorites; these forms have been given the name of 'Moissanite' (Moissan, 1905). The β form was also found naturally in some rocks (Leung *et al.*, 1990).

The production of silicon carbide on a large scale was performed for the first time using the Acheson process (Acheson, 1893). The simplicity of the process enables the production of large quantities of silicon carbide that is suitable to be used as an abrasive. The starting materials are made from silica (sand containing quartz) or quartzite minced (58–65 wt%), graphite or coke (35–42 wt%), sodium chloride (1–2 wt%), and also strips of wood.

The overall reaction of the process of synthesis of SiC in the temperature range 1510–1750°C is:

$$SiO_2(s) + 3C(s) = SiC(s) + 2CO(g). \tag{7.8}$$

Crystals, whiskers, or high purity powders of SiC are routinely synthesized starting from the constituent elements through the vapor phase reaction of silane or silicon tetrachloride (to generate gaseous Si) with carbon, carbon-based compounds, or hydrocarbons in inert or reducing atmosphere and in the temperature range 1200–1800°C. As in the case of Si_3N_4, nanopowders of silicon carbide can be produced by laser synthesis.

Silicon carbide is a crystalline compound in which carbon and silicon are linked by strong covalent bonds whose energy is about 318 kJ/mol (Huheey *et al.*, 1993). Silicon carbide is the only solid intermediate in the system Si-C which crystallizes in cubic and in hexagonal lattices in many polytypes. SiC and Si react eutectically at a temperature of 1405°C.

The units of the fundamental structure of the SiC lattice are the Si-C tetrahedra (Fisher and Barnes, 1990): Each edge of the tetrahedron is bound to a tetrahedral coordination with other atoms of Si or C. These tetrahedra are positioned in planes, have in common an apex and a corner with the tetrahedra located on adjacent plane. The cubic polytype (3C) is usually denoted by β-SiC, while all the hexagonal or rhombohedral polytypes (6H) are indicated by α-SiC. The structures of the crystalline cells of the more stable and frequently observed polytypes are shown in Figure 7-4.

It is generally observed that the cubic polytype 3C (β-SiC) is formed at moderate temperatures and turns at high temperatures into α-SiC. The 6H polytype is the most common at high temperatures (>1870°C) and the polytype transformation 3C$\rightarrow$6H is the most commonly observed. The transformation of $\beta \rightarrow \alpha$, during sintering or annealing processes, is generally associated with the formation of flat and elongated grains or to an anisotropic growth, which offers the possibility of *in situ* toughening by increasing the fracture

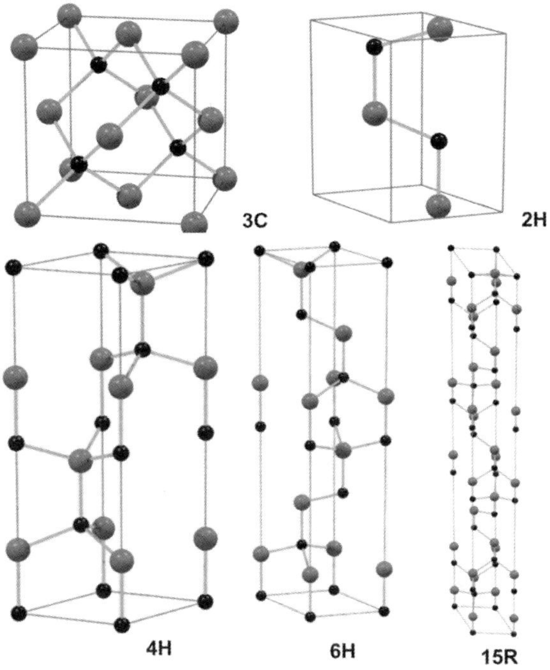

Figure 7-4. Crystallographic structures of some SiC polytypes.

toughness of the material (Cao *et al.*, 1996; Kim *et al.*, 1995; Padture, 1994; Sciti *et al.* 2001; Zhan *et al.*, 2001).

It is important to know the conditions of stability of the different polytypes in order to predict and prevent certain unwanted changes during the production process. Some important electronic properties, such as the band gap, depend upon the particular polytype and also in the case of structural applications the polytype transformations that occur during sintering can determine the variations of the mechanical characteristics (Telle, 1994).

3.1.2. *Sintering, microstructure, and mechanical properties of SiC*

As in the case of Si_3N_4, the sintering of SiC is generally performed with the use of sintering aids and various methods such as sintering without pressure (PLS), HP, HIP, sintering in gas pressure (GPS) can be used. Silicon carbide can be densified by solid state sintering (SSS) and LPS.

At industrial level, silicon carbide is sintered in the solid state at 2100 and 2200°C in argon atmosphere or vacuum, possibly applying pressure in the final stage of densification. The sintering aids are generally boron and carbon. The effectiveness of B and C as sintering additives was reported for the first time by Prochazka (Prochazka, 1975; Prochazka and Scanlan, 1975).

The amount of B necessary to obtain materials with a density close to the theoretical one is rather small, about 0.3 wt%. Boron can be added not only in elemental form but also as a compound such as B_4C (Lange and Groupta, 1976).

SSS-SiC presents outstanding high temperature resistance but poor mechanical properties (toughness 2–2.5 $MPa{\cdot}m^{1/2}$, bending strength 300–350 MPa) due to an unrefined microstructure (mean grain size of about 20–25 μm) (Tanaka, 1991).

LPS allows the material to densify at temperatures between 1800 and 2000°C, with or without external pressure. The most used additive system is made from alumina (Al_2O_3) and yttria (Y_2O_3) or yttrium aluminum garnet, YAG ($Al_5Y_3O_{12}$) in different ratios, the amount varying from 5 to 15 wt% (Dressler and Riedel, 1997; Mulla and Krstic, 1991). Thanks to the lower process temperatures compared to SSS-SiC, LPS-SiC generally has a much higher mechanical strength and fracture toughness (4–5 $MPa{\cdot}m^{1/2}$) due to a change in fracture mode from transgranular to intergranular (van Dijen and Mayer, 1996). The reason for this change lies in the weakening of the SiC/SiC grain boundaries, which can be put in relation with the presence of secondary phases. The fracture is deflected along grain boundaries and dissipates more energy following this tortuous path.

As reported for Si_3N_4, the anisotropic growth of the grains of α-SiC can significantly improve the fracture toughness through different mechanisms such as crack bridging, crack deflection, or pull-out (Padture, 1994). The most common procedure to introduce elongated grains into the microstructure is based on the $\beta \rightarrow \alpha$ phase transformation at high temperature, through an annealing treatment (Figure 7-5). If SiC powder consists of single β-phase, a

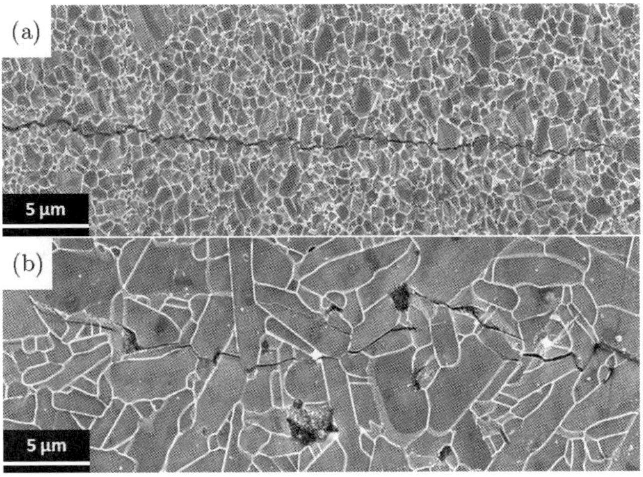

Figure 7-5. SEM micrographs of crack paths in a LPS-SiC before (a) and after (b) annealing treatment showing the increasing of crack tortuosity due to the formation of elongated α-SiC grains. *Courtesy of Dr. Diletta Sciti.*

fine and homogeneous microstructure (400–500 nm) is obtained by hot-pressing (Figure 7-5a) (Sciti and Bellosi, 2000; Sciti *et al.*, 2001). High values of flexural strength (750 MPa) and very high hardness (20–23 GPa) are obtained with compositions containing 10 wt% additives (4 wt% Y_2O_3-6 wt% Al_2O_3).

Because dwell temperature and time prevent the $\beta \rightarrow \alpha$ phase transformation, HP-sintered materials are thermally treated at temperatures between 1900 and 2000°C after sintering to obtain a final microstructure with high values of grain aspect ratio (3.5 and 4.5) (Figure 7-5b). Lee (1998) and Kim *et al.* (1998) reported fracture toughness values up to 9 MPa·m$^{1/2}$. By using other sintering aids such as Al, B, and C (Cao *et al.*, 1995) similar fracture toughness values were obtained with a flexural strength around 650 MPa, but without annealing after HP. Weibull modulus of sintered α-SiC has an average value of 11 ± 3 in the temperature range 25–1500°C (Munro, 1997).

Finally, it should be mentioned that some mechanical properties of ceramics can be improved by the reduction of grain size. In particular, the wear resistance of ceramic-on-ceramic couplings

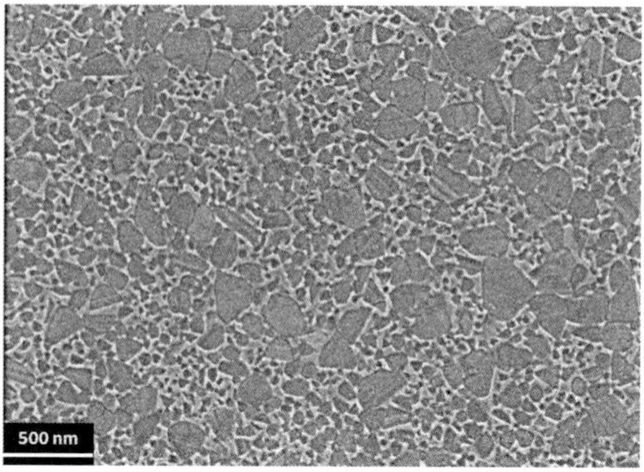

Figure 7-6. SEM micrograph showing the microstructures of a nano-structured SiC. *Courtesy of Dr. Diletta Sciti.*

was shown to increase when nano-ceramics were used (Bellosi *et al.* 2004; Guicciardi *et al.*, 2005, 2007). An example of nano-sized SiC is shown in Figure 7-6. The advantages of nano-ceramics are attributed either to the higher grain boundary strength, as in the case of the nano-composites, or to different deformation mechanisms with respect to the micro-sized SiC materials (Bellosi *et al.*, 2004). In nano-composites where SiC has been added as secondary phase to matrices of Al_2O_3, no evident improvement in strength and toughness was associated with nano-sized microstructures in comparison to micro-sized microstructures (Bellosi *et al.*, 2004). However, Al_2O_3 nano-composites with the addition of just 5 vol% of SiC have lower friction coefficient and higher wear resistance (almost three orders of magnitude) than the pure alumina (Bellosi *et al.*, 2004, Guicciardi *et al.*, 2005).

4. Si_3N_4 and SiC Ceramics as Prosthetic Materials

As orthopedic bearings must remain stable *in vivo* during use, enduring two million or more gait-related cycles of loading each year (Heisel *et al.*, 2004; Skinner, 1999) any synthetic material for joint replacement should possess the following characteristics (Rahaman *et al.*, 2007):

— mechanical reliability (low risk of failure) and resistance to deformation when subjected to biomechanical loading. The biomechanical loads vary from three times the body weight (~3 kN) for normal walking to eight times the body weight (~8 kN) for jogging or stumbling (Willmann, 2001). Beside high strength, the material should also possess high elastic modulus and high fracture toughness;
— long-term wear resistance (low wear) and low friction;
— good lubrication in the body; this is assured by the good wetting (low contact angle) between the bearing surface and the synovial fluids (that is a proteinaceous polar fluid); and,
— bioinertness and biocompatibility *in vivo*; high corrosion resistance is needed and properties of self-healing of the surface layer when scratched in an environment with very low oxygen partial pressure (high affinity for oxygen).

Ceramics fulfill almost all the requirements listed above and several of their remarkable properties have fueled excitement about their potential applications in the biomedical field. Oxide ceramics such as Al_2O_3 and stabilized ZrO_2 have a long history in prosthetic hip and knee replacements and the favorable outcomes and the limitations of these ceramics are all well known (Chevalier and Cremillard, 2009; Rahaman *et al.*, 2007). Today, Al_2O_3 is the most common ceramic bearing used in orthopedic surgery. Alumina composites containing ZrO_2 (namely zirconia-toughened alumina, ZTA) have been designed to provide tougher orthopedic bearings with low wear properties. The best known of these composites is BIOLOX®delta by CeramTec, which has been in clinical use since 2002 (Heimke *et al.*, 2002; Rahaman *et al.*, 2007).

In the following, the behavior of Si_3N_4 and SiC will be discussed in comparison with oxide ceramics, taking into account the essential characteristics listed above. Table 7-1 summarizes the most important mechanical and physical properties of metallic and ceramic materials for orthopedic bearings.

Table 7-1. Mechanical and physical properties of metallic and ceramic materials for orthopedic bearings.

	Si_3N_4	SiC	Al_2O_3	ZTA	BIOLOX® delta	CrCo	Ti-alloy
Density, $g{\cdot}cm^{-3}$	3.15–3.26	3.20	3.99	5.02	4.37	8.5	4.43
Hardness, GPa	13–16	27	14–20	19–20	18.5	3–4	3.4
Elastic modulus, GPa	300–320	410	400–450	285	358	210–250	105–115
Flexural strength, MPa	800–1100	550–750	400–600	1000	1150	—	—
Toughness, $MPa{\cdot}m^{1/2}$	8–11	3–9	4–5	6.5	8.5	50–100	75
Weibull modulus	19–50	11–14	5	7	13	—	—
Thermal conductivity, $W{\cdot}m^{-1}{\cdot}K^{-1}$	30–40	100–120	25–30	17	17	100	6.7
Wettability in water, contact angles,°	46.5[a] 58.7[b] 61.4[c]	77–110[d]	71.9	88.4	—	—	—
Wettability in bovine serum, contact angles,°	50.1[a] 40.3[b] 59.2[c]	—	58.7	54.1	—	—	

Notes: [a]Si_3N_4-bioctive glass, [b]Si_3N_4-MgO, [c]Si_3N_4-TiN (Mazzocchi *et al.*, 2008). [d]Present work.

It should be again noted that strength, toughness, and Weibull modulus (namely reliability) of non-oxide ceramics (especially Si_3N_4) are higher than or comparable with oxide ceramics. Bal *et al.* (2008; 2009) proposed for total hip arthroplasty a Si_3N_4 with 6 wt% Y_2O_3 and 4 wt% Al_2O_3 sintered by combining pressureless sintering and post-HIPing. The flexural strength was 923 ± 70 MPa, with a Weibull modulus of 19 and a fracture toughness of 10 ± 1 $MPa{\cdot}m^{1/2}$.

Silicon nitride has been proposed as the most superior bearing material among ceramic materials for applications requiring high performance in severe conditions (Takebayashi, 2003). The results of a rolling life testing, in which a thrust-type bearing tester was used with oil lubrication, indicate the load resistance and the rolling life increasing in the order: Alumina <silicon carbide <zirconia <silicon nitride, making the performance of Si_3N_4 equal or better than those of bearing steels (Takebayashi, 2003). On the other hand, SiC is recognized as a ceramic material (especially when nano-sized) with superior wear properties thanks to high hardness and elastic modulus. It was reported by Guicciardi *et al.* (2007) that the wear resistance of a ceramic-on-ceramic coupling measured by a pin-on-disc test was improved when nano-sized SiC was matched to micro-sized Si_3N_4.

Some other important properties must be now mentioned. Si_3N_4 and SiC (but also Al_2O_3 and ZrO_2 ceramics) are partially radiolucent, which means that the implant, adjacent bone, and the implant–bone interface can be visualized easily on plain radiography. This is not the case with metal implants, which, being radio-opaque, can block radiographic visualization of the underlying tissue. Furthermore, as pointed out by Bal and Rahaman (2012), Si_3N_4 is a non-magnetic material which enables magnetic resonance imaging (MRI) examination of soft tissues proximal to Si_3N_4 implants with no artifact.

Another attractive property of non-oxide ceramics is their ability to be formulated into both a porous substrate and a hard bearing surface retaining high mechanical properties (Bal and Rahaman, 2012; Gonzales *et al.*, 2003; Mazzocchi *et al.*, 2013). Porous Si_3N_4 (see the example in Figure 7-7) can support direct, appositional bone ingrowth that is necessary for durable biological fixation to the skeleton (Bal and Rahaman, 2012). Si_3N_4 could therefore be used to make orthopedic implants with a smooth articulating surface on one plane and a porous ingrowth surface on another plane within the same implant (Bal and Rahaman, 2012). This could be an interesting option for hip resurfacing, which differs from hip replacement in that the arthritic host femoral head is resurfaced with a prosthetic cap,

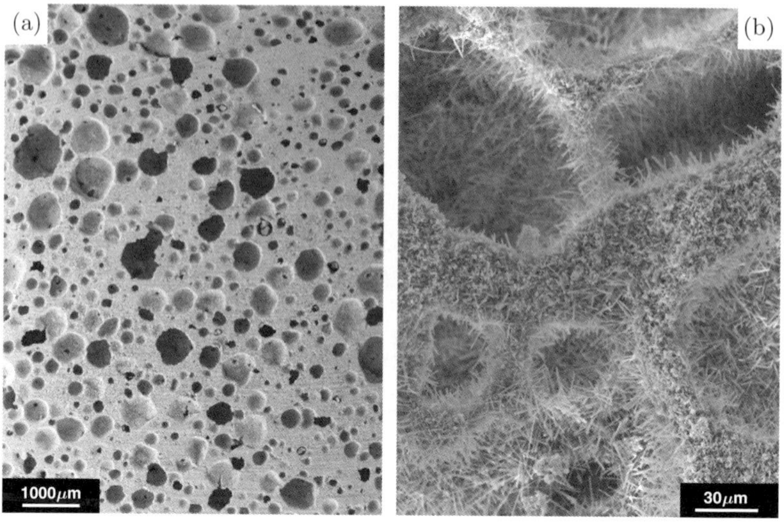

Figure 7-7. SEM micrographs (a, b) of a porous MgO-Si_3N_4 showing in (b) elongated β-Si_3N_4 grains grown on the porous surface. (Courtesy of Dr. Mauro Mazzocchi.)

rather than being surgically excised and replaced *Bal and Rahaman, 2012; Zhang et al., 2010*. As well, the use of Si_3N_4 in load-bearing hip resurfacing components is supported by finite element analyses (Zhang *et al.*, 2010).

As for silicon nitride, the possibility of realizing SiC ceramics with complex shapes and functional porosity is extremely appealing. In this context, the development of biomorphic SiC ceramics (Gonzales *et al.*, 2003) has attracted a lot of interest. These materials have an excellent mechanical properties/density relationship and are obtained following a near net shaping process. Pre-shaping is performed in the selected wood (chosen on the basis of its intrinsic characteristics of porosity in term of pore size, distribution, amount, etc., which in turn influence the mechanical properties), which is then converted by pyrolysis into C preform, losing about 60% of its volume and 75% of its weight. Final shape is given to the C template, which is infiltrated with Si, forming SiC without undergoing significant dimensional changes. These abilities of non-oxide ceramics open the door to several novel skeletal applications.

4.1. *Wettability and Biocompatibility of Si_3N_4 and SiC*

The wetting properties of the surfaces are important for the broad issue of biocompatibility. They influence solid–liquid interaction, lubrication, and tissue adhesion. All these features are important parameters for biological effects at cell level, like affinity, adhesiveness, and protein adsorption (Mazzocchi *et al.*, 2008). In a basic approximation, the more wettable the material, the better the human body tolerates it (Agathopoulos and Nikolopoulos, 1995; Amaral *et al.*, 2002; Annarelli *et al.*, 1999; Lampin *et al.* 1997).

Technical ceramics have crystalline structures in which the atoms are held together by a combination of strong ionic and covalent bonds (Carter and Norton, 2013). Strong atomic bonding between the crystals gives rise to the desirable mechanical properties of ceramics (high strength, elastic modulus, and hardness) and their chemical inertness *in vivo*. The biocompatibility of Al_2O_3 and ZrO_2 ceramics is related to the high chemical stability of these materials, which confers resistance to corrosion and reliable *in vivo* behavior over time (Rahaman and Yao, 2007). The surfaces of these oxides have polar hydroxyl (–OH) groups that promote interaction with the aqueous body fluids to provide a lubricating layer (Rahaman and Yao, 2007) (wettability). Similarly, the surfaces of Si_3N_4 (Hah *et al.*, 1999) and SiC (Rahaman *et al.*, 1986; 1987) ceramics present a nanometric SiO_2-rich oxide layer produced by exposure to ambient air. The natural oxidation layer of silicon nitride at room temperature is no more than 2.5–3.0 nm and it is composed of a monolayer of adventitious carbon, 0.2–0.5 nm of SiO_2, and 1.0–1.5 nm of SiO_xN_y on the Si_3N_4 substrate (Du *et al.*, 1989; Hah *et al.*, 1999), while the SiC surface is close to a SiO_2 composition (Rahaman *et al.*, 1986; 1987).

Thanks to the presence of the surface oxide, significantly lower contact angles of water on Si_3N_4 ceramics (Table 7-1) have been observed in comparison with those observed on alumina and zirconia, confirming a more hydrophilic character of the Si_3N_4 based ceramics (Mazzocchi *et al.*, 2008). The water contact angles were found to decrease with an increase in the amount of glassy silicatic grain boundary phases. The different values in the contact angles can be attributed to the surface charges and related physicochemical phenomena, since the morphologies (mean surface roughness R_a = 0.03–0.07 μm) of the materials' surfaces were not significantly different (Mazzocchi *et al.*, 2008). The polarity can be regarded as an indicator of hydrophilicity. The different behaviors between alumina, zirconia, and silicon nitride (and among different silicon nitride ceramics; see Table 7-1) can be imputed to the polar surface energy component (compared to the dispersive one) governing the surface tension of the SiO_2-containing phases Si_3N_4-based ceramics.

The nature of the intermolecular forces established between the solid surface and the aqueous biological liquids depends on the surface chemical composition. In the case of Si_3N_4 powders, it was demonstrated that the surface reactivity of silicon nitride induces the formation of a few nanometers-thick layer composed of Si_2N_2O and containing mainly silanol (Si–OH) and secondary amine groups (Si_2–NH) (Bondanini *et al.*, 2001). As a result, the surface charge of Si_3N_4 powder in aqueous media is negative above the isoelectric point. The Si_3N_4 surface charge is the result of the preferential equilibria between the surface functional groups and Si–O unsaturated bonds, governed by the presence of –OH (Mazzocchi *et al.*, 2008). Instead, the behavior of SiC in water is similar to SiO_2 (Balbo *et al.*, 2007) and due to the different chemical composition of the oxide surface, the water contact angle results are higher in SiC than in Si_3N_4 (the present authors have recorded values of 77° and 110° respectively on polished and unpolished surfaces of the same SiC sample; see Table 7-1).

Similar wettability trends among different Si_3N_4 ceramics were obtained (Mazzocchi *et al.*, 2008) when bovine serum was used as wetting liquid (Table 7-1). In this case the decrease of the contact angle is correlated with the transport of albumin to the surface of the drop with a consequent decrease of the surface tension. The protein adhesion on different ceramics is related to the surface charge. Silicon nitride is characterized by a negative charge and high adsorption of albumin, although other chemical and physical factors influence the phenomena.

Concerning biocompatibility, and as expected in agreement with the wettability assessment, Si_3N_4 ceramics are non-toxic, but in addition, the material is found to encourage cell adhesion, normal proliferation, and differentiation when tested *in vitro* with mouse fibroblast cells (L929), rabbit marrow stromal cells, human osteoblast-like MG-63 cell line, or human mesenchymal stem cells (Kue *et al.*, 1999). Promising results were obtained *in vivo* in a rabbit model (Bal and Rahaman, 2012, Cappi *et al.*, 2009). An excellent cytocompatibility *in vitro* of SiC ceramics was demonstrated by Cappi *et al.* (2009) with mouse fibroblast cells (L929) and human mesenchymal stem cells, as for silicon nitride. In addition, Yakimova *et al.* (2007) reported that α-SiC is well tolerated in the cortex and more stable in physiological saline fluid than Si_3N_4.

In vitro and *in vivo* studies have indicated that SiC is biocompatible depending on particle size for phagocytosis (Yakimova *et al.*, 2007). SiC particles were well tolerated by rabbit bone, causing no aggregation of macrophages and were apparently harmless (Aspenberg *et al.*, 1996). Cytotoxicity tests showed that $5\,\mu$m SiC particles inhibited colony outgrowth by one third (Yakimova *et al.*, 2007). These results suggest that SiC debris could be well tolerated *in vivo*.

The preliminarily assessed biocompatibility for the electro-conductive Si_3N_4–TiN composite is promising for the production of high strength electro-conductive composite non-oxide ceramics that can be machined by electrical discharge machining to obtain complex shapes or functional surface topographies (Mazzocchi and Bellosi, 2008). In particular, the study included the cytotoxicity assessment, according to the ISO 10093-part 5 normative, of dense sintered ceramics and of the raw materials including therefore, the Si_3N_4 phases, the formed intergranular phases, and the TiN electro-conductive phase. In addition, the tests included analysis of the toxicity of possible contaminations from the different processing steps: Powder mixing, drying, sieving, sintering, etc. The results demonstrated the non-cytotoxicity of the materials, either dense silicon nitride or Si_3N_4-sintering aids powder mixtures. Therefore, neither the raw powders of Si_3N_4, TiN, and the sintering aids, nor possible contaminations from the processing affect the biocompatibility of the electro-conductive ceramic.

Significantly, recent work has shown that Si_3N_4 is highly resistant to bacterial biofilm formation, colonization, and growth (McEntire *et al.*, 2012) without resorting to the use of antibiotics (Gorth *et al.*, 2012a). The results were linked to the differential surface chemistry and surface nanostructure which lead to differential adsorption of physiologic proteins. In particular, in contrast to Ti and PEEK, the surface of Si_3N_4 is hydrophilic, with a net positive charge (Gorth *et al.*, 2012b). In a rat model, anti-infective properties of silicon nitride has been also evidenced (Webster *et al.*, 2012) three months after surgery and bacterial infection injection: No live bacteria adjacent to Si_3N_4 were observed, differently from PEEK (88%) and Ti (21%). Independently of a specific role eventually played by bacterial biofilm in biotribology, the resistance to bacterial biofilm formation is important since infection is the most common reason for repeat surgery after otherwise successful prosthetic joint replacement.

4.2. *Bio-Tribological Behavior of Si_3N_4 and SiC*

Total joint replacements require materials with low friction and wear rate. The surface wettability (discussed in Section 4.1) has a significant influence on the friction and wear behavior of a tribological system, as in the direct contact between ceramic bearing surfaces (Mazzocchi *et al.*, 2008). A good lubrication is assured by the good wetting (low contact angle) between the bearing surface and the synovial fluids (Rahaman *et al.*, 2007). Ceramics promote the formation of a lubricating layer thanks to the interaction between the surface oxides with the aqueous body fluid (Rahaman and Yao, 2007). However, it must be considered that a low contact angle is not the only discriminant parameter for a good lubrication. In fact, the thermal conductivity is proposed to be an additional very important parameter for lubrication (Willmann *et al.*, 2001). Experiments in hip-simulator and *in vivo* showed that the temperature rise of the wear couple zirconia-on-zirconia (Z/Z) was higher than of zirconia-on-alumina, which was higher than of alumina-on-alumina (Willmann *et al.*, 2001). The thermal conductivity of high-purity alumina is about 25 W/m·K, and for zirconia it is about 2 W/m·K. Further, the determined contact temperature was far above 40°C.

The synovial fluid, being protein-based, can degenerate at such temperatures. Thus, materials or material combinations with low thermal conduction do not offer satisfactory requirements for low friction in joint replacement. From this point of view, SiC ceramics would outperform Si_3N_4 ones, since the thermal conductivity values are ~100 W/m·K and ~30 W/m·K, respectively (Table 7-1).

According to several studies (Akazawa and Kato, 1988; Jahanmir and Fisher, 1988), silicon nitride–silicon nitride coupling seems to satisfy friction and wear requirements because under some test conditions the contact surface of silicon nitride becomes ultra-smooth due to tribochemical polishing and the friction becomes very low at increasing sliding distances. Particularly if the surface is rendered ultra-smooth by the fine machining or running-in, the tribological properties of silicon nitride against itself in water is excellent (Zhou *et al.*, 1997a, 1997b). The *in vivo* environment should be more favorable yet, since human synovial fluid is an excellent lubricant, regardless of the bearing material used (Bal and Rahaman, 2012; Blewis *et al.*, 2007; Iliev, 2010).

Mazzocchi *et al.* (2008) set up a disc-on-ball test in dilute bovine serum at 37°C (using an alumina ball as static element) under different experimental conditions and on different Si_3N_4-based ceramics, namely Si_3N_4-bioglass, Si_3N_4-MgO, and electro-conductive Si_3N_4-TiN. The results clearly indicated the independence of the low (0.10–0.18) friction coefficients from load, linear speed, and covered distance, with almost undetectable surface modifications and wear tracks in the monolithic Si_3N_4 materials tested (Figure 7-8a). The wear track was instead observed in the Si_3N_4-TiN composite (Figure 7-8b), with a preferential removal of grain boundary phases associated with a slight oxidation of TiN and material removal by friction, maybe due to the lower hardness of TiN in comparison to alumina (Mazzocchi *et al.*, 2008).

Considerable controversy is found in the literature with friction coefficient ranging from 0.001 (Ohashia *et al.*, 1997) to 0.6–0.8 (Saito *et al.*, 1997; Xu and Kato, 2000) and wear properties of Si_3N_4 articulating against itself (Bal and Rahaman, 2012). Since Si_3N_4 has two principal wear modes, mechanical and tribochemical (Bal and

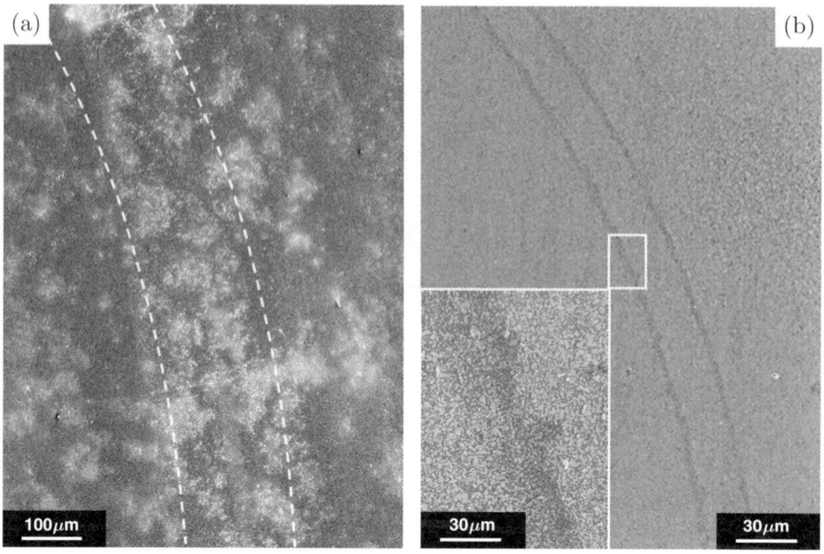

Figure 7-8. SEM micrographs of the tracks on the surfaces of (a) the Si_3N_4–bioactive glass disc and of (b) the Si_3N_4–TiN disc produced during the ball-on-disc wear test. *Adapted from Mazzocchi et al. (2008).*

Rahaman, 2012), the discordant results in friction and wear are dependent upon which mechanism is dominant (Xu and Kato, 2000).

Mechanical wear occurs under high loads, low speeds, and stop–start conditions, which typically results in high friction, high wear, and debris generated by fracture of the oxide surface and Si_3N_4 grains (Bal and Rahaman, 2012). Tribochemical wear, meanwhile, is an issue at lower loads, higher speeds, and under continuous motion (Bal and Rahaman, 2012). The chemical dissolution in the aqueous environment of Si_3N_4 generates very smooth articulating surfaces and a hydrated silicon oxide lubricating film between the articulating components, which results in the low friction and wear of the material (Akazawa and Kato, 1988; Amutha Rani *et al.*, 2005; Jahanmir and Fisher, 1988).

It should be reported that most of the results regarding the wear behavior (such as those mentioned above) were obtained by screening devices, or 'quick-tests' (Affatato and Traina, 2011). As such, they are claimed not to well represent a good estimate of the wear rate observed *in vivo*, mainly because they fail to accurately reproduce the specimen geometry which can influence the lubrication and the contact stress (Affatato *et al.*, 2008; Rahaman *et al.*, 2007). More reliable results, well correlated to clinical observations, are obtained by using hip and knee wear simulators. However, also in this case, the influence of several experimental variables must be taken into account such as: Number of stations, loading (physiological or simplified), degrees of freedom, anatomical or inverted configuration, and temperature-controlled test fluid baths for each hip joint assembly (Affatato and Traina, 2011).

For SiC ceramics, there are no reports on hip simulator tests even if some experimental results seem to indicate its suitability as load-bearing bioceramic either as bulk material (Li *et al.*, 2005) or coating (Pettersson *et al.*, 2013).

Instead, when Si_3N_4 was tested on a hip simulator where the Paul-type physiologic load profile was used (Bal *et al.*, 2008, 2009), Si_3N_4 acetabular cups produced low-volumetric wear whether articulating against Si_3N_4 or cobalt–chromium (Biomet) femoral heads. The wear rates were comparable to those of the well-assessed Al_2O_3-Al_2O_3 bearings (Figure 7-9; Bal *et al.*, 2008, 2009). Tribochemical

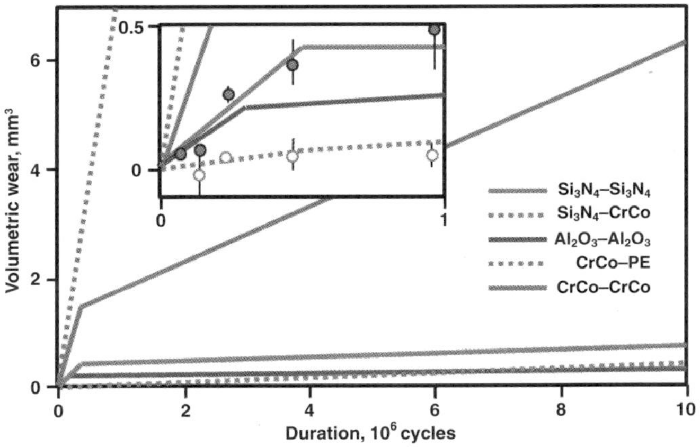

Figure 7-9. Volumetric wear of Si3N4 hip joint bearings tested in a hip simulator, compared with Al_2O_3–Al_2O_3, CoCr–CoCr, and CoCr–PE bearing couples. *Adapted from Bal et al.* (2009).

wear is probably the dominant mode for *in vitro* hip simulator tests using self-articulating Si_3N_4 (Bal and Rahaman, 2012) as the inspection of the Si_3N_4 surfaces after wear testing showed a smooth, glossy finish, with no scratching or wear marks (Bal *et al.*, 2009). However, debris is generated by transgranular or intergranular fracture of the oxide surface and Si_3N_4 grains in mechanical wear, which is also active during testing in a hip simulator (Bal and Rahaman, 2012). Si_3N_4 debris consists of rounded micron and submicron particles ($0.7 \pm 0.6\,\mu$m) (Bal *et al.*, 2009; Williams *et al.*, 2006), similar to Al_2O_3 debris (Stewart *et al.*, 2003).

Accumulation of wear particles of ultra-high molecular weight PE at the implants can be linked to osteolysis, which leads to bone loss and ultimately aseptic implant loosening. There is a consensus that ceramics offer the best way to reduce the wear rate and eliminate the problem of osteolysis and consequent surgery (Willmann, 2001). Ceramic particles are inert and less bioreactive than PE particles (Bal *et al.*, 2008; Ingham and Fisher, 2000). Further, particles of Si_3N_4 produced by mechanical wear are predicted to slowly dissolve in polar liquids and they have therefore the potential to be resorbed *in vivo*, potentially reducing the risk for aseptic loosening. A study has shown that α-Si_3N_4 powder can dissolve in physiological body solution at pH values of 4.8, 6.5, and 7.4 (the pH value in the vicinity of an implant can vary between 4.4 and 7.7), thus supporting the hypothesis that wear particles could be resorbed *in vivo* (Olofsson *et al.*, 2012).

However, it should be reported that there is still controversy over the suitability of silicon nitride and silicon carbide for bearing surfaces in knee and hip joint replacements (Bal *et al.*, 2012, Mazzocchi and Bellosi, 2008). Willmann (2001; 2002) expressed a major concern by claiming that Si_3N_4 and SiC would not be suitable because of the corrosive wear (Wright and Goodman, 2002) related to the formation of SiO_2 on the surface, which could chip off during the motion of the articulation, inducing catastrophic third-body wear. In another work, the same author affirmed the non-biocompatibility of Si_3N_4 and SiC due to the insufficient corrosion resistance in the body environment (Willmann *et al.*, 2001). As reported in Section

4.1, surface oxidation of Si_3N_4 and SiC is always active (already in ambient air) and when the oxide layer is removed through erosion or wear, the surface rapidly repairs itself through re-oxidization thereby limiting its degradation (Rahaman *et al.*, 2007). The presence of surface oxidation has been proved to be fundamental for wettability and biocompatibility, while tribochemical wear results in low friction and wear because of the presence of a hydrated silicon oxide film that acts as a lubricant (Bal and Rahaman, 2012). Si_3N_4 with a chemically inert material composition and a controlled microstructure in term of grain morphology and grain boundary phases (see Section 2.1.3) should be an excellent material for prosthetic hip and knee bearings as some studies have demonstrated (Bal *et al.*, 2009; Mazzocchi *et al.*, 2008), without any evidence of catastrophic third-body wear.

5. Conclusion

The current life expectancy for a successfully implanted hip joint can nowadays be estimated to be 15 years. However, with the development of alternative low-wear bearings, achievement of longer lifetimes are hopefully expected.

Non-oxide ceramics and particularly silicon nitride materials certainly exhibit better mechanical behavior as compared to oxide bioceramics, which would certainly represent a benefit, explicitly in terms of an improved safety factor. Besides the high fracture strength (comparable with that of composite oxides), the most appealing property is the high fracture toughness due to a microstructure containing elongated grains with a remarkable toughening effect due to crack bridging. Moreover, these engineered microstructures allow a very high reliability of Si_3N_4-based ceramics. With such interesting characteristics, one may wonder why non-oxide bulk ceramics were not widely used in orthopedics before.

As pointed out by Chevalier and Cremillard (2009), first of all, the validation of a new material by sanitary authorities is long and costly. Second, non-oxide ceramics must be sintered at higher temperatures than oxides and under inert atmosphere, requiring more effort during processing. Moreover, being very hard, they are also

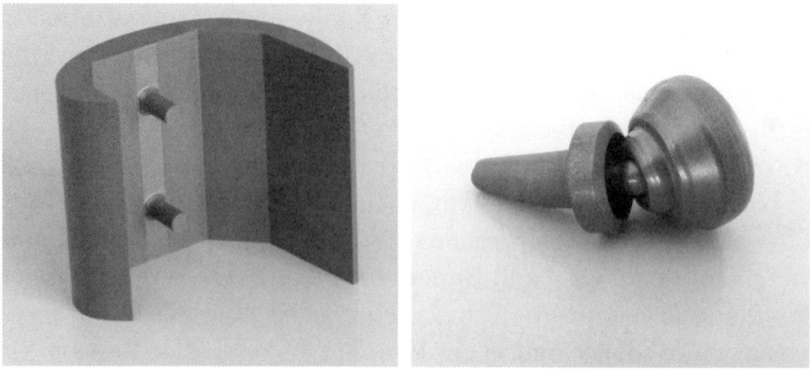

(a) (b)

Figure 7-10. Examples of knee prosthesis (a) and elbow prosthesis (b) obtained by EDM of Si_3N_4-35 vol% TiN.

difficult (and expensive) to machine. However, non-oxide ceramics are now approved also in terms of biocompatibility and the use of nano-powders, together with innovative sintering methods, will allow non-oxide ceramics to be sintered under moderate conditions and near net-shape sintering to be developed to overcome existing technological barriers.

Electro discharge machining is a highly cost-effective machining technique and allows the large bearing surfaces to be customized with complex topographies and shapes through CAD-CAM rendering. The use of an electro-conductive ceramic composite such as Si_3N_4–TiN opens the possibility of new design for articular bearing joints prosthesis (Figure 7-10) in relation to the required performances and to customize the devices without additional processing costs. As a consequence, from a technological point of view, fast development of silicon nitride in orthopedics can be expected in the next future (Chevalier and Cremillard, 2009).

However, more factors ranging from the scientific to the socio-economical must be taken into account, as outlined by Pezzotti and Yamamoto (2014).

The long-term failure probability of non-oxide ceramics remains an issue to be clarified, in terms of the delayed failure behavior of the materials or, more precisely, to their resistance to the subcritical growth of internal cracks propagating from pre-existing defects under the combined actions of static/dynamic load and environmental attack. The achievement of reliable tribological results on non-oxide ceramics, well correlated to clinical observations, is still needed. They can be obtained first by using hip and knee wear simulators. However, also in this case, the influence of several experimental variables must be taken into account and a standardization of the experiment should be set up in order to make results from different studies comparable each other. The controversy present in the literature about the oxide layers on silicon nitrides and carbides, which is hypothesized (but not demonstrated) to chip off over time due to corrosive wear, should be definitively solved in this way. On the other hand, many of the valuable characteristics (such as wettability, lubrication, biocompatibility) of silicon nitride and carbide are due to the oxidized surface.

Finally, an appropriate design is required to realize the optimum lubrication of ceramic joint prostheses and to avoid severe wear (Mabuchi *et al.*, 2004). Advances in technology, including not only the development of improved materials, related production processes, and characterization, but also improved surgical procedures and better understanding of natural tissue reactions, could certainly result in breakthroughs in both bioceramics and implant selections. However, new best performing bioceramics could be a necessary but not sufficient prerequisite to obtain a breakthrough in the hip arthroplastic field, which is driven not only by scientific but also by economic and social concerns. Unfortunately, manufacturers could choose to obtain easier profits by spreading old technologies in developing countries rather than taking the risks to push innovative technologies in affluent societies.

Acknowledgments

The authors gratefully acknowledge Dr. Andrea Balbo for his valuable contribution on silicon carbide and Dr. Stefano Guicciardi for his help in mechanical properties discussion.

References

Acheson, E.G. (1893). Production of artificial crystalline carbonaceous material, *U.S. Patent 492,767.*

Affatato, S., Spinelli, M., Zavalloni, M., Mazzega-Fabbro, C. and Viceconti, M. (2008). Review. Tribology and total hip joint replacement: Current concepts in mechanical simulation, *Med Eng Phys*, **30,** 1305–1317.

Affatato, S. and Traina, F. (2011). Bio and medical tribology, in Davim, J. P. (ed.), *Tribology for Engineers: A practical guide*, Woodhead Publishing, Philadelphia, p. 243.

Agathopoulos, S. and Nikolopoulos, P. (1995). Wettability and interfacial interactions in bioceramic-body-liquid systems, *J Biomed Mater Res*, **29**, 421–429.

Akazawa, M. and Kato, K. (1988). Wear properties of Si_3N_4 in rolling-sliding contact, *Wear*, **124**, 123–132.

Amaral, M., Lopes, M.A., Santos, J.D. and Silva, R.F. (2002).Wettability and surface charge of Si_3N_4-bioglass composites in contact with simulated physiological liquids, *Biomaterials*, **23**, 4123–4129.

Amutha Raini, D., Yoshizawa, Y., Jones, M.I., Hyuga, H., Hirao, K. and Yamauchi, Y. (2005). Comparison of tribological behavior between a-Sialon/Si_3N_4 and Si_3N_4/Si_3N_4 sliding pairs in water lubrication, *J Am Ceram Soc*, **88**, 1655–1658.

Annarelli, C.C., Fornazero, J., Cohen, R., Bert, J. and Besse, J.L. (1999). Colloidal protein solutions as a new standard sensor for adhesive wettability measurements, *J Colloid Interface Sci*, **213**, 386–394.

Aspenberg, P., Anttila, A., Konttinen, Y.T., Lappalainen, R., Goodman, S.B., Nordsletten, L. *et al.* (1996). Benign response to particles of diamond and SiC: Bone chamber studies of new joint replacement coating materials in rabbits, *Biomaterials*, **17**, 807–812.

Back, D.L., Dalziel, R., Young, D. and Shimmin A. (2005). Early results of primary Birmingham hip resurfacings. An independent prospective study of the first 230 hips, *J Bone Joint Surg Br*, **87**, 324–329.

Bal, B.S. and Rahaman, M.N. (2012). Orthopedic applications of silicon nitride ceramics, *Acta Biomater*, **8**, 2889–2898.

Bal, B.S., Khandkar, A., Lakshminarayanan, R., Clarke, I., Hoffman, A.A. and Rahaman, M.N. (2008). Testing of Silicon Nitride Ceramic Bearings for Total Hip Arthroplasty, *J Biomed Mater Res B Appl Biomater*, **87**, 447–454.

Bal, B.S., Khandkar, A., Lakshminarayanan, R., Clarke, I., Hoffman, A.A. and Rahaman, M.N. (2009). Fabrication and testing of silicon nitride bearings in total hip arthroplasty, *J Arthroplasty*, **24**, 110–116.

Balbo, A., Sciti, D., Costa, A.L. and Bellosi, A. (2007). Effects of powder processing on colloidal and microstructural characteristics of β-SiC powders, *Mater Chem Phys*, **103**, 70–77.

Becher, P.F., Sun, E.Y., Plucknett, K.P., Alexander, K.B., Hsueh, C.H., Lin, H.T. *et al.* (1998). Microstructural design of silicon nitride with improved fracture toughness: I, effects of grain size and shape, *J Am Ceram Soc*, **81**, 2821–2830.

Becher, P.F., Painter, G.S., Shibata, N., Satet, R.L., Hoffmann, M.J. and Pennycook, S.J. (2006). Influence of additives on anisotropic grain growth in silicon nitride ceramics, *Mater Sci Eng*, **422**, 85–91.

Bellosi, A., Sciti, D. and Guicciardi, S. (2004). Synergy and competition in nano- and micro-design of structural ceramics, *J Eur Ceram Soc*, **24**, 3295–3302.

Belmonte, M., González-Julián, J., Miranzo, P. and Osendi, M.I. (2010). Spark plasma sintering: A powerful tool to develop new silicon nitride-based materials, *J Eur Ceram Soc*, **30**, 2937–2946.

Bergman, B. (1984). On the estimation of the Weibull modulus, *J Mater Sci Letters*, **3**, 689–692.

Bernero, J., Khandkar, A., Lakshminarayanan, R. and Hofmann, A. (2006). Knee prosthesis with ceramic tibial component, *U.S. Patent US20060052875*.

Berzelius, J.J. (1824). II. Untersuchungen über Flussspathsäure und deren merkwürdigsten Verbindungen, *Ann Phys*, **77**, 169–230.

Blewis, M.E., Nugent-Derfus, G.E., Schmidt, T.A., Schumacher, B.L. and Sah, R.L. (2007). A model of synovial fluid lubricant composition in normal and injured joints, *Eur Cells Mater*, **13**, 26–39.

Bowen, L.J., Weston, R.J., Carruthers, T.G. and Brook, R.J. (1978). Hot-pressing and the β-phase transformation in silicon nitride, *J Mater Sci*, **13**, 341–350.

Bracisiewicz, M., Medri, V. and Bellosi, A. (2002). Factors inducing degradation of properties after long term oxidation of Si_3N_4-TiN electroconductive composites, *Appl Surf Sci*, **202**, 139–149.

Bondanini, A., Monteverde, F. and Bellosi, A. (2001). Influence of powder characteristics and powder processing routes on microstructure and properties of hot pressed silicon nitride materials, *J Mater Sci*, **36**, 4851.

Bucciotti, F., Mazzocchi, M. and Bellosi, A. (2010). Perspectives of the Si_3N_4-TiN ceramic composite as a biomaterial and manufacturing of complex-shaped implantable devices by electrical discharge machining (EDM), *J Appl Biomater Biomech*, **8**, 28–32.

Cannon, W.R., Danforth, S.C., Flint, J.H., Haggerty, J.S. and Marra, R.A. (1982). Sinterable ceramic powders from laser-driven reactions: I, process description and modeling, *J Am Ceram Soc*, **65**, 324–330.

Carter, C. B. and Norton, M. G. (2013). *Ceramic Materials: Science and Engineering*, Springer, New York.

Cao, G. Z. and Metselaar, R. (1991). α'-Sialon Ceramics: A Review, *Chem Mater*, **3**, 242–252.

Cao, J.J., MoberlyChan, W.J., De Jonghe, L.C., Gilbert, C.J. and Ritchie, R.O. (1996). *In situ* toughened silicon carbide with Al–B–C Additive, *J Am Ceram Soc*, **79**, 461–69.

Cappi, B., Neuss, S., Salber, J., Telle, R., Knuchel, R. and Fischer, H. (2010). Cytocompatibility of high strength non-oxide ceramics, *J Biom Mater Res A*, **93**(1), 67–76.

Chevalier, J., and Gremillard, L. (2009). Ceramics for medical applications: A picture for the next 20 years, *J Eur Ceram Soc*, **29**, 1245–1255.

Dressler, W. and Riedel, R. (1997). Progress in silicon based non oxide structural ceramics, *Int J Refract Met Hard Mat*, **15**, 13–47.

Du, H., Tressler, R. E. and Spear K. E. (1989). Thermodynamic and of Si–N–O system and kinetic of oxidation of Si_3N_4, *J Electrochem Soc*, **136**, 3210–3215.

Ely, K., Khandkar, A., Lakshminarayanan, R. and Hofmann, A. (2005). Hip prosthesis with monoblock ceramic acetabular cup, *US Patent US20050273176.*

Fisher, G.R. and Barnes, P. (1990). Toward a unified view of polytypism in silicon carbide, *Philos Mag*, **61**, 217–236.

Gogotsi, Y.G. (1994). Particulate silicon nitride based composites (Review), *J Mat Sci*, **29**, 2541–2556.

Gorth, D.J., Puckett, S., Ercan, B., Webster, T.J., Patel, A.A. and Lakshminarayanan, R. (2012a). Decreased bacterial biofilm formation and function associated with silicon nitride (Si_3N_4) materials used in interbody fusion cages (IBF) compared to titanium and polyetheretherketone (PEEK) (unpublished scientific presentation), *Ann N Am Spine Soc Meet 2012*, Dallas.

Gorth, D.J., Puckett, S., Ercan, B., Webster, T.J., Rahaman, M. and Bal, B.S. (2012b). Decreased bacteria activity on Si_3N_4 surfaces compared with PEEK or titanium, *Int J Nanomed*, **7**, 4829–4840.

Goursat, P. and Foucaud, S. (2007). Non-oxide ceramics, in Boch, P. and Nièpce, J.C. (eds.), *Ceramic Materials: Processes, Properties and Application*, ISTE Ltd., 231–260.

Guicciardi, S., Melandri, C., Medri, V. and Bellosi, A. (2003). Effect of testing temperature and thermal treatments on some mechanical properties of a Si_3N_4–TiN composite, *Mater Sci Eng*, **360**, 35–45.

Guicciardi, S., Sciti, D., Melandri, C. and Bellosi, A. (2005). Dry sliding wear behavior of Al2O3–SiC submicro- and nano-composites, *J Am Ceram Soc*, **88**, 179–183.

Guicciardi, S., Sciti, D., Melandri, C. and Pezzotti, G. (2007). Dry sliding wear behavior of nano-sized SiC pins against SiC and Si_3N_4 discs, *Wear*, **262**, 529–535.

Hah, S., Burk, C.B. and Fischer, T.E. (1999). Surface quality of tribochemically polished silicon nitride. *J Electrochem Soc*, **146**, 1505–1509.

Hampshire, S. (2007). Silicon nitride ceramics — review of structure, processing and properties, *J Ach Mat Man Eng*, **24**, 43–50.

Heimke, G., Leyen, S. and Willmann, G. (2002). Knee arthoplasty: Recently developed ceramics offer new solutions, *Biomaterials*, **23**, 1539–1551.

Heisel, C., Silva, M. and Schmalzried, T.P. (2004). Bearing surface options for total hip replacement in young patients, *Instr Course Lect*, **53**, 49–65.

Hirosaki, N., Akimune, Y. and Mitomo, M. (1993). Effect of grain growth of β-silicon nitride on strength, weibull modulus and fracture toughness, *J Am Ceram Soc*, **76**, 1892–1894.

Huheey, J.E., Keiter, E.A. and Keiter, R.L. (1993). *Inorganic Chemistry*, Harper Collins College Publisher, New York.

Iturriza, I., Castro, F. and Fuentes, M. (1989). Sinter and sinter-HIP of silicon nitride ceramics with yttria and alumina additions, *J Mater Sci*, **24**, 2047–2056.

Jahanimir, S. and Fisher, T.E. (1988). Friction and wear of silicon nitride lubricated by. humid air, water, hexadecane + 0.5 percent stearic acid, *STLE Trans*, **31**, 32–43.

Kalnins, U., Erglis, A., Dinne, I., Kumsars, I. and Jegere, S. (2002). Clinical outcomes of silicon carbide coated stents in patients with coronary artery disease, *Med Sci Monit*, **8**, PI16–PI20.

Kamijo, E., Honda, M., Higuchi, M., Takeuchi, H. and Tanimura, T. (1985). Electrical discharge machinable Si_3N_4 ceramics, Sumitomo *Electr Tech Rev*, **24**, 183–190.

Khandkar, A. (2010). Ceramic–ceramic articulation surface implants, *US Patent US20100049331 A1.*

Khandkar, A., Brodke, D. and Lakshminarayanan, R. (2008). Total disc implant, *US Patent US20080033563 A1.*

König, W., Dauw, D.F., Levy, G. and Panten, U. (1988). EDM-future steps towards the machining of ceramics, *CIRP Ann-Manuf Techn*, **37**, 623–631.

Kim, Y.W., Mitomo, M. and Hirotsuru, H. (1995). Grain growth and fracture toughness of fine-grained silicon carbide ceramics, *J Am Ceram Soc*, **78**, 3145–3148.

Kim, Y.W., Mitomo, M., Emoto, H. and Lee, J.G. (1998). Effect of initial α-phase content on microstructure and mechanical properties of sintered silicon carbide, *J Am Ceram Soc*, **81**, 3136–3140.

Kue, R., Sohrabi, A., Nagle, D., Frondoza, C. and Hungerford, D. (1999). Enhanced proliferation and osteocalcin production by human osteoblast-like MG63 cells on silicon nitride ceramic discs. *Biomaterials*, **20**, 1195–1201.

Iliev, C. (2010). On the wear behaviour of silicon nitride sliding against metals in water, *Ind Lubr Tribol*, **62**, 32–36.

Ingham, E. and Fisher, J. (2000). Biological reactions to wear debris in total joint replacement. *Proc Inst Mech Eng H*, **214**, 21–37.

International Organization for Standardization. (1992). *ISO/TC 206 — Fine ceramics.* Available at: http://www.iso.org [Accessed 31 March 2014].

Lange, F.F. (1979). Fracture toughness of Si_3N_4 as a function of the initial α-phase content, *J Am Ceram Soc*, **62**, 428–430.

Lange, F.F. and Groupta, T.K. (1976). Sintering with boron compound, *J Am Ceram Soc*, **11–12**, 537–538.

Lee, C.S. (1998). Microstructure and mechanical properties of self reinforced α-silicon carbide, *Ceram Int*, **24**, 489–495.

Lampin, M., Warocquier-Clerout, R., Legris, C., Degrange, M. and Sigot-Luizard, M.F. (1997). Correlation between substratum roughness and wettability, cell adhesion, and cell migration, *J Biomed Mater Res*, **36**, 99–108.

Leung, I., Guo, W., Friedman, I. and Gleason, J. (1990). Natural occurrence of silicon carbide in a diamondiferous kimberlite from Fuxian, *Nature*, **346**, 352–354.

Li, C.W., Lui, S.C. and Goldacker, J. (1995). Relation between strength, microstructure, and grain-bridging characteristics in *in situ* reinforced silicon nitride, *J Am Ceram Soc*, **78**, 449–459.

Li, X., Wang, X., Bondokov, R., Morris, J., An, Y. H. and Sudarshan, T. S. (2005). Micro/nanoscale mechanical and tribological characterization of SiC for orthopedic applications, *J Biomed Mater Res B Appl Biomater*, **72**, 353–361.

Mabuchi, K., Sakai, R., Ota, M. and Ujihira, M. (2004). Appropriate radial clearance of ceramic-on-ceramic total hip prostheses to realize squeeze-film lubrication, *Clin Biomech*, **19**, 362–369.

Martin, C., Cales, B., Vivier, R. and Mathieu, R. (1989). Electrical discharge machinable ceramic composites, *Mater Sci Eng*, **109**, 351–356.

Mazzocchi, M. and Bellosi, A. (2008). On the possibility of silicon nitride as a ceramic for structural orthopaedic implants. Part I: Processing, microstructure, mechanical properties, cytotoxicity, *J Mater Sci Mater Med*, **19**, 2881–2887.

Mazzocchi, M., Medri, V. and Bellosi, A. (2013). Functionalized silicon nitride for bio-applications. *Conf Eur Ceram Soc 2013*, Limoges.

Mazzocchi, M., Gardini, D., Traverso, P.L., Faga, M.G. and Bellosi, A. (2008). On the possibility of silicon nitride as a ceramic for structural orthopaedic implants. Part II: Chemical stability and wear resistance in body environment, *J Mater Sci Mater Med*, **19**, 2889–2901.

McEntire, B.J, Lakshminarayanan, A, Bal, B.S. and Webster, T.J. (2012). An overview of silicon nitride as a novel biomaterial (unpublished scientific presentation), *Innovation Biomedical Materials Meeting*, Raleigh.

McMinn, D., Treacy, R., Lin, K. and Pynsent, P. (1996). Metal on metal surface replacement of the hip. Experience of the McMinn prostheses, *Clin Orthop Relat Res*, **329**, S89–S98.

Moissan, H. (1905). Etude de Siliciure de Carbone de la Meteorite de Canon Diablo, *Compt Rendu*, **CXL**, 45–46.

Monnink, S., van Boven, A., Peels, H., Tigchelaar, I., de Kam, P., Crijns, H. *et al.* (1999). Silicon carbide coated coronary stents have low platelet and leukocyte adhesion during platelet activation, *J Invest Med*, **47**, 304–310.

Mulla, V.D. and Krstic, M.A. (1991). Low-temperature pressureless sintering of β-Silicon carbide with aluminium oxide and yttrium oxide additions, *Amer Ceram Soc Bull*, **70**, 439–443.

Munro, R.G., (1997). Material properties of a sintered a-SiC, *J Phys Chem Ref Data*, **26**, 1195–1203.

Ohashia, M., Zhoua, Y.S., Tomitaa, N., Ikeuchia, K. and Takashimaa, K. (1997). Study on the possibility of Si_3N_4- Si_3N_4 as a material for hip prostheses, *Mat Sci Eng C*, **5**, 125–127.

Padture, N.P., (1994). *In situ* toughened silicon carbide, *J Am Ceram Soc*, **77**, 519–23.

Pettersson, M., Tkachenko, S., Schmidt, S., Berlind, T., Jacobson, S., Hultman, L. *et al.* (2013). Mechanical and tribological behavior of silicon nitride and silicon carbon nitride coatings for total joint replacements, *J Mech Behav Biomed*, **25**, 41–47.

Petzow, G. and Herrmann, M. (2002). Silicon nitride ceramics, in Jansen, M. (ed), *High performance non-oxide ceramics II*, Springer, Berlin, pp. 47–167.

Petzow, G., Telle, R. and Danzer, R. (1991). Microstructural defects and mechanical properties of high-performance ceramics, *Mater Charact*, **26**, 289–302.

Pezzotti, G. and Yamamoto, K. (2014). Artificial hip joints: The biomaterials challenge, *J Mech Behav Biomed*, **31**, 3–20.

Prochazka, S. (1975). The role of boron and carbon in the sintering of silicon carbide, in Popper, P. (ed), *Special Ceramics*, British Ceramic Research Association, Manchester, pp. 171–182.

Prochazka S. and Scanlan, R. M. (1975). Effect of boron and carbon on sintering of SiC, *J Am Ceram Soc*, **58**, 72.

Rahaman, M.N. and De Jonghe, L. C. (1987). Angle-resolved XPS analysis of oxidized polycrystalline SiC surfaces, *Am Ceram Soc Bull*, **66**(5), 783–785.

Rahaman, M.N., Boiteux, Y. and De Jonghe, L.C. (1986). Surface characterization of silicon nitride and silicon carbide powders, *Am Ceram Soc Bull*, **65**(8), 1171–1176.

Rahaman, M.N., Yao, A., Bal, B.S., Garino, J.P. and Ries, M.D. (2007). Ceramics for prosthetic hip and knee joint replacement, *J Am Ceram Soc*, **90**(7), 1965–1988.

Ramirez-Rico, J., Torres-Raya, C., Hernandez-Maldonado, D., Garcia-Garian, C., Martinez-Femandez, J. and de Arellano-Lopez, A.R. (2010). Porous biomorphic SiC for medical implants processed from natural and artificial precursors, in Narayan, R. and Colombo, P. (eds.), *Advances in Bioceramics and Porous Ceramics 11*, The American Ceramic Society, 203–214.

Ray, R. (1993). Fundamental research in structural ceramics for service near 2000°C, *J Am Ceram Soc*, **76**(9), 2147–2174.

Saito, T., Imada, Y. and Honda, F. (1997). An analytical observation of the tribochemical reaction of silicon nitride sliding with low friction in aqueous solutions, *Wear*, **205**, 153–159.

Satet, R.L., Hoffmann, M.J. and Cannon, R.M. (2006). Experimental evidence of the impact of rare-earth elements on particle growth and mechanical behaviour of silicon nitride, *Mater Sci Eng A*, **422**, 66–76.

Sciti, D. and Bellosi, A. (2000). Effects of additives on densification, microstructure and properties of liquid phase sintered silicon carbide, *J Mat Sci*, **35**, 3849–3855.

Sciti, D., Guicciardi, S. and Bellosi, A. (2001). Effect of annealing treatments on microstructure and mechanical properties of liquid-phase sintered silicon carbide, *J Eur Ceram Soc*, **21**, 621–632.

Skinner, H. B. (1999). Ceramic bearing surfaces, *Clin Orthop Relat R*, **369**, 83–91.

Sonntag, R., Reinders, J. and Kretzer, J.P. (2012). What's next? Alternative materials for articulation in total joint replacement, *Acta Biomater*, **8**, 2434–2441.

Stewart, T.D., Tipper, J.L., Insley, G., Streicher, R.M., Ingham, E. and Fisher, J. (2003). Long-term wear of ceramic matrix composite materials for hip prostheses under severe swing phase microseparation, *J Biomed Mater Res B Appl Biomater*, **66**, 567–573.

Sun, E.Y., Becher, P.F., Plucknett, K.P., Hsueh, C.-H., Alexander, K. B., Waters, S.B. *et al.* (1998). Microstructural design of silicon nitride with improved fracture toughness: II, effects of yttria and alumina additives, *J Am Ceram Soc*, **81**, 2831–2840.

Takebayashi, H. (2003). Ceramic Bearing, in Somiya, S., Aldinger, F., Claussen, N., Spriggs, R.M., Uchino, K., Koumoto, K. and Kaneno, M., (eds), *Handbook of Advanced Ceramics Vol. I: Materials Science*, Elsevier, Amsterdam, pp. 313–331.

Tanaka, H. (1991). Sintering of silicon carbide, in Somiya, S., Inomata, Y. (eds.), *Silicon Carbide Ceramics-1*, Elsevier, New York, 213–238.

Telle, R. (1994). Boride and carbide ceramics, in Cahn, R.W., Haasen, P. and Kramer, E.J. (eds.), *Materials Science and Technology — Structure and properties of ceramics*, VCH, Weinheim, pp. 163–266.

Themelin, L., Desmaison-Brut, M. and Billy, M. (1993). Oxidation behaviour of a hot isostatically pressed silicon nitride material, *J Phys IV*, **3**, C9-C5-881-C9-C5-888.

Thompson, D.S. and Pratt, P.L. (1966). The structure of silicon nitride, *Sci Ceramics*, **3**, 33.

Varela-Feria, F.M., Martinez-Fernandez, J., de Arellano-Lopez, A.R. and Singh, M. (2002). Low density biomorphic silicon carbide: Microstructure and mechanical properties, *J Eur Ceram Soc*, **22**, 2719–2725.

Van Dijen, F.K. and Mayer, E. (1996). Liquid phase sintering of silicon carbide, *J Eur Ceram Soc*, **16**, 413–420.

Van Dijen, F.K., Kerber, A., Vogt, U., Pfeiffer, W. and Schultze, M. (1994). A comparative study of three silicon nitride powders obtained by three different syntheses, *Key Eng Mater*, **89–91**, 19–28.

Wagner, C. (1961). Theory of Ostwald ripening, *Z Electrochem*, **65**, 581–591.

Webster, T.J., Patel, A.A., Rahaman, M.N. and Bal, B.S. (2012). Anti-infective and osteointegration properties of silicon nitride, poly(ether ether ketone), and titanium implants, *Acta Biomater*, **8**, 4447–4454.

Weibull, W. (1939). Ingen Ors Vetenskapsakademiens Handlingar, **151**, 45.

Wild, S., Grieveson, P. and Jack, K.H. (1972). The crystal structures of alpha and beta silicon and germanium nitrides, in Popper, P. (ed), *Special Ceramics*, British Ceramic Research Association, Manchester, 385–395.

Williams, P.A., Lakshminarayanan, R., Khandkar, A., Green, D.D. and Clarke, I.C. (2006). Wear debris morphology of silicon-nitride generated from a hip simulator model, *Proc Ann Meet Soc Biomat*, Pittsburgh, 553.

Willmann, G. (2001). Improving bearing surfaces of artificial joints, *Adv Eng Mater*, **3**, 135–141.

Willmann, G. (2002). Bioceramics in joint replacement: State-of-the-art and future options, CFI, *Ceram Forum Int*, **79**(5), E27–E31.

Willmann, G., von Chamier, W., Pfaff, H.G. and Rack, R. (2001). Biocompatibility of a new alumina matrix biocomposite AMC, *Key Eng Mater*, **192–195**, 569–572.

Wright, T. M. and Goodman, S. B. (2002). *Implant Wear in Total Joint Replacement: Clinical and Biological Issues, Material and Design Considerations*, American Academy of Orthopaedic Surgeons (AAOS), Rosemont.

Xu, J. and Kato, K. (2000). Formation of tribochemical layer of ceramics sliding in water and its role for low friction, *Wear*, **245**, 61–75.

Yakimova, R., Petoral Jr., R.M., Yazdi, G.R., Vahlberg, C., Lloyd Spetz, A. and Uvdal, K. (2007). Surface functionalization and biomedical applications based on SiC, *J Phys D Appl Phys*, **40**, 6435–6442.

Zhan, G.D., Xie, R.J., Mitomo, M. and Kim, Y.W. (2001). Effect of β to α transformation on the microstructural development and mechanical properties of fine grained silicon carbide ceramics, *J Am Ceram Soc*, **84**, 945–950.

Zhang, W., Titze, M., Cappi, B., Wirtz, D.C., Telle, R. and Fischer, H. (2010). Improved mechanical long-term reliability of hip resurfacing prostheses by using silicon nitride, *J Mater Sci Mater Med*, **21**, 3049–3057.

Zhou, Y.S., Ikeuchi, K. and Ohashi, M. (1997a). Comparison of the friction properties of four ceramic materials for joint replacements, *Wear*, **210**, 171.

Zhou, Y.S., Tomita, N., Ikeuchi, K., Ohashi, M. and Takashima, K. (1997b). Study on the possibility of silicon nitride-silicon nitride as a material for hip prostheses, *Mater Sci Eng C*, **5**, 125–129.

Chapter 8

Poly-Ether–Ether–Ketone (PEEK)

Markus A. Wimmer[a], Michel P. Laurent[a], Irene Sinz[b] and Sandra Utzschneider[c]

[a]*Department of Orthopedic Surgery, Rush University Medical Center, Chicago, USA*

[b]*Invibio Ltd., Lancashire, United Kingdom*

[c]*Department of Orthopaedic Surgery, University Hospital of Munich (LMU), Campus Großhadern, Munich, Germany*

1. Introduction

Poly-ether–ether–ketone, commonly referred to as 'PEEK', belongs to the polymer family of poly-aryl-ether–ketones (PAEKs). Commercial manufacturing of PEEK started as early as 1978 in the United Kingdom (Victrex, 2008). Approximately eight years later, a report on fiber-reinforced PEEK as a potential candidate for tribological applications marked the first scientific publication on PEEK as a bearing material (Voss and Friedrich, 1987). In the medical field, the first peer-reviewed publication of PEEK dates back to the late eighties, when Williams *et al.* (1987) confirmed its biocompatibility and potential for use in long-term implants. Driven by the idea of replacing relatively rigid metals with polymers to approximate bone stiffness and avoid stress shielding, PEEK and its modifications were applied to various musculoskeletal problems as an isoelastic solution (Skinner, 1988). Interest grew rapidly in orthopedics (Liao, 1994; Maharaj and Jamison, 1993), trauma (Corvelli *et al.*, 1997; Klesey *et al.*, 1997), and spine (Brantigan and Lauryssen, 2006), until PEEK was offered as an implantable biomaterial for the first time in 1998 by Invibio Ltd. (Thornton Cleveleys, UK). So far, PEEK has had its biggest success in the area of spine, where the properties of this polymer outperform metal and ceramics by allowing physiological loading concepts and enhanced imaging. However, its corrosion and wear resistance, strength and durability, combined with a low elastic modulus, make it an interesting candidate for joint replacement as well. Previous reviews about PEEK in orthopedics were spearheaded by Kurtz and colleagues (Kurtz and Devine, 2007; Kurtz and Nevelos, 2012). This chapter builds on this knowledge.

2. What is PEEK?

PEEK is a high-performance thermoplastic polymer with an average molecular weight of 80,000–120,000 g/mol. Its molecular structure consists of a chain of stable aromatic rings connected by ether and ketone functional groups (Figure 8-1). One molecule of PEEK comprises approximately 100 repeat units. The PEEK molecule is relatively stiff due to the presence of the aromatic rings, but can rotate around the ether and ketone groups to form chain folds and create higher order domains: So-called crystals. Typically, PEEK consists of amorphous and crystalline domains forming a two-phase semicrystalline microstructure (May, 1988). Having a bond angle of 125°, the PEEK molecular chain has a zigzag conformation within the crystallites (Figure 8-2) (Dawson and Blundell, 1980). PEEK crystals consist of very fine lamellae, which can organize into larger spherulites (Kumar and Anderson, 1986). The thickness of the lamellae and size

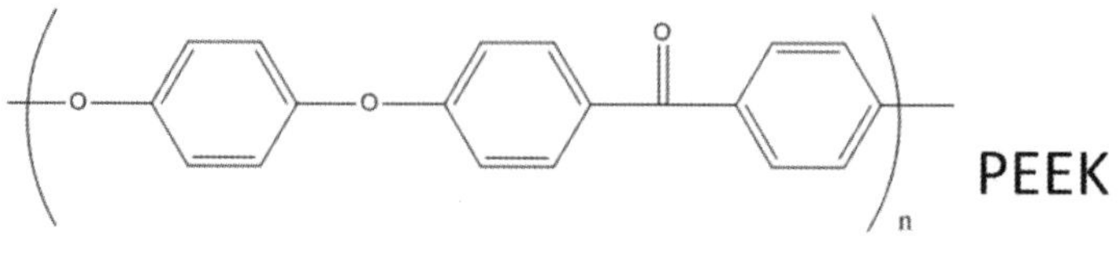

Figure 8-1. Chemical formula of poly-ether–ether–ketone (PEEK).

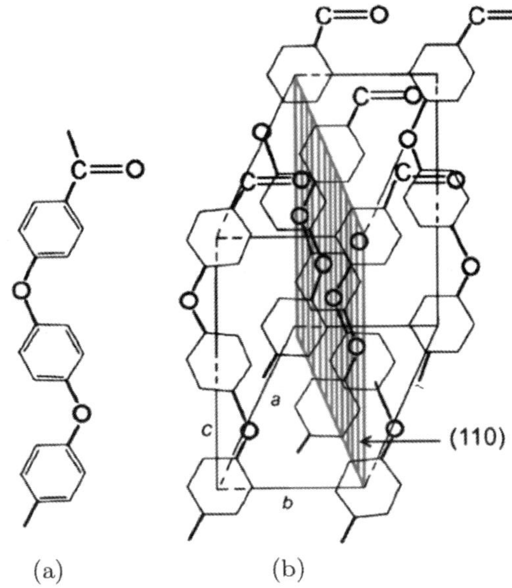

Figure 8-2. (a) Chain formation of PEEK and (b) orthorhombic crystal unit cell of PEEK.

of spherulites and density are dependent on the processing parameters, which can be very complex. Typically, the crystalline content of injection molded PEEK is between 30% and 35%.

PEEK combines several advantageous properties as a biomaterial, such as high strength, stiffness, ductility, abrasion resistance, thermal stability, as well as resistance to chemical hydrolysis and radiation. Hydrolysis and radiation resistance in particular are favorable properties to minimize chemical alterations and subsequent aging during common sterilization techniques. In addition, being radiolucent and non-magnetic, PEEK is compatible with all standard imaging technologies without blocking the field of view and/or creating image artifacts. This makes PEEK particularly attractive as a biomaterial in the area of spine.

PEEK is the dominant member of the PAEK polymer family due to its balanced range of properties and economic production. Other family members that have been considered for implant production are PEK (poly-ether–ketone), PEKK (poly-ether–ketone–ketone),

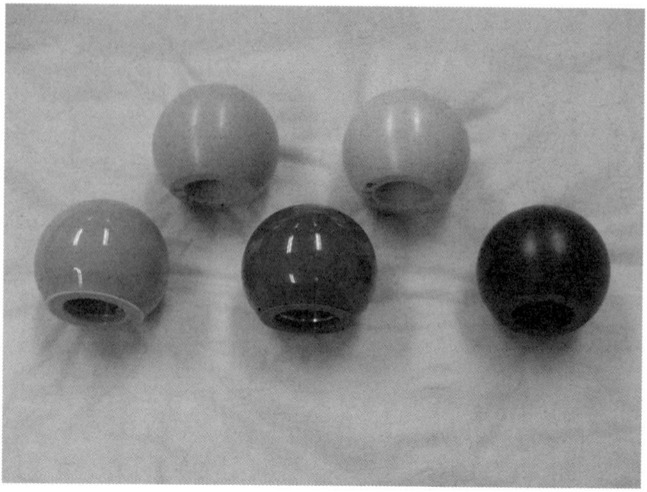

Figure 8-3. Color differences in PEEK, PEK (top, from left to right), and PEKK, GFR-PEEK, CFR-PEEK (bottom).
Notes: GFR = glass fiber-reinforced,
CFR = carbon fiber-reinforced.

and PEKEKK (poly-ether-ketone-ether–ketone–ketone). Depending on the functional groups within the molecule, the respective family members differ in material properties and color (Figure 8-3). Two of the important properties that change based on functional PAEK groups are the glass transition and melt temperatures, which are in the range of 134–160°C and 335–441°C, respectively.

2.1. *PEEK Composite Materials*

In order to fulfill the mechanical requirements for load bearing applications, PEEK has been blended with glass and carbon fibers of different type, length, and content. By reinforcing PEEK with carbon fibers (CFR-PEEK), the elastic modulus can be enhanced by a factor of 4–5, closely matching that of cortical bone (15–18 MPa) (Skinner, 1988). In addition, the tensile strength of these materials can be increased to reach those of metals (Green, 2012). Commercially available carbon fibers vary in terms of tensile modulus and strength. Also processing routes differ using either the high strength polyacrylonitrile (PAN) fiber or the softer coal tar pitch (pitch).

Hence, available carbon composite materials are often differentiated based on the inclusion of PAN and pitch fibers.

Carbon fibers have interesting tribological properties and have been investigated for various bearing applications. The strength of the fiber/matrix interface is of paramount importance, as painfully experienced by the use of Poly II for total knee arthroplasty. Here, 'Poly II' refers to ultra-high molecular weight polyethylene (UHMWPE) blended with carbon fibers, a material used for artificial bearings in the 1980s. Fatigue of the tibial insert was a typical clinical failure scenario at the time. Because of the weak adhesion between fiber and matrix, fiber pull-out and matrix delamination were commonly observed in a retrieval analysis conducted by Birken (2003). Since the interfacial shear strength of CFR-PEEK is with 72–200 MPa at least an order of magnitude stronger than that of Poly II (Green, 2012), a similar failure scenario for PEEK appears unlikely but should be carefully monitored. In particular, it has been observed that processing parameters, especially the cooling rate, have significant effects on the ductility and interlaminar fracture resistance of PEEK composites (Gao and Kim, 2000, 2001). While a slow cooling rate improves both the adhesion between fiber and matrix as well as the strength/stiffness of the PEEK matrix, a fast cooling enhances the ductility of the matrix and gives rise to a high interlaminar fracture toughness. These two properties, fiber–matrix adhesion and matrix ductility, do not act synergistically but often counteract each other as identified in the study by Gao and Kim (*ibid.*).

3. Clinical History of PEEK in Joint Arthroplasty

Interestingly, the first application of PEEK in joint arthroplasty was to replace metal surfaces in a finger joint. Only later did PEEK replace UHMWPE in some applications. Recognizing that excessive wear debris may cause osteolysis and subsequent prosthetic loosening, carbon fiber-reinforced PEEK was considered as a substitute material to articulate against ceramics (and metals). Although several positive attributes of PEEK in replacing UHMWPE have been recognized, the now nearly 15 years of successful clinical experience with highly crosslinked polyethylenes will inevitably slow down such developments. However, PEEK may replace metallic bearing surfaces in the future. Its radiolucent and artifact-free behavior during imaging, its elastic properties avoiding excessive stress shielding of bone, the absence of metal ion release, and the access to polymer mass production technologies that allow the manufacture of more economically friendly implants make PEEK an interesting candidate for future joint replacements.

The first clinically utilized bearing application, the PEEK RM finger joint, was introduced in 1999 by Mathys Ltd., Switzerland. Using a typical polymer processing technology, i.e. injection molding, components that were previously manufactured from metal were now manufactured from PEEK. A thin titanium coating on the distal and proximal stem enhanced bone ingrowth. Meanwhile, thousands of patients have received RM finger joints showing promising results (Förster *et al.*, 2003; Richter *et al.*, 2003). Although the articulation appears to be working fine, there has been a report about mal-rotation of RM finger prostheses in patients with rheumatoid arthritis (RA) (Middleton *et al.*, 2011). Since only 1 device out of 15 was associated with osteolysis, the authors ruled out wear as the cause and attributed the failure to insufficient rotational stability of the prosthesis within the medullary canal in RA patients.

Since March 2003, the Mutars Modular Knee Tumor System (Implantcast, Germany) has used a PEEK lock to connect femur and tibia parts, replacing the previously utilized UHMWPE lock which had a relatively high failure rate and was responsible for nearly 20% of revisions (Kinkel *et al.*, 2009). By comparison, only one single PEEK lock (accounting for 1% of revisions) was found defective in the above study.

The first PEEK-on-PEEK articulating spinal implant — the Nubac^{TM} Disc Arthroplasty system (Pioneer Surgical Technology, USA) — was introduced in 2005 to treat low-back pain caused by degenerative disc disease. The clinical outcome after two years demonstrated that Nubac^{TM} can relieve symptoms of discogenic back pain without intra- and postoperative complications (Balsano *et al.*, 2011).

After several years of material and implant design development, and as an outcome of two clinical pilot studies (Cambridge Cup and ABG™ II cup: Howmedica International Inc., Limerick, Ireland), the MITCH PCR™ Monobloc hip cup (Stryker, Mawah, New Jersey) using CFR-PEEK was first implanted in January 2007. The Mitch cup design — a flexible, horseshoe-shaped acetabular cup — was based on the findings of the Cambridge Cup project, which showed no evidence of migration or osteolysis during a ten-year clinical study. Several pre-clinical and clinical studies led to the choice of a CFR-PEEK shell instead of a UHMWPE shell running against a ceramic femoral head (Field *et al.*, 2012; Latif *et al.*, 2007; Pace *et al.*, 2004). Unfortunately, the clinical trial with 25 enrolled patients was stopped after three years (personal communication). Details on the clinical and tribological findings during this trial period are reported in Section 4.1.1.

In 2008 the NuNec spinal disc prosthesis (Pioneer Surgical Technology, Inc. DBA RTI Surgical; Figure 8-4) was first implanted, as a novel cervical total disc replacement device made of PEEK-OPTIMA® from Invibio® Biomaterial Solutions and using a unique rotating CAM mechanism for endplate fixation. The self-mating PEEK bearing components have the advantage of being radiolucent

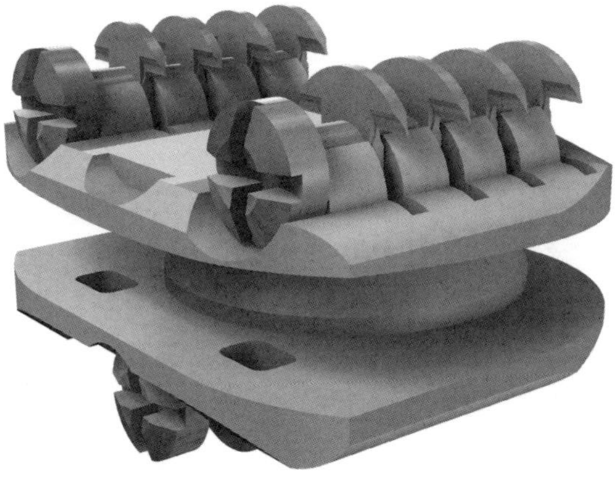

Figure 8-4. The NuNec™ Cervical Arthroplasty Disc: The first PEEK cervical disc replacement launched in Europe (picture courtesy of RTI Surgical, Inc.).

with minimal MRI artifact. To date, the clinical outcome is similar to other cervical disc arthroplasty devices (Karpe *et al.*, 2013; Yuan *et al.*, 2009).

The EnduRo Rotational Knee System (Aesculap AG, Germany) uses CFR-PEEK in all hinge mechanisms. It is used in the treatment of severe bone defects and ligamentous insufficiency. Since January 2010, it has been commercially available in Europe and received FDA clearance in December 2010. Over 2000 implantations have now been carried out with good clinical outcome. The knee system has been described as having "low wear and no macroscopic surface fatigue" (Grupp *et al.*, 2012).

The first medial interpositional knee implant — the PEEK Mobility™ (ABS Corporation, USA) — articulates against cartilage or denuded bone and is made from neat PEEK. It received CE Mark approval in September 2010 (Crosbie *et al.*, 2013). First implantations have been carried out successfully in Europe (Figure 8-5).

Recent developments in the upper extremity have involved finger and wrist joints. Poor bone quality and limited space are characteristics where PEEK often provides more design flexibility than traditional materials. For example, a novel spreading design for the proximal interphalangeal joints was realized in the Zrinski PIP prosthesis (Zrinski, Germany). The replacement of metal-on-metal articulations was addressed by Bioimplant Scandinavia AB (Sweden) with their BioSpring® System. The latter has been in clinical use

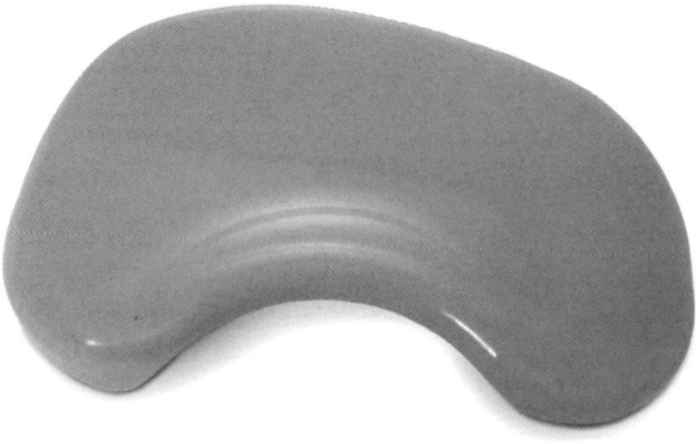

Figure 8-5. The PEEK Mobility™ medial knee implant system (picture courtesy of ABS Corporation, USA).

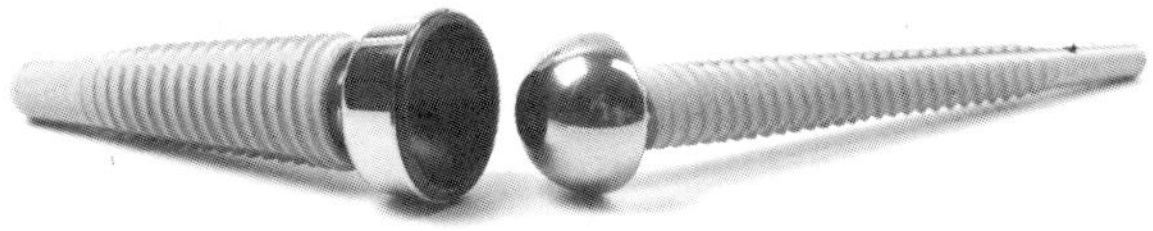

Figure 8-6. The PEEK Motec® Wrist Prostheses (picture courtesy of Swemac Orthopaedics AB, Sweden).

since 2010 and uses neat PEEK as an articulating material. The Motec® Wrist and Basal Thumb Prostheses (Swemac, Sweden), with the former showing promising mid-term results (Reigstad *et al.*, 2012), also use PEEK wear grades (PEEK-OPTIMA© Wear Performance — formerly MOTIS© from Invibio Biomaterial Solutions, UK) as an alternative to metal-on-metal and have been available since 2012 (thumb) and 2013 (wrist) (Figure 8-6).

The latest and perhaps most novel development of PEEK as a bearing surface is being explored in total knee arthroplasty and is geared towards an all-polymer implant. Wear tests of neat PEEK against UHMWPE were run successfully (East *et al.*, 2013; Wang *et al.*, 2011), and PEEK emerged as a promising candidate to articulate against UHMWPE. Besides being softer than metal, thus lowering stress shielding of bone in contact with the artificial bearing (de Ruiter *et al.*, 2014), PEEK is also economically more efficient due to using polymer mass processing technologies, resulting in less expensive implants.

The focus will now turn to the biotribological properties of PEEK and the larger PAEK family in the following sections.

4. Biotribology of PEEK and its Composites

Interest in using PEEK polymers as an artificial bearing surface began when the search for alternatives to conventional UHMWPE bearings still had some urgency because polyethylene wear remained one of the major limitations in the service life of joint prostheses. CRF-PEEK composites were already successfully being used in bearing surfaces subjected to severe conditions in industrial applications (Friedrich *et al.*, 1995; Lancaster, 1986), and PEEK and carbon fibers had been found to be biocompatible (Moore *et al.*, 1997). Outside the medical device field, basic wear and friction investigations on carbon fiber-reinforced PEEK polymers were published in the 1980s and 1990s and included the influence of metal counterface roughness (Friedrich *et al.*, 1991), temperature (Friedrich *et al.*, 1991), fiber reinforcement (Lu and Friedrich, 1995; Voss and Friedrich, 1987), and type of fiber (Flöck *et al.*, 1999). Other variants of fiber-reinforcement, such as glass fiber (GFR), were also studied. However, under water boundary lubrication, GFR-PEEK showed little improvement in friction and wear over neat PEEK (Yamamoto and Hashimoto, 2004).

4.1. *Screening Tests*

It is noteworthy that the first biotribological studies of PEEK entailed wear tests in hip simulators by (Wang *et al.*, 1998, 1999) rather than in basic configurations, such as a pin-on-disk, normally used to screen materials. Rieker *et al.* (2003) as well as Joyce *et al.* (2006) evaluated PEEK in a Joyce Finger Simulator, before Scholes and Unsworth (2007) published the first orthopedically focused screening tests of CFR-PEEK against ceramics. Using a pin-on-plate machine, multi-directional sliding was realized through reciprocating motion of the plates and superimposed rotation of the pins. Both pitch- and PAN-based carbon fiber-reinforced (CFR) PEEK OPTIMA® pins (Invibio, Ltd.), 5 mm in diameter and flat ended, were tested against ceramic BIOLOX® Forte and BIOLOX® Delta plates (CeramTec GmbH). All four possible material combinations were tested up to 2 million cycles at 1 Hz in 25% bovine serum at a 40 N contact load and compared with metal-on-metal couples. The lowest total wear was obtained with pitch-based CFR-PEEK against BIOLOX® Forte plates, but all four CFR-PEEK wear factors were within the same range ($0.15–0.23 \times 10^{-6}\,\text{mm}^3/\text{Nm}$). The authors noted that this was considerably lower than the previously determined wear of self-mating high-carbon CoCrMo pins and plates on the same screening apparatus ($0.84 \times 10^{-6}\,\text{mm}^3/\text{Nm}$).

At about the same time (2006), the MAW laboratory conducted screening tests with CFR-PEEK using the AMTI Ortho-POD. Pins

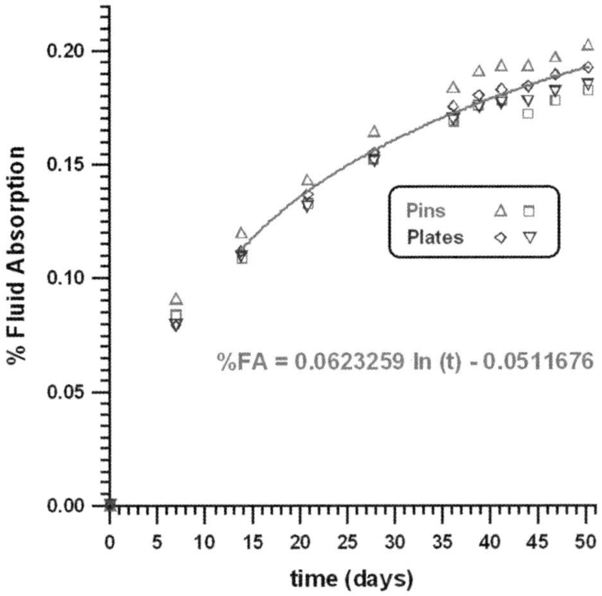

Figure 8-7. Passive fluid uptake of CFR-PEEK in aqueous solution.

were 9.5 mm in diameter with a 100 mm tip radius and articulated against a plate following a 5×5 mm square motion pattern. The investigational material combinations were CFR-PEEK against ceramics (BIOLOX® Delta), and CFR-PEEK against itself. Self-mating CoCrMo served as control. The contact load was adjusted to 80 N and tests were conducted for 1 million cycles at 1 Hz. 25% bovine serum was used as the lubricant. The lowest total wear was found with CFR-PEEK against ceramics (0.073×10^{-6} mm^3/Nm), followed by CFR-PEEK against itself (0.18×10^{-6} mm^3/Nm), and metal-on-metal (0.54×10^{-6} mm^3/Nm). The reported data were compromised by a relatively high fluid absorption of the CFR-PEEK (in excess of more than an order of magnitude when compared to UHMWPE samples; see Figure 8-7). Furthermore, samples were not completely saturated when the test was started. Because the wear rates were on the same order of magnitude as the passive fluid absorption, and it is known that mechanical interaction due to wear can further increase the fluid uptake, actual material loss may have been masked by weight gain and the presented data should be read with care, despite the use of a soak control sample. Friction was high in all investigated bearing couples, in particular when compared to UHMWPE. The lowest average coefficient of friction was measured for CFR-PEEK versus ceramics (0.16), followed by self-mating PEEK (0.21) and metal-on-metal (0.23). This is considerably higher than the typically measured friction factors of 0.04–0.07 for UHMWPE/CoCrMo couples on the OrthoPod in the MAW laboratory. In addition, the friction factor of self-mating CFR-PEEK increased from 0.18 to 0.24 over time, with the maximum value occurring at 0.6 million cycles before dropping again. The evolution of friction seemed to coincide with the measured wear, which may be attributed to an adhesive mechanism involving polymer transfer and break-away.

Following the study by the present authors, Austin *et al.* (2009) investigated self-mating PEEK pairings more closely. Using identical sample dimensions and applying similar environmental conditions (but a different motion pattern), the investigators incrementally increased the load on the AMTI Ortho-POD from 80 to 400 N to create 'adverse' contact conditions. The CFR all-polymer couples had a lower wear rate than the neat PEEK bearing couples throughout the test. After 1 million cycles and 80 N contact load, the wear factor of the neat PEEK couple was approximately 5.0×10^{-6} mm^3/Nm. Once the normal load was increased beyond 200 N, neat PEEK showed increased adhesive wear and failed at 300 N. The self-mating CFR version resisted catastrophic failure and withstood loads up to 400 N. After 3 million cycles (and various loads) the average wear factor was 0.074×10^{-6} mm^3/Nm.

In 2010, Scholes and Unsworth (2010) followed up with a full paper on self-mating wear couples of the PAEK family. Using the identical pin-on-plate configuration and testing environment as described above for CFR–PEEK against ceramics, the lowest average steady-state wear factors were found for self-mating PAN and pitch CFR–PEEK (0.30×10^{-6} mm^3/Nm and 0.92×10^{-6} mm^3/Nm, respectively). Neat PAEK couples showed up to one order of magnitude higher wear factors (1.6, 4.5, and 5.4 $\times$ 10^{-6} mm^3/Nm for PEK, PEEK, and PEKEKK, respectively).

CFR–PEEK also demonstrated low wear factors in the articulation against CoCrMo in the range of 0.13 ... 0.23 $\times$ 10^{-6} mm^3/Nm (Turell *et al.*, 2003). This is comparable to its wear factors against alumina. In contrast, neat PEEK paired with CoCrMo showed a very high wear rate. Scholes and Unsworth (2009b) measured 7.4 $\times$ 10^{-6} mm^3/Nm. This is considerably higher than for polyethylene. Wear factors of UHMWPE against CoCrMo obtained using the OrthoPOD (under similar environmental conditions but different sample geometries and loads as described above) are in the range of 1.0 $\times$ 10^{-6} mm^3/Nm (Wimmer *et al.*, 2003). This is comparable to, although lower than, the values of 2.2 $\times$ 10^{-6} mm^3/Nm (Turell *et al.*, 2003), 1.6 $\times$ 10^{-6} mm^3/Nm (Saikko, 2005), 2.7 $\times$ 10^{-6} mm^3/Nm (Saikko, 2006), and 1.2 $\times$ 10^{-6} mm^3/Nm (Korduba and Wang, 2011) found in the literature.

Of the basic biotribological studies that followed (Borruto, 2010; Marques and Davim, 2012; Rasheva *et al.*, 2010), a noteworthy one is that of Geringer *et al.* (2011) because it provides some initial insights into the wear mechanism of PAEK polymers against metal counterfaces. Using a pin-on-disk configuration, they investigated the wear and friction of PEEK, PEKK, and CFR–PEKK (30% carbon fibers) pins against CoCrMo, 316L stainless steel, and Ti_6Al_4V disks. All the polymer surfaces underwent an abrasive wear mechanism. The PEEK and PEKK surfaces also underwent local delamination, but not the CFR–PEKK. The metal counterfaces experienced corrosion with the PAEK polymers, but not with UHMWPE, which is of particular significance for implant bearing applications. The effect was more extensive with the CFR–PEKK, for which all the metal pins exhibited corrosion and significant abrasive damage, attributed tentatively to hard carbon fiber-containing debris. A major limitation of this study is that the effect of multidirectional sliding motion was not investigated, which may explain why their wear rankings for the non-carbon fiber-reinforced materials do not agree with the previous studies described above.

4.1.1. *Hip*

As mentioned above, Wang *et al.* (1998, 1999) were the first to report on a comprehensive set of hip wear tests performed on cups manufactured from three variants of a commercial grade PEEK: (1) neat; (2) reinforced with PAN carbon fiber; and, (3) reinforced with pitch carbon fiber. Fiber content was 30 wt% for both of the fiber-reinforced materials. These cups were articulated against three different types of femoral heads: Forged CoCrMo, alumina, and zirconia. UHMWPE, gamma-sterilized in air with a nominal dose of 2.5 Mrad was used as a control. The pitch-based CFR–PEEK/zirconia combination was found to be the best combination, with a wear rate of 0.39 mm^3/Mc, or only 1.1% of the corresponding UHMWPE/zirconia couple. CoCrMo heads were found to be unsuitable for articulation against the composite PEEKs, because they yielded significantly higher wear rates than the ceramic heads and they exhibited severe scratching. Interestingly, the neat PEEK cups exhibited a wear rate eight times greater than the UHMWPE cups, validating the screening tests and underscoring the extreme dependence of PEEK on carbon fiber reinforcement to achieve excellent tribological properties.

A decade later, Scholes *et al.* (2008) and Latif *et al.* (2008) presented results of wear tests for a new horseshoe cup design (Figure 8-8). The motivation for this design was to take advantage of the higher strength and lower wear rate of CRF–PEEK compared to UHMWPE to produce a flexible acetabular cup that distributed stresses more physiologically than the standard hemispherical cups, thus mitigating stress shielding effects (*ibid.*). Over the 25 million cycle (Mc) duration of the wear test, the mean wear rate was 1.16 mm^3/Mc (range: 0.81–1.39 mm^3/Mc) (Scholes *et al.*, 2008), which is much lower than typical wear rates for conventional gamma-irradiated UHMWPE (see e.g. Geerdink *et al.*, 2006; Laurent *et al.*, 2008; McKellop *et al.*, 1999a, 1999b; Muratoglu *et al.*, 2001; Wang *et al.*, 1998), and comparable to wear rates reported for highly crosslinked UHMWPE (Dumbleton *et al.*, 2006; Johnson *et al.*, 2014; Laurent *et al.*, 2008; McKellop *et al.*, 1999b). Brockett *et al.* (2012) recently reported a mean wear rate of $0.30 \pm 0.07\,mm^3$/Mc

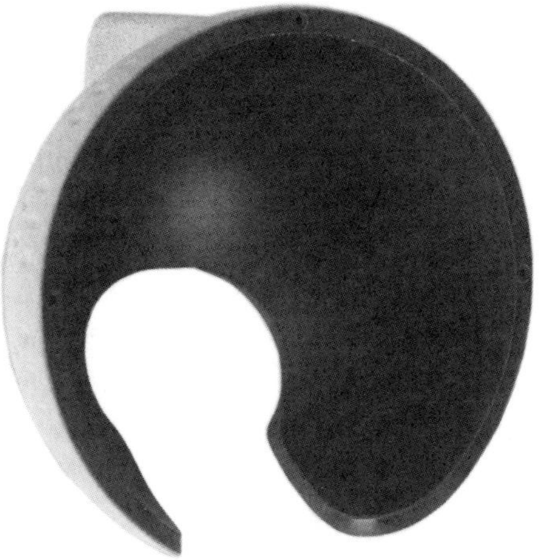

Figure 8-8. Horseshoe shaped MITCH CFR-PEEK cup. The backside has an outer coating of hydroxyapatite with a thickness of 90 ± 30 μm and surface roughness of 12 μm Ra. Two polar fins are placed in the load-bearing segment of the acetabulum. (Picture courtesy of Stryker Orthopaedics, USA.)

for pitch-based carbon fiber-reinforced standard cups (MOTIS^{TM} polymer from Invibio Biomaterial Solutions, UK), 36 mm in diameter, articulating against zirconia-toughened alumina (Biolox Delta, CeramTec GmbH, Germany) heads. This wear rate is comparable to that reported by Wang *et al.* (1998) for a similar bearing couple, but 28 mm in diameter, mentioned above. In addition, Brockett *et al.* (2012) observed a very interesting step-like wear behavior throughout the 10 Mc of testing, with periods of higher wear followed by periods of lower wear. They suggested these phases of wear correspond to loss of PEEK matrix material alternating with loss of carbon fiber material (*ibid.*). Of equal significance, this CRF-PEEK bearing combination exhibited a significantly higher friction factor (approximately 0.35) than the highly crosslinked polyethylene control (approximately 0.05). In another recent hip simulator study of the same bearing couple, but 40 mm in diameter, Wang *et al.* (2012), reported wear rates of $0.551 \pm 0.115\,\text{mm}^3/\text{Mc}$ and $0.493 \pm 0.107\,\text{mm}^3/\text{Mc}$ using two types of soak controls. They also reported high friction factors, ~0.25–0.35, using lubricants based on 25% diluted bovine serum mixed with carboxy methyl cellulose to have viscosities of 0.001–0.003.

There is little clinical data on the performance of PEEK-based materials for hip arthroplasty. As of April 2014, only two reports and one case study could be found. The earliest report is that of Pace *et al.* (2004) in a brief abstract from the European Hip Society meeting of 2004. It outlined an ongoing clinical trial of a CFR-PEEK acetabular liner incorporated in the ABG^{TM} II total hip system (Stryker SA, Montreux, Switzerland). Thirty CFR-PEEK acetabular inserts were implanted in 30 patients. At a mean follow-up of 30 months (range 23–37 months), they reported that "we have not had material intolerance complications". No subsequent follow-up was found. The second report is that of Field *et al.* (2012), describing the results of a three-year prospective two-center clinical trial of the cementless MITCH PCR cup (Stryker SA, Montreux, Switzerland), that has the horseshoe-shape cup design, as described above. The cup was implanted in 12 men and 13 women with a mean age of 67.9 years (range 57.4–74.9). Taking advantage of the greater strength and lower wear rate of the CFR-PEEK, the cup is only 3 mm thick in the polar region, tapering off to a thickness of 2 mm at the extremity of the horseshoe arms. The cup is cementless, using a coating of hydroxyapatite for fixation and osteointegration. In keeping with the philosophy of approximating physiological stresses and range of motion, the bearing surface diameters were large, 42–52 mm. The results from this trial were disappointing, with five cases of acetabular component migration and calcar resorption observed at three years, and a survivorship of 96% at three years and 88% at four years. The cause of the osteolysis is being investigated (Field *et al.*, 2012). In the same vein, the recently reported evaluation of CRF-PEEK cup and stem fixation in an ovine model by Nakahara *et al.* (2013) may have some bearing. Of the five cementless, hydroxyapatite-coated cups they implanted, only two were found to be well-fixed on manual examination and were observed to exhibit bony ongrowth fixation. Interestingly, all the stems, whether cementless or cemented, exhibited stable fixation.

4.1.2. *Knee*

Little work has been done on PEEK polymers for knee applications. In one of the initial biotribological studies, Wang *et al.* (1999)

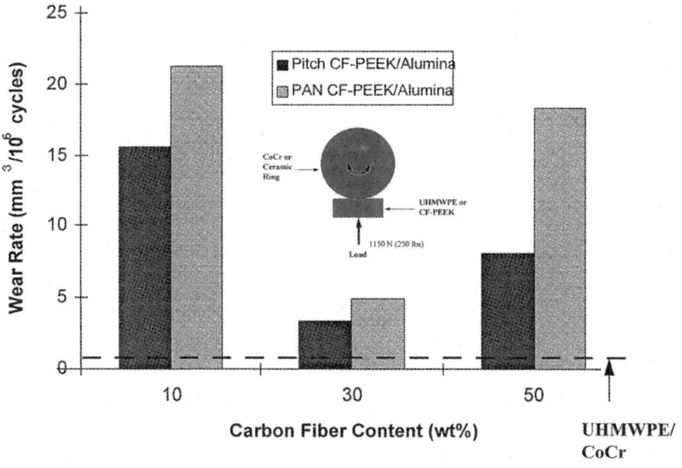

Figure 8-9. Wear rate of CFR-PEEK for various carbon fiber contents, tested in a high stress line contact configuration (inset). The corresponding wear rate for UHMWPE is shown with a dashed line (Wang *et al.*, 1999; Reproduced with permission).

found that both the pitch and CFR-PEEK PAN gave much higher wear rates than UHMWPE when subjected to a high stress non-conforming contact (Figure 8-9). They therefore concluded that these PEEK composites would not be suitable for tibial components in TKR, given their non-congruent contacts (*ibid.*). A decade later, Scholes and Unsworth (2009a) reported on a study in which actual tibial components were tested in a knee simulator. They tested a unicondylar knee based on the Oxford® Partial Knee (Biomet UK Ltd, Bridgend, UK) in which a pitch-based CFR PEEK OPTIMA® mobile tibial meniscal bearing was sandwiched between a CoCrMo femoral component and a CoCrMo tibial component with a flat articular surface. They obtained a mean wear rate of 1.70 mm^3/Mc for the medial bearing and of 1.02 mm^3/Mc for the lateral bearing. The combined medial plus lateral mean wear rate of 2.73 mm^3/Mc compares favorably with the wear rates of metal-on-UHMWPE knee prostheses tested similarly on the same simulator: 3.23 mm^3/Mc for the Kinematic knee and 4.06 mm^3/Mc for the Kinemax knee. However, a comparison with the identical knee design but with an UHMWPE meniscal bearing tested alongside as a control would have been more conclusive. Interestingly, the individual wear curves (wear volume versus cycles) exhibit a step-like wear behavior, as also observed by Brockett *et al.* (2012) when testing CFR-PEEK acetabular cups in a hip wear simulator (see above, under Hip Bearings), suggesting the alternating increase/decrease in wear rates may be an inherent tribological characteristic of CFR-PEEK polymers connected with differential fiber-matrix wear properties.

In contrast to the study by Scholes and Unsworth (2009a), the study by Grupp *et al.* (2010b) focused on the wear performance of a unicondylar knee with a low congruency CFR-PEEK fixed bearing. This knee design (Univation® F, Aesculap AG, Tuttlingen, Germany) was already in clinical use with an UHMWPE tibial insert articulating against a CoCrMo alloy femoral condyle. Performing wear tests in a hip simulator according to ISO 14243-1:2002 (E), Grupp *et al.* (2010b) compared three versions of the unicondylar knee that differed only in the composition of the tibial insert, which was either the intended UHMWPE, pitch CFR-PEEK (CFR-PEEK-Optima LT1 CP 30, Invibio Ltd), or CFR-PEEK PAN (CFR-PEEK-Optima LT1 CA 30, Invibio Ltd). The resulting tibial wear rates were $5.1 \pm 2.3\,\text{mm}^3/\text{Mc}$ for the pitch CFR-PEEK knee, $5.2 \pm 6.9\,\text{mm}^3/\text{Mc}$ for the CFR-PEEK PAN knee, versus $8.6 \pm 2.2\,\text{mm}^3/\text{Mc}$ for the UHMWPE knee. However, the decrease in the wear rates with the CFR-PEEK materials versus UHMWPE achieved only weak statistical significance ($p \geq 0.067$) and the relative variability of the wear rates was higher for the CFR-PEEK materials than for UHMWPE. They also observed the staircase-type wear, in which periods of high and low wear alternated, for nearly every individual CFR-PEEK tibial component. Interestingly, this staircase pattern correlated with the degree of darkening of the serum lubricant. The authors hypothesized that the CRF-PEEK composites are subject to threshold loading conditions that take them from a low wear to a high wear regime, as supported by the large increase in CFR-PEEK wear rates in going for the low stress, high conformity contact of a hip bearing to a high stress line contact, as reported by Wang *et al.* (1999) and described above. Grupp *et al.* (2010b) thus concluded that the CFR-PEEK PAN is unsuitable for low congruency knee bearing applications, and that the pitch CFR-PEEK cannot be recommended because its wear reduction relative to UHMWPE was unconvincing.

In line with the concept that CFR-PEEK composites perform well in conforming contacts, Grupp *et al.* (2012, 2013) subsequently reported on a study evaluating the wear of CFR-PEEK PAN bushings and flanges in a rotating hinge knee EnduRo® AS, Aesculap AG, Germany. Testing in a wear simulator according to ISO 14243-1:2002 (E), the volumetric wear of the CFR-PEEK PAN bushings and flanges articulating against CoCrMo surfaces was 2.3 ± 0.48 mm^3/Mc. The wear decreased to 0.21 ± 0.02 mm^3/Mc when the CoCrMo surfaces were coated with zirconium nitride (ZrN). No macroscopic surface fatigue was observed on CFR-PEEK components. The wear particles generated against the ZrN surface had a larger mean diameter (1.89 ± 2.54 μm) and lower elongation (2.23 ± 1.60 μm) than those generated against the CoCrMo surface (mean diameter 0.82 ± 1.80 μm, elongation 3.29 ± 2.52 μm), but the authors concluded that these differences were not significant, presumably based on statistical considerations. Data for a control using UHMWPE bushings and flanges was not provided.

4.1.3. *Spine*

Arthroplasty of spinal motion segments entails the replacement of the disk (or nucleus) between two vertebrae with artificial devices to recreate the normal kinematics and biomechanics of the degenerated segment. It is considered an alternative treatment for patients who would otherwise require spinal fusion (Uschold *et al.*, 2012). The proposed advantage of arthroplasty over standard fusion techniques is the preservation of motion, which is thought to reduce the development of adjacent level disk disease. Although cadaveric testing has provided compelling evidence for such hypothesis, definitive conclusions are limited due to insufficient clinical evidence (*ibid.*).

Disk arthroplasty devices mimic the kinematics of the motion segment but not the biomechanics of the natural disk. Attempts to simulate the natural disk by a flexible elastomeric device failed clinically and led to its removal from the market (Fraser *et al.*, 2004). Hence, an alternative approach has been to borrow the concept of sliding rotational bearings from joint replacement. From a biotribological perspective, it is important to recognize that the intervertebral disk space provides a different biological environment than that of synovial joints, which may impact lubrication and wear. Also, the proximity to neurological structures calls for particular attention to wear debris and its biologic reactions.

Articular surfaces of disk replacement devices include a variety of materials. Sekhon *et al.* (2007) found that devices composed of CoCrMo alloy obscured imaging compared with titanium or polymer alternatives. This may explain the popularity of PEEK in the area of disk arthroplasty. In 2006, on behalf of Pioneer Surgical Technology (Marquette, USA), a series of wear experiments were conducted on self-mating PEEK nucleus replacement devices in the MAW laboratory. The NUBAC™ prosthesis is a semi-constrained, two-piece inner articulating ball-and-socket joint manufactured from PEEK OPTIMA® (Invibio, Ltd.). Six prostheses were mounted on a servo-hydraulic Endolab spine simulator (Figure 8-10), and tested in close agreement with ISO/DIS 18192-1:2007(E) in a bovine serum (20 g/l) testing fluid. The parameter which differed from ISO was the

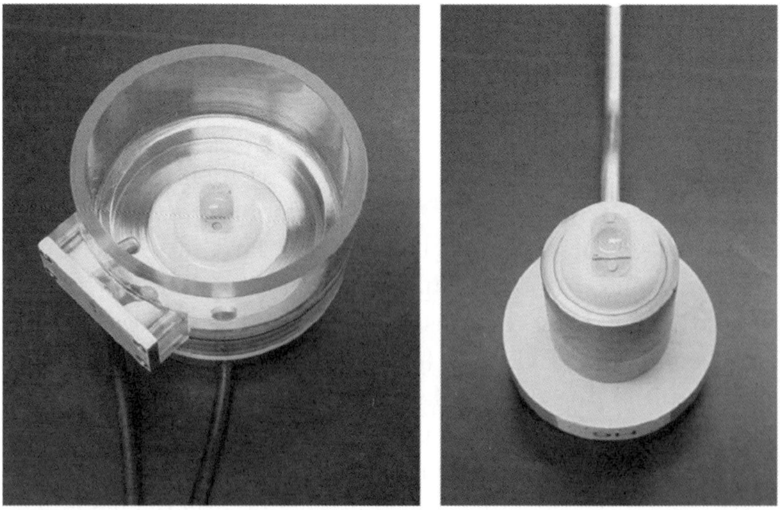

Figure 8-10. Fully assembled and potted NUBAC™ prosthesis, ready for testing.

maximum load, which was reduced from 2000 to 1024 N to represent the physiological load sharing mechanism between the annulus and nucleus in the lumbar intervertebral disk. Tests were run at 2 Hz up to 10 Mc and stopped every 0.5 Mc to measure weight loss. Wear-in behavior was observed for all specimens from 0 to 1 Mc. Thereafter, the implants experienced a constant average total wear rate of 0.40 ± 0.03 mm^3/Mc. The contact surfaces showed evidence of highly polished areas, mild burnishing, and light surface scratches. No delamination or pitting was observed, and signs of major adhesive wear were absent (Schwenke *et al.*, 2007).

In a second experiment, the same parameter setting was applied, except for a slight frequency shift, which guaranteed changing motion trajectories on the articulating surfaces (Nechtow *et al.*, 2006). With 0.46 ± 0.01 mm^3/Mc the generated wear rate was only slightly higher and was not significantly different from the one with fixed crossing motion trajectories reported above.

Finally, in a third test, the susceptibility of PEEK wear to aging was investigated (Wimmer *et al.*, 2008). The simulated aging process was similar to ASTM F2003-02, which has been developed to measure accelerated degradation of UHMWPE packaged in air, except that the aging time within the oxygen bomb (5 atm at 70°C) was extended from 14 to 40 days. As expected (because of the known chemical stability of PEEK), the wear rate was not much affected by aging and increased to approximately 0.8 mm^3/Mc during the first 5 Mc but reached levels of unaged PEEK during the subsequent 5–10 Mc interval. The state of soaking actually seemed to play a bigger role than aging, as suggested by the decrease in wear after a compulsory break at 5 Mc (Figure 8-11). Brown *et al.* (2010) published the above data in a peer-reviewed journal. The authors concluded that the wear rates were quite insensitive to changes in testing parameters and "compare well with the reported wear rates of other material combinations used in nucleus replacement and total disc arthroplasty". Using the same simulator, UHMWPE/CoCrMo and CoCrMo/CoCrMo ball-in-socket disk arthroplasty devices were also measured. Following the ISO protocol, wear rates of 4 mm^3/Mc and 0.2 mm^3/Mc were obtained. Of course, this comparison has to be

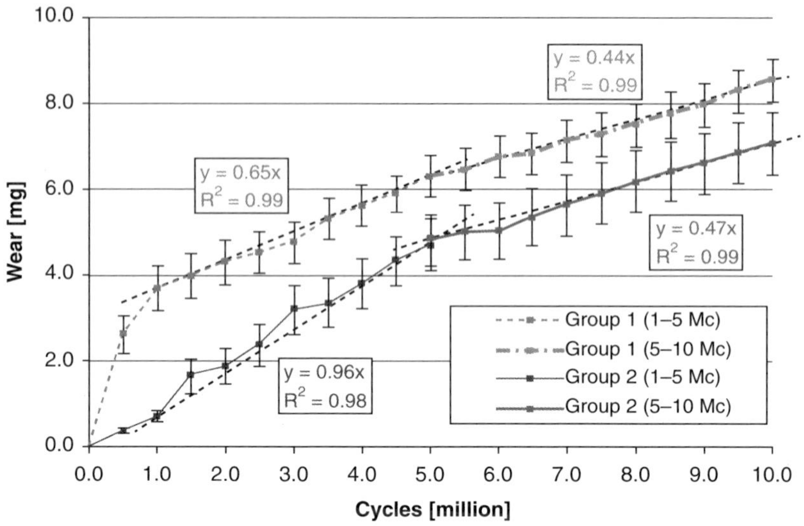

Figure 8-11. Weight loss plots (in mg) of 30 kGy sterilized (Group 1) and 200 kGy sterilized plus aged (Group 2) PEEK NUBAC^{TM} components. Wear tests were interrupted at 5 million cycles and paused for 28 weeks. Components were stored in 37°C saline solution until testing was resumed. Regression slopes for each group and respective wear interval are plotted suggesting a slight wear decrease with soaking state.

taken with a pinch of salt, since the latter devices have seen the actual ISO testing parameters and thus about twice the amount of load.

Brown and Bao (2012) also published about self-mating PEEK for cervical disk arthroplasty. The compressive loads in the cervical spine are much lower and are applied in the range of 0–150 N using ASTM and ISO testing profiles. Applying different test frequencies and protein levels (0–20 g/l) in the test medium, the authors found that both lower test frequencies and lower protein contents increased wear. Except in the case of a pilot test, where the test medium contained no EDTA, all five testing groups showed relatively benign material loss (range 0.26–1.23 mm^3/Mc). The specimens in the pilot group failed after just 0.5 MC with significant surface destruction. The authors speculated that due to the absence of EDTA, Ca^{2+}/protein complexes may have formed and were trapped inside the bearing, which ultimately caused its failure.

A similar study was performed by Kraft *et al.* (2012). Using a similar ball-and-socket bearing as the one explored in the above study, Kraft and colleagues tested PEEK-on-PEEK bearing couples with large and small radial clearances using the ISO standard 18192-1. Load and motion profiles of both cervical and lumbar disks were explored. The lubricant contained 30 g/l protein and 20 mmol/l EDTA. To the surprise of the investigators, the bearings failed with severe surface damage. While thermal effects were ruled out in the course of the experiment, an explanation why these results differed from those of Brown *et al.* (2010) was not provided. Interestingly, a change of the wear test parameters from cervical to lumbar conditions (i.e. a ten-fold load increase and a decrease in motion) lessened wear and degradation of the bearing surfaces.

Grupp *et al.* (2010a) also found that neat PEEK-on-PEEK has a tendency towards pitting and delamination when tested according to ISO guidelines as a cervical disk replacement. However, not all tested samples developed that problem and, as a group, the wear rate of the PEEK-on-PEEK prototype was insignificantly higher than that of the currently clinically used device (active® C, Aesculap AG) with a UHMWPE/CoCrMo ball and socket joint. In contrast, self-mating PAN carbon fiber-reinforced PEEK prototypes showed excellent tribological characteristics and "have a high potential for next generation disk replacements" (*ibid.*).

5. Biologic Response of Wear Particles

PEEK and PEEK composite materials have been found to be biocompatible and bioinert in bulk form, as determined through implantation in animal models (Jockisch *et al.*, 1992; Williams *et al.*, 1987), and the interaction of the surfaces of these materials with cells, typically fibroblasts and/or osteoblasts (Hunter *et al.*, 1995; Lin *et al.*, 1997; Sagomonyants *et al.*, 2008; Scotchford *et al.*, 2003; Wenz *et al.*, 1990). Extracts from bulk PEEK (Morrison *et al.*, 1995; Wenz *et al.*, 1990) or finely cut PEEK material (Katzer *et al.*, 2002) have also been found to have low to negligible cytoxicity. For example, Morrison *et al.* (1995) examined the effect of extracts from disks made of PEEK with and without carbon fiber reinforcement on cultured fibroblasts and osteoblasts, and concluded that the PEEK material did not exhibit overt signs of cytotoxicity, and actually increased osteoblast cell protein content. As this chapter examines tribological aspects, the focus will be on the bioactivity of wear debris particulates from PEEK biomaterials. For the interested reader, comprehensive reviews on the biocompatibility of PEEK biomaterials can be found elsewhere (Toth *et al.*, 2012; Medical PEEK Lexicon, available at: http://www.medicalpeek.org/lexicon/bearings).

In an *in vitro* study to investigate the biological response to wear debris from various carbon-based composite materials, Howling *et al.* (2003) found that wear particles from 30% CFR-PEEK PAN were not cytotoxic to L929 fibroblasts and U937 monocytic cells in culture. The wear particles were generated by sliding the polymer pins against a smooth alumina counterface in a pin-on-flat configuration, with 25% bovine serum as the lubricant. Unfortunately, the particle size and morphology were not specified. In a study of innate immune reactions to particle challenges, Hallab *et al.* (2012) evaluated the responses of human monocyte and macrophage cells subjected to PEEK–OPTIMA, UHMWPE, and highly crosslinked UHMWPE (HXPE) particles. They used particles of three mean sizes (0.7 μm, 2 μm, and 10 μm), generated by cryopulverization, and subjected the cells to a dose of 20 particles/cell and exposures of 24 to 48 hours. Cell responses were measured using cytotoxicity, viability and proliferation assays, and cytokine analysis. They found that PEEK–OPTIMA particles were less cytotoxic to macrophages than UHMWPE and HXPE particles, with the 0.7 μm UHMWPE particles being the most cytotoxic. The PEEK–OPTIMA particles were significantly less inflammatory than UHMWPE and HXPE at the 24-hour point, whereas no significant differences were observed at 48 hours. Interestingly, for HXPE, the smaller, 0.7 μm particles elicited a lower cytokine response than the 2 and 10 μm particles. Perhaps this large particle effect is connected with the particle dosing method used in this study, which is based on a constant number of particles per cell, rather than based on a constant total volume of particles, as found in some other studies (Lorber *et al.*, 2014;

Utzschneider *et al.*, 2010). While cautioning on the limitations of *in vitro* analysis, the authors conclude that PEEK–OPTIMA (R) debris does not present a greater inflammatory risk than UHMWPE debris.

The biological response of cells to particles is complex and at present insufficiently understood (Purdue *et al.*, 2007). Many cells like T-lymphocytes, fibroblasts, mast cells, macrophages, plasma cells, neutrophils, endothelial cells, osteoclasts, and osteoblasts are involved in the reaction to wear particles. For this reason, not only cell studies but also *in vivo* studies are needed to analyze the complex cellular interactions with wear particles. As part of a comprehensive set of pre-clinical studies to validate the MITCH PCR cup, Latif *et al.* (2008) reported on the biocompatibility of CFR-PEEK particles evaluated in a rat-pouch model. Although inflammation in the pouches subjected to CFR-PEEK particles exceeded that of the control pouches, it was less than in the pouches subjected to polyethylene particles. However, the three treatments (CFR-PEEK, polyethylene, and control) did not differ significantly with respect to the thickening of the fibrous tissue and macrophage infiltration. The authors concluded that the effect of the CFR-PEEK and polyethylene particles were similar, but pointed out that the wear rate of CFR-PEEK is an order of magnitude less than that of polyethylene, as determined from hip simulator wear tests (*ibid.*), and therefore the biological load from the PEEK debris is presumably correspondingly less.

In one study by the present authors, the inflammatory reaction of two different kinds of CFR-PEEK and UHMWPE wear particles in the murine knee joint was quantified (Utzschneider *et al.*, 2010). Particles were generated using a cryopulverization process under liquid nitrogen. Particle size and shape distribution was matched with those from a knee simulator experiment. In this test, the tibial inserts were made from UHMWPE (GUR 1020) and PEEK (PEEK-Optima LT1, Invibio Ltd. Thornton-Cleveleys, UK) with either a carbon fiber reinforcement of 30% pitch- or 30% PAN-based carbon fibers. The experimental inserts were then articulated in 24 UnivationF® knee prostheses (Aesculap, Germany) on a four-station knee simulator (EndoLab GmbH, Germany) for over 5 million cycles according to ISO 14243-1:2002. Wear particles were separated from the lubricant using acid digestion and imaged by scanning electron microscopy. Based on the determined particle size and shape, sterile polymer particles were generated using the above described cryopulverization process, avoiding side effects due to endotoxin. Then, a 50 μl particle suspension of the particulate biomaterials in phosphate-buffered saline (PBS) was injected intra-articularly in the left knee joints of female BALB/c mice under sterile conditions. For the control group, only PBS was injected. Intravital fluorescence microscopy as well as histological evaluation of the synovial layer was performed to assess the synovial microcirculation seven days after particle injection. Enhanced leukocyte-endothelial cell interactions, an increase of functional capillary density as well as histological investigations revealed that all tested biomaterials cause a significantly increased inflammatory reaction compared to the control animals, but without any significant difference between tested biomaterials (Utzschneider *et al.*, 2010).

To validate these results, the cytokine expression (IL-1β, IL-6, TNF-α) in the synovial layer, the adjacent bone marrow of the femur and tibia as well as the articular cartilage was analyzed (Lorber *et al.*, 2014). Considering the use of unicompartmental knee replacements, the analysis of cartilage is particularly important, as intact remaining cartilage is mainly responsible for any long-term success. While there was no difference between CFR-PEEK pitch, CFR-PEEK-PAN, and UHMWPE with regards to the leucocyte–endothelial cell interactions and histological parameters, elevated cytokine secretions were detectable (*ibid.*). Especially in the adjacent bone of the two CFR-PEEK varieties, significantly increased cytokine expressions compared to the control and UHMWPE group were found. Furthermore, the data showed that CFR-PEEK pitch caused a significantly higher level of cytokine expression in the articular cartilage (Figure 8-12). As potential bearing material in unicondylar knee replacements, CFR-PEEK pitch wear particles might provoke the destruction of the remaining cartilage. However, these data need further investigation.

Elevated levels of IL-1β and TNF-α found in the adjacent bone indicate that wear particles reacted with these cells within one week.

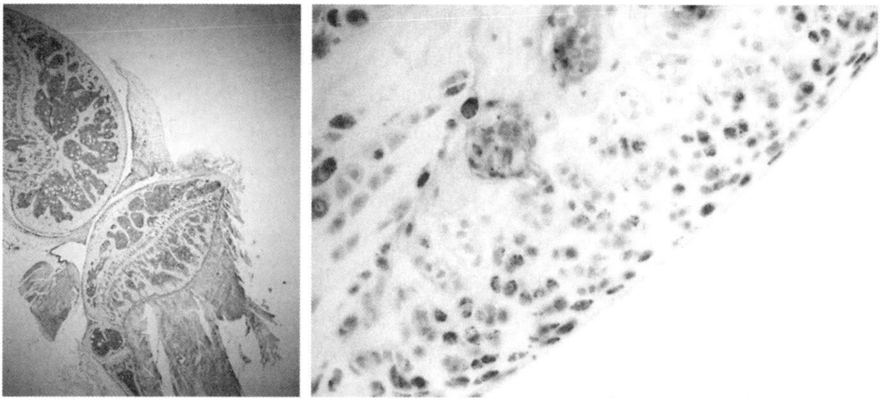

Figure 8-12. Overview of the inflammatory reaction in a murine knee joint after injection of CFR-PEEK pitch particles (left), and detail of the femoral condyle (right). Reddish appearing cells inside the cartilage stained positively for IL-6 expression.

Since the wear particles were injected intra-articularly, the particles had to migrate or were actively being transported into the bone. Concerning the mechanism of migration or transport of wear particles to the implant-bone-interface, there are various theories (Libouban *et al.*, 2009; Massin *et al.*, 2004; Schmalzried *et al.*, 1997), but this would need further investigation for this particular model. Compared to the UHMWPE group, the CFR-PEEK pitch and the CFR-PEEK PAN group caused a higher degree of inflammation in the adjacent bone. The reasons for this are not fully understood, but it is important to take note of the proinflammatory potential of PEEK wear debris. The specific *in vivo* model was introduced to measure leucocyte–endothelial cell interactions concerning inflammatory reactions to wear particles using intravital-fluorescence microscopy. Direct effects on the bone metabolism cannot be assessed with this model. This is a major limitation of the study, including that all conclusions are drawn based on inflammatory cytokine expressions. Nevertheless, knowing these mediators are the key factors in aseptic loosening (Chiu *et al.*, 2009; Holt *et al.*, 2007), such an approach seems to be justified.

The study by Lorber *et al.* (2014), is a reminder of the difficulty in thoroughly assessing biocompatibility outside human *in vivo* conditions. This difficulty is inevitable because biocompatiblity, like wear, is a system property, and thus must be ultimately evaluated in the actual system. Although these *in vitro* and *in vivo* studies are crucial first steps toward establishing the clinical suitability of using the PEEK bearing surfaces, the biocompatiblity of the PEEK materials can only be assessed definitively through clinical trials and sustained follow-up of PEEK devices after limited release. Based on recent experience with the large head metal-on-metal hips, such follow-up should have a duration of at least five years before the device is introduced on a widespread scale.

References

Austin, H., Powell, M., Medley, J. and Langohr, D. (2009). Exploring the wear of a PEEK all-polymer articulation for spinal applications, *Trans Soc Biomater*, San Antonio, 77.

Balsano, M., Zachos, A., Ruggiu, A., Barca, F., Tranquilli-Leali, P. and Doria, C. (2011). Nucleus disc arthroplasty with the NUBAC^{TM} device: 2-year clinical experience, *Eur Spine J*, **20**(Suppl 1), 36–40.

Birken, L. (2003). *Verschleißverhalten eigenfaserverstärkter Polyethylenwerkstoffe für tibiale Komponenten nicht-konformer totaler Knieendoprothesen*, Shaker, Aachen.

Borruto, A. (2010). A new material for hip prosthesis without considerable debris release, *Med Eng Phys*, **32**(8), 908–913.

Brantigan, J.W. and Lauryssen, C. (2006). *Intervertebral Fusion Using Carbon Fiber reinforced Polymer Implants*, CRC Press, St. Louis.

Brockett, C.L., John, G., Williams, S., Jin, Z., Isaac, G.H. and Fisher, J. (2012). Wear of ceramic-on-carbon fiber-reinforced poly-ether ether ketone hip replacements, *J Biomed Mater Res Part B*, **100**, 1459–1465.

Brown, T. and Bao, Q.B. (2012). The use of self-mating PEEK as an alternative bearing material for cervical disc arthroplasty: A comparison of different simulator inputs and tribological environments, *Eur Spine J*, **21**(Suppl 5), 717–726.

Brown, T., Bao, Q.B., Kilpela, T. and Songer, M. (2010). An *in vitro* biotribological assessment of NUBAC, a polyetheretherketone-on-polyetheretherketone articulating nucleus replacement device: Methodology and results from a series of wear tests using different motion profiles, test frequencies, and environmental conditions, *Spine*, **35**, 774–781.

Chiu, R., Ma, T., Smith, R.L. and Goodman, S.B. (2009). Ultrahigh molecular weight polyethylene wear debris inhibits osteoprogenitor proliferation and differentiation *in vitro* , *J Biomed Mat Res*, Part A, **89**(1), 242–247.

Corvelli, A.A., Biermann, P.J. and Roberts, J.C. (1997). Design, analysis, and fabrication of a composite segmental bone replacement implant, *J Adv Mater*, **28**, 2–8.

Crosbie, S.H., Felt, J.C., Mehawej, J.P., Markman, D.A. and Rydell, M.A. (2013). Particulate and gravimetric wear rate analysis and flexural fatigue testing of a PEEK medial knee interpositional arthroplasty implant, *Int PEEK Meet 2013*, Philadelphia.

Dawson, P.C. and Blundell, D.J. (1980). X-ray data for Poly(aryl-ether-ketones), *Polymer*, **21**(5), 577–578.

Dumbleton, J.H., D'Antonio, J.A., Manley, M.T., Capello, W.N. and Wang, A. (2006) The basis for a second-generation highly cross-linked UHMWPE, *Clin Orthop Relat R*, **453**, 265–71.

East, R., Briscoe, A., Jarman-Smith, M., Simpson, D., Collins, S. and Unsworth, A. (2013). The wear of CFR-PEEK and PEEK OPTIMA articulating against HXLPE, *Int PEEK Meet 2013*, Philadelphia.

Field, R.E., Rajakulendran, K., Eswaramoorthy, V.K. and Rushton, N. (2012). Three-year prospective clinical and radiological results of a new flexible horseshoe acetabular cup, *Hip Int*, **22**(6), 598–606.

Flöck, J., Friedrich, K. and Yuan, Q. (1999). On the friction and wear behaviour of PAN- and pitch-carbon fiber reinforced PEEK composites, *Wear*, **225–229**, 304–311.

Förster, A., Große, L. and Melzer, C. (2003). Ergebnisse des endoprothetischen Ersatzes der MCP-sowie PIP-Gelenke durch zementfreie Fingerendoprothesen der Firma MATHYS, *DGOOC*, Berlin (available at: http://www.egms.de/en/meetings/dgu2003/03dgu0746.shtml) [Accessed July 26, 2014].

Fraser, R.D., Ross, E.R., Lowery, G.L., Freeman, B.J. and Dolan, M. (2004). AcroFlex design and results, *Spine J*, **4**(6 Suppl), 245–251.

Friedrich, K., Karger-Kocsis, J. and Lu, Z. (1991). Effects of counterpart roughness and temperature on friction and wear of PEEK-composites, *Wear*, **148**, 235–247.

Friedrich, K., Lu, Z. and Hager, A.M. (1995). Recent advances in polymer composites' tribology, *Wear*, **190**, 139–144.

Gao, S.L. and Kim, J.K. (2000). Cooling rate influences in carbon fibre/PEEK composites. Part I. Crystallinity and interface adhesion, *Composites A*, **31**, 517–530.

Gao, S.L. and Kim, J.K. (2001). Cooling rate influences in carbon fibre/PEEK composites. Part II: Interlaminar fracture toughness, *Composites A*, **32**, 763–774.

Geerdink, C.H., Grimm, B., Ramakrishnan, R., Rondhuis, J., Verburg, A.J. and Tonino, A.J. (2006). Crosslinked polyethylene compared to conventional polyethylene in total hip replacement: Pre-clinical evaluation, *in vitro* testing and prospective clinical follow-up study, *Acta Orthop*, **77**(5), 719–725.

Geringer, J., Tatkiewicz, W. and Rouchouse, G. (2011). Wear behavior of PAEK, poly (aryl-ether-ketone), under physiological conditions, outlooks for performing these materials in the field of hip prosthesis, *Wear*, **271**, 2793–2803.

Green, S. (2012). Compounds and Composite Materials. Chapter 3, in Kurtz, S.M. (ed), *PEEK Biomaterials Handbook*, Elsevier, Boston, 23–48.

Grupp, T.M., Giurea, A., Miehlke, R.K., Hintner, M., Gaisser, M., Schilling, C. *et al.* (2013). Biotribology of a new bearing material combination in a rotating hinge knee articulation, *Acta Biomater*, **9**(6), 7054–7063.

Grupp, T.M., Meisel, H.J., Cotton, J.A., Schwiesau, J., Fritz, B., Blömer, W. *et al.* (2010a). Alternative bearing materials for intervertebral disc arthroplasty, *Biomaterials*, **31**(3), 523–531.

Grupp, T.M., Utzschneider, S., Giurea, A., Miehlke, R.K., Schwiesau, J., Fritz, B. *et al.* (2012). *In vitro* and *in vivo* characterisation of a new bearing material for a rotating hinge knee, *J Biomech*, **45**(Suppl 1), 80.

Grupp, T.M., Utzschneider, S., Schröder, C., Schwiesau, J., Fritz, B., Maas, A. *et al.* (2010b). Biotribology of alternative bearing materials for unicompartmental knee arthroplasty, *Acta Biomater*, **6**(9), 3601–3610.

Hallab, N.J., McAllister, K., Brady, M. and Jarman-Smith, M. (2012). Macrophage reactivity to different polymers demonstrates particle size- and material-specific reactivity: PEEK-OPTIMA® particles versus UHMWPE particles in the submicron, micron, and 10 micron size ranges, *J Biomed Mater Res B*, **100**, 480–492.

Holt, G., Murnaghan, C., Reilly, J. and Meek, R.M. (2007). The biology of aseptic osteolysis, *Clin Orthop Relat R*, **460**, 240–252.

Howling, G.I., Sakoda, H., Antonarulrajah, A., Marrs, H., Stewart, T.D., Appleyard, S. *et al.* (2003). Biological response to wear debris generated in carbon based composites as potential bearing surfaces for artificial hip joints, *J Biomed Mater Res B*, **67**(2), 758–764.

Hunter, A., Archer, C.W., Walker, P.S. and Blunn, G.W. (1995). Attachment and proliferation of osteoblasts and fibroblasts on biomaterials for orthopaedic use, *Biomaterials*, **16**(4), 287–295.

International Standard ISO 14243 (2002). *Implants for surgery — wear of total knee-joint-prostheses — Part 1: Loading and displacement parameters for wear-testing machines with load control and corresponding enviromental conditions for tests.*

Jockisch, K.A., Brown, S.A., Bauer, T.W. and Merritt, K. (1992). Biological response to chopped-carbon-fiber-reinforced PEEK, *J Biomed Mater Res*, **26**(2), 133–146.

Johnson, A.J., Loving, L., Herrera, L., Delanois, R.E., Wang, A. and Mont, M.A. (2014) Short-term wear evaluation of thin acetabular liners on 36 mm femoral heads, *Clin Orthop Relat R*, **472**(2), 624–629.

Joyce, T., Rieker, C. and Unsworth, A. (2006). Comparative *in vitro* testing of PEEK and UHMWPE capped metacarpophalangeal prostheses, *Biomed Mat Eng*, **16**, 1–10.

Karpe, P., Purushothaman, B., Berg, A., Reddy, G., Bhatia, C. and Friesem, T. (2013). Randomized control trial comparing prestige and nunec cervical disc arthroplasty, *ISASS 2013*, Vancouver.

Katzer, A., Marquardt, H., Westendorf, J., Wening, J.V. and von Foerster, G. (2002). Polyetheretherketone-cytotoxicity and mutagenicity *in vitro*, *Biomaterials*, **23**(8), 1749–1759.

Kinkel, S., Lehner, B., Kleinhans, J.A., Jakubowitz, E., Ewerbeck, V. and Heisel, C. (2009). Medium to long-term results after reconstruction of bone defects at the knee with tumor endoprostheses, *J Surg Oncol*, **101**, 166–169.

Klesey, D.J., Springer, C.S. and Goodman, S.B. (1997). Composite implants for bone replacement, *J Compos Mater*, **31**(16), 1593–1632.

Korduba, L.A. and Wang, A. (2011). The effect of cross-shear on the wear of virgin and highly-crosslinked polyethylene, *Wear*, **271**, 1220–1223.

Kraft, M., Koch, D.K. and Bushelow, M. (2012). An investigation into PEEK-on-PEEK as a bearing surface candidate for cervical total disc replacement, *Spine J*, **12**, 603–611.

Kumar, S. and Anderson, D.P. (1986). Crystallisation and morphology of poly(aryl-ether-etherketone), *Polymer*, **27**, 329.

Kurtz, S.M. and Devine, J.N. (2007). PEEK biomaterials in trauma, orthopedic, and spinal implants, *Biomaterials*, **28**, 4845–4869.

Kurtz, S.M. and Nevelos, J. (2012). Arthroplasty Bearing Surfaces, Chapter 16, in Kurtz, S.M. (ed), *PEEK Biomaterials Handbook*, Elsevier, Boston, 261–275.

Lancaster, J.K. (1986). Composites for aerospace dry bearing applications, in Friedrich, K. (ed), *Friction and Wear of Polymer Composites*, Elsevier, Amsterdam, 363–396.

Latif, A.M., Mehats, A., Elcocks, M., Rushton, N., Field, R.E. and Jones, E. (2008). Pre-clinical studies to validate the MITCH PCRTM Cup: A flexible and anatomically shaped acetabular component with novel bearing characteristics, *J Mater Sci Mater Med*, **19**(4), 1729–1736.

Laurent, M.P., Johnson, T.S., Crowninshield, R.D., Blanchard, C.R., Bhambri, S.K. and Yao, J.Q. (2008). Characterization of a highly cross-linked ultra-high molecular-weight polyethylene in clinical use in total hip arthroplasty, *J Arthroplasty*, **23**(5), 751–761.

Liao, K. (1994). Performance characterization and modeling of a composite hip prosthesis, *Exp Techniques*, **18**, 33–38.

Libouban, H., Massin, P., Gaudin, C., Mercier, P., Basle, M.F. and Chappard, D. (2009). Migration of wear debris of polyethylene depends on bone microarchitecture, *J Biomed Mater Res B Appl Biomater*, **90**(2), 730–737.

Lin, T.W., Corvelli, A.A., Frondoza, C.G., Roberts, J.C. and Hungerford, D.S. (1997). Glass peek composite promotes proliferation and osteocalcin production of human osteoblastic cells, *J Biomed Mater Res*, **36**(2), 137–144.

Lorber, V., Paulus, A.C., Buschmann, A., Schmitt, B., Grupp, T.M., Jansson, V. and Utzschneider, S. (2014). Elevated cytokine expression of different PEEK wear particles compared to UHMWPE *in vivo*, *J Mater Sci Mater Med*, **25**(1), 141–149.

Lu, Z.P. and Friedrich, K. (1995). On sliding friction and wear of PEEK and its composites, *Wear*, **181–183**, 624–631.

Maharaj, G.R. and Jamison, R.D. (1993). Intraoperative impact: Characterization and laboratory simulation on composite hip prosthesis, in Jamison, R.D. and Gilbertson, L.N. (eds), *STP 1178: Composite materials for implant applications in the human body; characterization and testing*, ASTM, Philadelphia, 98–108.

Marques, N. and Davim, J.P. (2012). Tribological behaviour of peek (poly-ether-ether-ketone) materials to biomedical applications, in Davim, J.P. (ed), *Biomedical Tribology*, Nova Science Publishers, New York, 159–168.

Massin, P., Chappard, D., Flautre, B. and Hardouin, P. (2004). Migration of polyethylene particles around nonloosened cemented femoral components from a total hip arthroplasty-an autopsy study, *J Biomed Mater Res B Appl Biomater*, **69**(2), 205–215.

May, R. (1988). Polyetheretherketones, in Mark, H.K., Bikales, N.M., Overberger, C.G., Menges, G. and Kroschiwitz, J.I. (eds), *Encyclopedia of Polymer Science and Engineering*. Wiley, New York, 313–320.

McKellop, H.A., Shen, F., Campbell, P. and Ota, T. (1999a). Effect of molecular weight, calcium stearate, and sterilization methods on the wear of ultra high molecular weight polyethylene acetabular cups in a hip joint simulator, *J Orthop Res*, **17**(3), 329–339.

McKellop, H., Shen, F.W., Lu, B., Campbell, P. and Salovey, R. (1999b). Development of an extremely wear-resistant ultra high molecular weight polyethylene for total hip replacements, *J Orthop Res*, **17**(2), 157–167.

Middleton, A., Lakshmipathy, R. and Irwin, L.R. (2011). Failures of the RM finger prosthesis joint replacement system, *J Hand Surg Eur*, **36**(7), 599–604.

Moore, R., Beredjiklian, P., Rhoad, R., Theiss, S., Cuckler, J., Ducheyne, P. *et al.* (1997). A comparison of the inflammatory potential of particulates derived from two composite materials, *J Biomed Mater Res*, **34**(2), 137–147.

Morrison, C., Macnair, R., MacDonald, C., Wykman, A., Goldie, I. and Grant, M.H. (1995). *In vitro* biocompatibility testing of polymers for orthopaedic implants using cultured fibroblasts and osteoblasts, *Biomaterials*, **16**(13), 987–992.

Muratoglu, O.K., Bragdon, C.R., O'Connor, D., Perinchief, R.S., Estok, D.M., Jasty, M. *et al.* (2001). Larger diameter femoral heads used in conjunction with a highly cross-linked ultra-high molecular weight polyethylene: A new concept, *J Arthroplasty*, **16**(Suppl 1), 24–30.

Nakahara, I., Takao, M., Bandoh, S., Bertollo, N., Walsh, W.R. and Sugano, N. (2013). *In vivo* implant fixation of carbon fiber-reinforced PEEK hip prostheses in an ovine model, *J Orthop Res*, **31**(3), 485–492.

Nechtow, W., Hintner, M., Bushelow, M. and Kaddick, C. (2006). IVD replacement mechanical performance depends strongly on input parameters, *Transactions ORS*, **31**, 118.

Pace, N., Spurio, S. and Rizzato, G. (2004). Clinical trial of a new CF16-PEEK acetabular insert in hip arthroplasty, *Hip Int*, **14**(2), 132–133.

Purdue, P.E., Koulouvaris, P., Potter, H.G., Nestor, B.J. and Sculco, T.P. (2007). The cellular and molecular biology of periprosthetic osteolysis, *Clin Orthop Relat R*, **454**(1), 251–261.

Rasheva, Z., Zhang, G. and Burkhart, T. (2010). A correlation between the tribological and mechanical properties of short carbon fibers reinforced PEEK materials with different fiber orientations, *Tribol Int*, **43**, 1430–1437.

Reigstad, O., Lütken, T., Grimsgaard, C., Bolstad, B., Thorkildsen, R. and Røkkum, M. (2012). Promising one- to six-year results with the Motec wrist arthroplasty in patients with post-traumatic osteoarthritis, *J Bone Joint Surg Br*, **94**(11), 1540–1545.

Richter, K., Jäckle, T. and Ganzer, D. (2003). Vergleich zweier Endoprothesentypen bei der Versorgung der MCP- und PIP-Gelenke der Rheumatischen Hand, *DGOOC 2003*, Berlin.

Rieker, C.B., Joyce, T., Unsworth, A., Hagena, F.W. and Meuli, C. (2003). Tribologic investigation of a metacarpophalangeal prosthesis, *Orthopäde*, **32**, 784–788.

De Ruiter, L., Janssen, D., Briscoe, A. and Verdonschot, N. (2014). A biomechanical analysis of a PEEK-Optima® femoral component on implant fixation construct integrity and bone remodeling opportunities in total knee arthroplasty, *Trans ORS*, **39**, 860.

Sagomonyants, K.B., Jarman-Smith, M.L., Devine, J.N., Aronow, M.S. and Gronowicz, G.A. (2008). The *in vitro* response of human osteoblasts to polyetheretherketone (PEEK) substrates compared to commercially pure titanium, *J Biomaterials*, **29**(11), 1563–1572.

Saikko, V. (2005). A 12-station anatomic hip joint simulator, *Proc Inst Mech Eng H*, **219**, 437–448.

Saikko, V. (2006). Effect of contact pressure on wear and friction of ultra-high molecular weight polyethylene in multidirectional sliding, *Proc Inst Mech Eng H*, **220**, 723–731.

Schmalzried, T.P., Campbell, P., Schmitt, A.K., Brown, I.C. and Amstutz, H.C. (1997). Shapes and dimensional characteristics of polyethylene wear particles generated *in vivo* by total knee replacements compared to total hip replacements, *J Biomed Mat Res*, **38**(3), 203–210.

Scholes, S.C. and Unsworth, A. (2007). The wear properties of CFR-PEEK-OPTIMA articulating against ceramic assessed on a multidirectional pin-on-plate machine, *Proc Inst Mech Eng H*, **221**(3), 281–289.

Scholes, S.C. and Unsworth, A. (2009a). Pitch-based carbon-fibre-reinforced poly (ether-ether-ketone) OPTIMA assessed as a bearing material in a mobile bearing unicondylar knee joint, *Proc Inst Mech Eng H*, **223**(1), 13–25.

Scholes, S.C. and Unsworth, A. (2009b). Wear studies on the likely performance of CFR-PEEK/CoCrMo for use as artificial joint bearing materials, *J Mater Sci Mater Med*, **20**(1), 163–170.

Scholes, S.C. and Unsworth, A. (2010). The wear performance of PEEK-OPTIMA based self-mating couples, *Wear*, **268**, 380–387.

Scholes, S.C., Inman, I.A., Unsworth, A. and Jones, E. (2008). Tribological assessment of a flexible carbon-fibre-reinforced poly(ether-ether-ketone) acetabular cup articulating against an alumina femoral head, *Proc Inst Mech Eng H*, **222**(3), 273–283.

Schwenke, T., Brown, T., Bao, Q., Kilpel, T. and Wimmer, M.A. (2007). Wear assessment of a self-mating polymer for nucleus replacement devices, *Transaction ORS*, **32**, 1125.

Scotchford, C.A., Garle, M.J., Batchelor, J., Bradley, J. and Grant, D.M. (2003). Use of a novel carbon fibre composite material for the femoral stem component of a THR system: *In vitro* biological assessment, *Biomaterials*, **24**, 4871–4879.

Sekhon, L.H., Duggal, N., Lynch, J.J., Haid, R.W., Heller, J.G., Riew, K.D. *et al.* (2007). Magnetic resonance imaging clarity of the Bryan, Prodisc-C, Prestige LP, and PCM cervical arthroplasty devices, *Spine J*, **32**(6), 673–680.

Skinner, H.B. (1988). Composite technology for total hip arthroplasty, *Clin Orthop Relat R*, **235**, 224–236.

Toth, J.M. (2012). Biocompatibility of polyaryletheretherketone polymers, in Kurtz, S.M. (ed), *PEEK Biomaterials Handbook*, Elsevier, Boston, 81–92.

Turell, M., Wang, A. and Bellare, A. (2003). Quantification of the effect of cross-path motion on the wear rate of ultra-high molecular weight polyethylene, *Wear*, **255**, 1034–1039.

Uschold, T.D., Fusco, D., Germain, R., Tumialan, L.M. and Chang, S.W. (2012). Cervical and lumbar spinal arthroplasty: Clinical review, *AJNR Am J Neuroradiol*, **33**(9), 1631–1641.

Utzschneider, S., Becker, F., Grupp, T.M., Sievers, B., Paulus, A., Gottschalk, O. *et al.* (2010). Inflammatory response against different carbon fiber-reinforced PEEK wear particles compared with UHMWPE *in vivo*, *Acta Biomater*, **6**, 4296–4304.

Victrex, Ltd. (2008). *Victrex announces 30 years of VICTREX® PEEK polymer innovation.* Press release Nov 10, 2008. Available at: http://www.victrex.com/en/victrex-library/press-releases/detail/detail.php?id=230 [Accessed Feb 04, 2014].

Voss, H. and Friedrich, K. (1987). On the wear behaviour of short-fibre-reinforced peek composites, *Wear*, **116**, 1–18.

Wang, A., Lin, R., Stark, C. and Dumbleton, J.H. (1999). Suitability and limitations of carbon fiber reinforced PEEK composites as bearing surfaces for total joint replacements, *Wear*, **225–229**(2), 724–727.

Wang, A., Lawrynowicz, D., Zhang, Z., Korduba, L.A. and Herrera, L. (2011). Polyether ether ketone as an orthopaedic bearing surface against UHMWPE, *UHMWPE Int Meet 2011*, Philadelphia.

Wang, A., Lin, R., Polineni, V.K., Essner, A., Stark, C. and Dumbleton, J.H. (1998). Carbon fiber reinforced polyether ether ketone composite as a bearing surface for total hip replacement, *Tribol Int,* **31**(11), 661–667.

Wang, Q.Q., Wu, J.J., Unsworth, A., Briscoe, A., Jarman-Smith, M., Lowry, C. *et al.* (2012). Biotribological study of large diameter ceramic-on-CFR-PEEK hip joint including fluid uptake, wear and frictional heating, *J Mater Sci Mater Med*, **23**(6), 1533–1542.

Wenz, L.M., Merritt, K., Brown, S.A., Moet, A. and Steffee, A.D. (1990). In vitro biocompatibility of polyetheretherketone and polysulfone composites, *J Biomed Mater Res*, **24**(2), 207–215.

Williams, D.F., McNamara, A. and Turner, R.M. (1987). Potential of polyetheretherketone (PEEK) and carbon-fibre-reinforced PEEK in medical applications, *J Mater Sci Lett*, **6**, 188–190.

Wimmer, M.A., Sprecher, C., Hauert, R., Täger, G. and Fischer, A. (2003). Tribochemical reaction on metal-on-metal hip joint bearings: A comparison between *in vitro* and *in vivo* results, *Wear*, **255**, 1007–1014.

Wimmer, M.A., Schwenke, T., Brown, T., Kilpela, T. and Bao, Q. (2008). The effect of accelerated aging on the wear of PEEK for use in disc arthroplasty, *Trans ORS*, **33**, 1922.

Yamamoto, Y. and Hashimoto, M. (2004). Friction and wear of water lubricated PEEK and PPS sliding contacts. Part 2: Composites with carbon or glass fibre, *fibre*, *Wear*, **257**, 181–189.

Yuan, H., Coric, D., Yuan, P. and Zou, D. (2009). Early clinical experience of NuNec, a novel PEEK-on-PEEK artificial cervical disc, *Spine Arthroplasty Society 2009*, London.

Chapter 9

The Use of Polyurethanes in Joint Replacement

Jonathan J. Elsner[a,*], Noam Eliaz[b] and Eran Linder-Ganz[a]

[a]*Research and Development Center, Active Implants, Netanya, Israel*

[b]*Biomaterials and Corrosion Laboratory, School of Mechanical Engineering, Department of Materials Science and Engineering, Tel Aviv University, Tel Aviv, Israel*

1. Introduction

Polyurethane (PU) elastomers are among the highest performing medical-grade polymers. They have mechanical and biological properties that make them suitable for use in a diverse range of implantable medical devices, as they demonstrate a unique combination of toughness, durability, flexibility, biocompatibility, and biostability (Christenson *et al.*, 2007; Khan *et al.*, 2005). PUs possess more complex chemical structures than many of the most widely produced polymers such as PEs, polystyrenes, or polypropylenes, which are synthesized from one or two monomer units. PUs typically comprise three reactive components: (i) a diisocyanate, (ii) a soft segment (which is an oligomeric macromonomer); and, (iii) a chain extender. The three degrees of freedom available when planning PU syntheses provide a wide range of combinations that can potentially yield PUs with vastly differing physicochemical and mechanical properties, as

*Corresponding author.

well as varying biostability (Christenson *et al.*, 2007; Khan *et al.*, 2005). PU elastomers typically show a two-phase structure in which hard segment microdomains are dispersed in a matrix of soft segments. The hard segment microdomains mainly comprise the diisocyanate and the chain extender. Consequently, PUs are often referred to as 'segmented block copolymers'. The microphase separation of segmented PUs is driven by the thermodynamic incompatibility of the hard and soft segments. The soft segments form amorphous, rubbery domains, whereas the hard segments form semicrystalline domains that are stabilized by hydrogen bonding between urethane and urea groups. The predominant linkage in the soft segment identifies the type of PU, for example, poly-(esterurethanes) incorporate ester linkages, poly-(etherurethanes) (PEUs) incorporate ether moieties, and poly-(carbonateurethanes) (PCUs) incorporate carbonate linkages.

The first generation of biomedical polyurethanes, poly-(ester urethanes), were found to be unsuitable for long-term implantation due to the rapid hydrolytic degradation of the aliphatic polyester soft segment. Poly-(ether urethanes) were identified as a suitable replacement due to their excellent hydrolytic stability. However, unanticipated failure rates of devices containing softer grade polyurethanes led to the discovery that PEUs were subject to oxidative degradation including environmental stress cracking (ESC) and metal ion oxidation (MIO) (Stokes *et al.*, 1995; Wiggins *et al.*, 2001; Zhao *et al.*, 1990). Failure of polyurethane-based pacemaker leads and breast implant coatings in the late 1980s brought the long-term stability of these implants under scrutiny. More recently, PCUs were designed to remove the susceptible ester and ether linkages in the soft segment. These polymers were developed specifically and purposely to address the problem of cracking or degrading when implanted for a long period of time during which other types of polyurethanes would degrade or crack (Pinchuk, 1992, 1993). The inclusion of silicone in the backbone to create silicone copolymer chemistries (PCU-S) has also been found to improve the biostability of PCUs under some conditions. These materials are commercially available from DSM (Berkeley, California) under the trade name Bionate®.

Polycarbonate urethanes have shown great promise as long-term biostable elastomers that exhibit excellent resistance to hydrolysis, ESC, and MIO. The following section outlines the main findings that support long-term use of PCU in orthopedic applications.

2. Basic Characterization of Polyurethanes as Biomedical Materials

2.1. *Biostability*

Several groups around the world have conducted extensive *in vitro* tests to assess the biostability of biomedical PUs. In their work, the authors compared the effect of the main degradation mechanisms observed in PUs: Hydrolysis, ESC, MIO, and calcification on various types of commercially available PEU and PCU materials. The main findings are brought below.

2.1.1. *Hydrolytic degradation*

Resistance to slow, long-term hydrolytic degradation was assessed by Khan *et al.* (2005) by incubating samples of each material in phosphate-buffered saline (PBS) solution at 37°C for up to three years. No changes in the surface morphologies of the samples were observed by optical stereomicroscope or environmental electron scanning microscopy (E-SEM) after long-term incubation compared with dry control samples. The surfaces of the samples remained very smooth, with no evidence of degradation. Differential scanning calorimetry (DSC) analysis of the samples showed a decrease in their transition temperature (T_g) which indicates improved phase separation between the soft and hard microdomains of the polymer. Plasticization effects were found to promote a large decrease in the ultimate tensile strength (UTS) within the first three months, which then leveled over the remaining incubation time. Corethane® 80A (now Bionate® 80A) showed the smallest overall change (−20%). Nevertheless, the changes in the mechanical properties were mainly reversible when samples taken after three years were dehydrated, and thus related to hydration of the polymer and not to its degradation.

2.1.2. *Resistance to oxidative degradation*

The clinical success of PU is dependent not only on its susceptibility to oxidation but also to ESC, which has been observed in PU devices that come into direct contact with tissue. Stokes and Cobian (1982) compared these two mechanisms of PU degradation and defined ESC as the "generation of deep crazed cracks in response to residual stress and exposure to some chemical environment". They suggested that *in vivo* ESC of PUs is the result of critical interactions of residual stress, autoxidation of ether linkages, and a proteinaceous crack driver such as α2-macroglobulin. Since the next generation PCUs were designed to remove the susceptible ester and ether linkages incorporated in the soft segments, they are expected to show better biostability in the long-term.

Resistance to oxidative degradation of PUs under stressed condition has been the focus of investigation by several groups. Khan *et al.* (2005) incubated unstrained and pre-strained samples (using a fixed 200% uniaxial strain) for three months in an *in vitro* $H_2O_2/CoCl_2$ degradation system, which is based on the transition metal ion catalyzed decomposition of hydrogen peroxide. No cracking was observed in the unstrained PEUs, but severe cracking had developed in the strained samples. The cracking was accompanied by significant decreases in UTS and strain at failure, losses in the soft segment ether absorbance as seen by Fourier transform infrared (FTIR) spectroscopy, and decreases in molecular weight. The ether-free PCUs, Corethane® 80A and ChronoFlex® 80A, both showed excellent resistance to ESC. Chandy *et al.* (2008) investigated strained PU tubes using the same system but under higher strains (200% and 300%) and found that 200% strained PEU (Pellethane®) tubes showed substantial cracking of the surface layer with pitting within one month, and complete degradation within 45 to 60 days. Gel permeation chromatography (GPC) analysis of the Pellethane samples indicated 72% reduction in the number average molecular weight (Mn) and about 50% reduction in the weight average molecular weight (Mw), after one month. The PCU samples (Bionate® 80A) only exhibited minute surface erosion in the depth of 0.25–1 μm after 10 months under 300%

strain. There was no evidence of major cracking or pitting and the GPC analysis showed 18% and 8% reductions in their Mn and Mw, respectively. Overall, the PCU underwent less degradation and the degraded surface layer was much thinner than PEU. Christenson *et al.* (2007) investigated the effect of oxidation at even higher strains (400%), and also investigated Silicone-PU copolymers. To further elucidate the mechanism of ESC, the treated PU films were stretched to fracture and then imaged with SEM. Poly-(etherurethane) films exhibited extensive surface cracking perpendicular to the direction of strain. Cracking of the surface layer was attributed to a combination of factors including surface embrittlement due to crosslinking, chain scission, and surface pitting. In contrast to PEU, no cracking was observed on the stretched PCU films, despite the presence of surface pitting. Interestingly, a buckling pattern with a spacing of about 0.5–1 μm was evident on the material's surface at high magnification. This was explained by recovery of the elastomeric bulk after stretching, while the plastically deformed, crosslinked surface layer could not fully recover. The calculated thickness of the coating layer using a buckling model was found to be 0.25 μm, a finding that correlates well with the depth of erosion reported by Chandy *et al.* (2008). Pits on the PCU-S specimen were approximately the same size as those found on PCU. However, the silicone modification appeared to decrease the severity of surface pitting. Based on these results, the silicone modification was concluded to increase biostability of both PEU and PCU. In summary, ESC of PUs may be alleviated by reducing residual stress (e.g. by annealing), protecting the polymer from stress cracking media (incorporating antioxidants), or using ESC resistant (ether-free) PUs.

2.1.3. *Resistance to metal ion oxidation*

The MIO mechanism occurs predominantly in medical devices that contain metallic components whose corrosion products can catalyze bulk oxidation of the PU. Although superficially similar to ESC by involving oxidation of the soft segment, MIO is fundamentally different. ESC occurs in response to residual stresses in the sample, while MIO is initiated at the interface between metallic parts and the polymer. Stress is not a required condition for MIO, although it may be present. To test MIO, a cobalt foil is clamped to the polymer which is then immersed in H_2O_2 solution.

Khan *et al.* (2005) also investigated MIO and reported that PUs underwent superficial to severe MIO cracking with large decreases in mechanical properties (with Pellethane® 80A giving a 50% reduction in UTS). In contrast, PCUs such as Corethane® 80A and ChronoFlex® 80A showed some chemical degradation in the polycarbonate soft segment, with ChronoFlex showing no decrease in their UTS, and a 10% and 20% decrease, respectively, in their failure strains. However, neither of them exhibited any cracking, implying that the polyether soft segment is more susceptible to MIO cracking than the polycarbonate soft segment. The results of these tests also confirmed that strain (or stress) is not required to initiate MIO cracking. Of the test specimens, Corethane 80A (Bionate® 80A) showed the greatest stability and significantly better retention of mechanical properties and soft segment chemistry.

2.1.4. *Resistance to enzymatic degradation*

The degradation of PUs by candidate enzymes has been the subject of numerous studies (Labow *et al.*, 2002; Tang *et al.*, 2001, 2002). However, these studies generally focused on model PUs and did not include commercial materials. The hydrolytic enzyme cholesterol esterase (CE) has been recognized as the most active enzyme in PU degradation. Based on this finding, Christenson *et al.* (2006) conducted an enzymatic degradation study using concentrated CE solutions to accelerate the degradation of commercial PUs. They used unstrained PU films which were incubated in phosphate buffer solution or buffer containing cholesterol esterase (2000 units/mL which is considerably higher than the estimated physiological level to accelerate the effect) for a period of 36 days. Examination of the PU film surfaces after being treated showed that they were smooth and relatively free of defects. Although there was evidence of surface degradation of the treated PUs, there were no significant differences in molecular weight or polydispersity as compared to the untreated controls. Attenuated total reflectance (ATR)-FTIR analysis of the specimens, after 36 days only, showed a small loss in surface soft segment content. Degradation processes initiated by CE did not penetrate into the bulk or cause deterioration of bulk properties. The authors then compared the results of these controlled tests to similar films which were implanted in rats for 12 months. The analyses of these films showed that oxidation was the dominant mechanism of degradation and that it appeared that any action of CE was confined to the immediate surface, and the magnitude of the effect was too small to account for the changes observed on implanted films. It was concluded that the potential of hydrolytic enzymatic degradation of PU and PCU *in vivo* is negligible.

2.1.5. *Resistance to mineralization*

A number of studies have demonstrated that ventricles made from PEUs experience calcification when implanted for periods exceeding 100 days. The propagation of this biomaterial-associated calcification causes the PEU material to become hard and brittle, which can lead to the early failure of some devices. Yang *et al.* (1999) investigated the relative tendency of different commercial biomedical PU membranes to calcify, using an *in vitro* model. The experimental results demonstrated that all six types of PU included in the study were susceptible to calcification and that calcification occurred primarily at the surface of a PU membrane without involving the bulk microphase, The rate of calcification was found to be associated with the surface chemistry of the PU itself. After 60 days of incubation in a calcification solution, PEU specimens exhibited the highest degree of calcification as measured by SEM and electron spectroscopy for chemical analysis (ESCA), while Corethane 80A and 55D membranes registered a relatively lower propensity to calcify. The authors suggested that this may be due to the different chemical composition of their soft segments affecting their ability to attract Ca ions. In addition, the study showed that calcification occurs primarily at the surface of a polyurethane membrane without involving the bulk microphase. Khan *et al.* (2005) used the same system to test tensed samples (200%). E-SEM analysis of the morphology of the surface deposits and energy dispersive spectroscopy (EDS) analysis of the

PU surface showed that surface mineralization had occurred, however the level of calcification was too low for ATR/FTIR detection. The PEUs, particularly high-ether Pellethane, showed more surface deposits and greater levels of Ca than the PCUs.

2.2. *Mechanical Properties*

Replacements for diseased or damaged joints have traditionally relied upon hard metals or ceramics articulating against ultra-high molecular weight polyethylene (UHMWPE), and although these materials have served well it has always been appreciated that mismatches exist between their mechanical properties and those of the natural systems being replaced (Figure 9-1).

A fundamental set of mechanical tests including uniaxial tension, planar tension (shear), biaxial tension, and uniaxial compression was performed on samples of the PCU material to provide good understanding of its mechanical properties. The results of such tests can be used, for example, to extract parameters of the material for use in finite element analysis (FEA), or to determine safety limits when used in a certain application. For each test, 3 samples were used

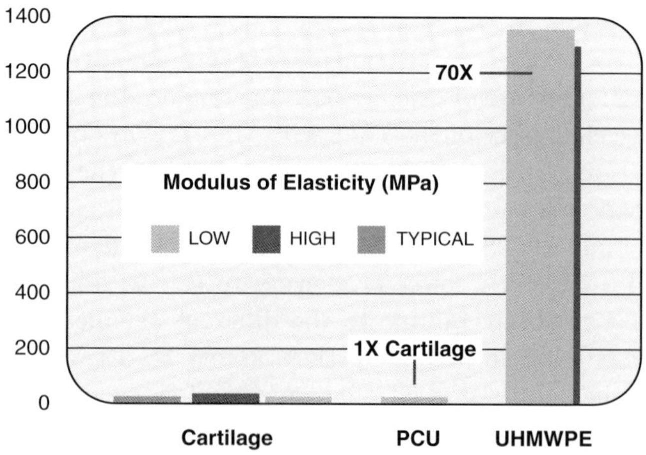

Figure 9-1. Comparison of the mechanical properties of polycarbonate urethane, cartilage and UHMWPE (McTighe *et al.*, 2009).

while kept in a 37°C environment, and stress-strain curves were constructed from the raw data. In addition, since PCU is best modeled as a hyper-elastic material, Mooney–Rivlin coefficients were calculated using data obtained from uniaxial tension, uniaxial compression, and planar uniaxial tension.

Figures 9-2(a)–9-2(d) depict the results of each test. As can be expected from a hyper-elastic material, the stress-strain curve resulting from uniaxial tension testing shows three distinct phases:

- *Phase A*: A linear phase in which the implant has a relatively high elastic modulus (E∼18 MPa).
- *Phase B*: A non-linear phase in the range 15–350% strains in which the elastic modulus drops before gradually stiffening.
- *Phase C*: A second linear phase in which the implant displays lower resistance to strain (E∼10 MPa), compared to that recorded in phase A (350–840% strain).

Similar behavior will be described in Section 3.2.2, in relation to a meniscus implant application made with PCU as its main bulk material. Under compression, the PCU material behaved linearly, with a compressive modulus of 20 MPa. This value is well matched to the instantaneous compressive modulus of cartilage which has been shown to be in the range of 5–19 MPa (Shepherd and Seedhom, 1999). The Mooney–Rivlin coefficients of PCU were calculated as: $C_1 = 2.912$ MPa, and $C_2 = -1.025$ MPa.

2.3. *Tribology*

Conventional total joint replacements typically operate between full fluid film lubrication (e.g. ceramic-on-ceramic) to a mixed (boundary and film) lubrication regime (e.g. PE-on-metal), which involves direct contact between the articulating surfaces (Scholes *et al.*, 2000). It is the contact between the asperities of a bearing's surfaces which creates wear debris. Soft bearings such as those based on PUs are designed to operate with full fluid film lubrication in which the two bearing surfaces are totally separated by a lubricating film, under continuous cyclic loading conditions. This is the same lubrication

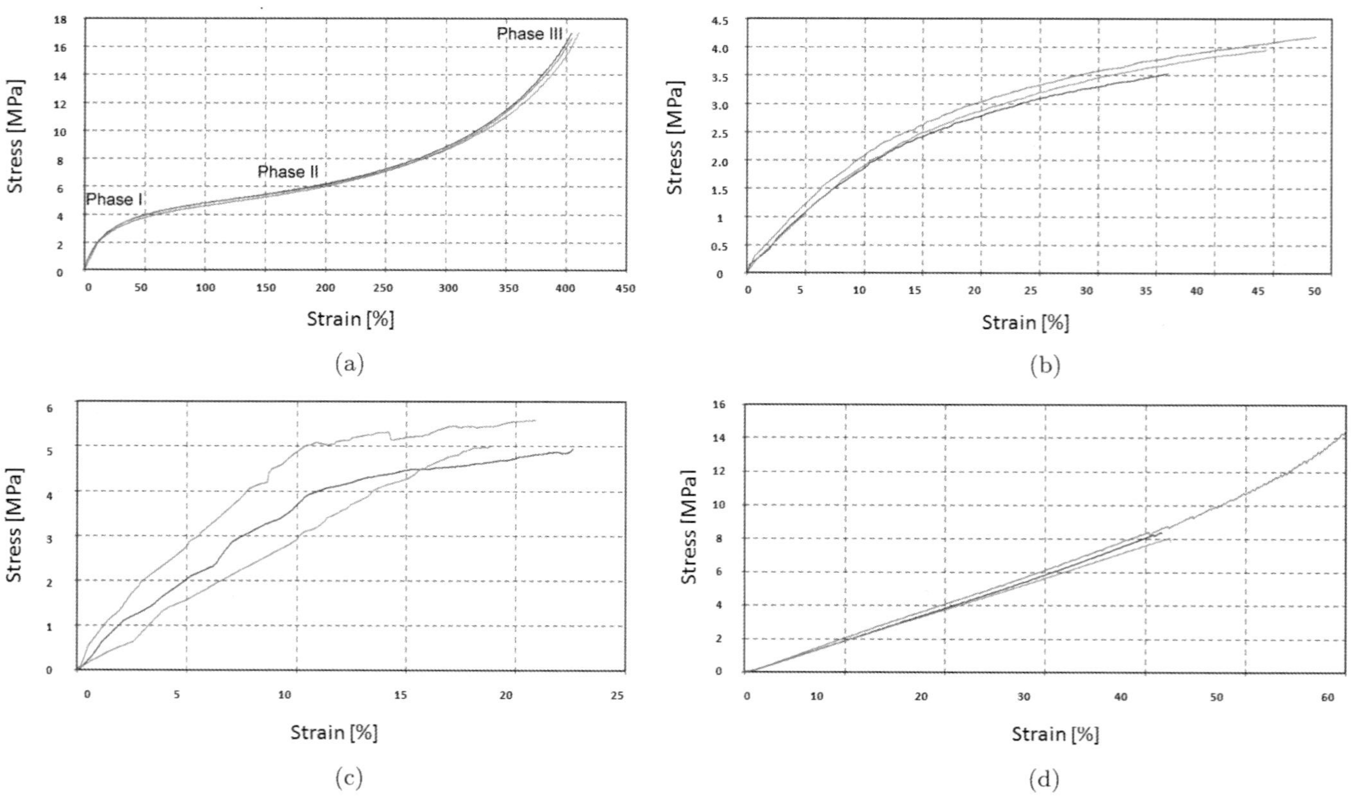

Figure 9-2. Stress-strain response of polycarbonate-urethane (Shore hardness 80A) to (a) tensile testing, (b) planar tension (shear) testing, (c) biaxial tensile testing, and (d) compression testing.

mechanism which occurs in the natural joint as a result of the pressure generated in the synovial fluid, relative motion of the two joint surfaces, and the elastic deformation of the cartilaginous joint surfaces (Unsworth, 1991). The improved tribology of soft bearings is expected to reduce both friction and wear. Various theoretical and experimental studies have confirmed that the tribology of soft bearings based on PUs is superior to that of traditional hard bearings. Early work by Dowson *et al.* (1991) and Auger *et al.* (1993) established that the mechanism responsible for successful tribology is a combination of elastohydroynamic (EHL) and microelastohydroynamic (μ-EHL) lubrication. The former is produced when the pressure developed in the lubricating film is sufficient to cause deformation of either surface, thus keeping them separated. The latter, meanwhile, is a localized form of EHL whereby pressure perturbations cause substantial flattening of asperities in the material's surface, thus assisting in the maintenance of a lubricious film.

Theoretical and experimental work which compared similar designs of soft and hard bearings of a hip joint showed that the friction factor of a PU hip bearing is much lower than in the equivalent UHMWPE cup (Scholes *et al.*, 2006; Smith *et al.*, 2000). Scholes *et al.* (2006) who conducted friction tests on acetabular cups made of Corethane 80A that articulated against standard, commercially available femoral heads, demonstrated friction factors approaching those for full fluid-film lubrication with only approximately 1% asperity contact. The mean and standard error of the wear rate reported by Smith *et al.* (2000) for the PU cups were 14.1 ± 4.3 mg per million cycles (Mc) ($12.0 \pm 3.6\,\text{mm}^3$ per Mc), compared to 44.8 ± 3.4 mg per Mc ($48.2 \pm 3.7\,\text{mm}^3$ per Mc) measured for UHMWPE cups.

In other studies of a cushion bearing in the knee joint, PU has been used in total and unicompartmental knee joint designs, where PU was used as the tibial component. In these studies it was found that the joint operated just within the mixed lubrication regime, but that it benefited from a substantial measure of fluid film lubrication and that μ-EHL lubrication was effective in preserving low friction and thin but effective lubricating films (Auger *et al.*, 1995a; Scholes *et al.*, 2006). Wear tests of the total knee prosthesis were carried out up to

5 million cycles, and no detectable wear debris was generated (Auger *et al.*, 1995b). Very low wear rates ($<1\,mm^3$/million cycles) were reported for the unicompartmental implant (Scholes *et al.*, 2006).

More recently, PU has also been the focus of research as a hemiarthroplasty material. Luo *et al.* (2009) investigated the use of PU against cartilage, as a potential hemiarthroplasty material in the knee instead of stainless steel. They tested in a simulator PU plates of different moduli in the range of 1.4–22 MPa against bovine cartilage samples. The lower-modulus PU caused reduced levels of contact stress and friction shear stresses, which resulted in reduced levels of opposing cartilage wear. The higher-modulus PU (22 MPa) demonstrated higher levels of friction shear stress, but the wear resulting on the opposing cartilage was not as severe as the wear from the stainless steel group. Similar results were reported in another tribological study by Pöllänen *et al.* (2011) who concluded that PU is a more compatible material than surgical steel in contact with living cartilage.

2.4. *In Vivo Studies*

There is a growing number of reports on *in vivo* use of PUs as bearing surfaces in orthopedics. In the second part of their study, Khan *et al.* (2005) tested the biostability of a PU soft bearing acetabular component from its theoretical design to a practical demonstration of the technology in an *in vivo* sheep model of hip arthroplasty. The most promising material of these tests in the laboratory–PCU Corethane 80A (Bioante 80A)–was chosen for the acetabular bearing component. No significant physical or chemical degradation was observed in the PCU after three years *in vivo*. Host variables such as weight, age, mobility, and implant duration produced little difference and there was remarkable consistency in the condition of the cups retrieved. There was no evidence of biodegradation such as ESC, which can result in the material becoming more opaque. The articular surfaces of the PCU bearing were in excellent condition, suggesting that there was a good joint function over the implant period. E-SEM and surface profilometry showed minimal normal wear. No significant soft tissue damage, wear particle generation or inflammatory tissue response were reported. The lack of third-body wear damage on most of the retrieved cups, and the absence of third-body particles in the articular surface, confirmed previous laboratory studies suggesting that the acetabular component can mimic the natural synovial joint by producing, promoting, and preserving an effective lubrication regime. The excellent condition of the articular surfaces of the compliant layer joints and the results from the material evaluation confirm that there was good joint function over the implant period.

Poly-(carbonateurethane) has also been tested as a bearing material in hemiarthroplasty. Turner *et al.* (2005) used a PCU femoral head against acetabular cartilage, and compared the results to a CoCr femoral head. Twelve adult male canines received a unilateral hemiarthroplasty of the hip using a cemented CoCr stem with either a PCU-covered femoral head, or a conventional CoCr head. The dogs were exercised daily, and limb usage was confirmed by comparing preoperative and terminal DEXA scans of both tibiae. It was found that articular cartilage damage, as measured by a reduction in cartilage thickness, was substantially less when using PCU compared to a CoCr head. In fact, the mean thickness of the articular cartilage articulating against PCU was no different from the thickness of cartilage thickness in the contralateral unopened hip. Particulates, consistent with wear debris, were not found in the acetabulum, joint capsules, joint fluid, or remote organs. No surface damage to the retrieved PCU bearing was observed. In another study of PCU against cartilage, a PCU meniscus was developed and implanted in sheep (Zur *et al.*, 2011). The PCU structure was reinforced internally with Kevlar fibers and implanted as an artificial meniscus following total medial meniscectomy, and evaluated at three and six months post-surgery. Macroscopic analysis and semi-quantitative histological analysis were performed on the cartilage of the operated knee and unoperated contralateral control joint. The PCU implant remained well secured throughout the experimental period and showed no signs of wear or changes in structural or material properties. Histological analysis showed relatively mild cartilage degeneration that was dominated by loss of proteoglycan content and cartilage structure. However, the total osteoarthritis score according to the modified Mankin score did not differ significantly between the control and operated knees, and there were no differences in the severity of degenerative changes between three and six months post-surgery. These findings provide preliminary evidence of the ability of an artificial PCU meniscal implant to delay or prevent osteoarthritic changes in the knee joint following a complete medial meniscectomy.

3. Applications in Joint Treatment

3.1. *Hip Replacement*

Throughout all the advancements and significant improvements that have been made to hip replacements over the past 50 years, the disparity between the material properties of hard-on-hard bearings and those of the natural tissue has not been addressed. The orthopedic community continues to face similar issues of wear, fatigue, squeaking, osteolysis, pseudotumors, and black sludge, problems that are associated with most current implant materials. Thus, the search for new and improved materials which can better mimic the function of the natural joint and provide long-term function continues. In 2006, PCU was applied for the first time in a commercial cushion-bearing system as an acetabular socket called the TriboFit® Acetabular Buffer (Active Implants, Memphis, TN) (Figure 9-3). This hip system, which pairs the PCU acetabular buffer with a CoCr femoral head, has been available on the European market for seven years. Since then, this system has undergone extensive testing in the lab and clinic. The following sections will introduce the system, preclinical testing, and experience gained during clinical use.

3.1.1. *Design rationale*

The TriboFit® Acetabular Buffer implant has significantly different design goals as compared to conventional PE, ceramic, and metal bearings. Soft compliant PCU is designed to function like the natural hip on the acetabular side of the hip joint. The PCU acetabular implant is 3 mm thick, thus it requires very little bone removal and enables the use of larger head sizes. It has a novel 'snap-fit' locking mechanism that provides ease of insertion and positive locking stability. In cases where it is needed, an acetabular metal shell backing

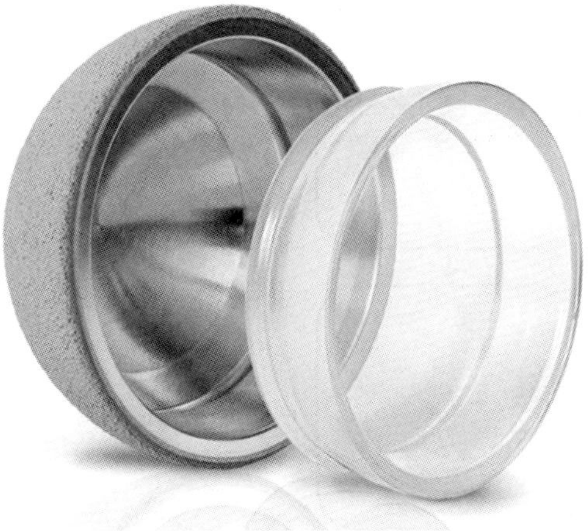

Figure 9-3. Side view of the TriboFit® PCU Buffer, and a hydroxyapatite coated metal shell. The buffer can be implanted directly against bone, or by fixation to the metal shell backing, by snap-fit mechanism based on a ring shaped flange.

is also available for use with the PCU as a snap-fit liner (Figure 9-3). This novel design provides versatility to be used as a stand-alone acetabular cartilage replacement or as a standard acetabular component, replacing the PE bearing surface. While it is too early in clinical evaluations to determine if one approach is better than the other over the long-term, it is certain that a PCU bearing used as a stand-alone cartilage implant has the advantage of less bone removal.

3.1.2. *Surgical technique*

The TriboFit® system is designed for all standard surgical approaches. If the buffer implant is to be used as a stand-alone cartilage replacement, it requires full bony containment so preparation and insertion techniques are significant factors. Light reaming can be done to ensure a hemispherical shaped socket, but it does not require reaching down to a bleeding bony bed (Figure 9-4(a), top). After reaming, a special groove reamer similar to the original Charnley grooved reamer is used to cut a locking channel into the acetabular wall (Figure 9-4(a), middle). The buffer implant is then snapped into place with finger pressure (Figure 9-4(a), bottom).

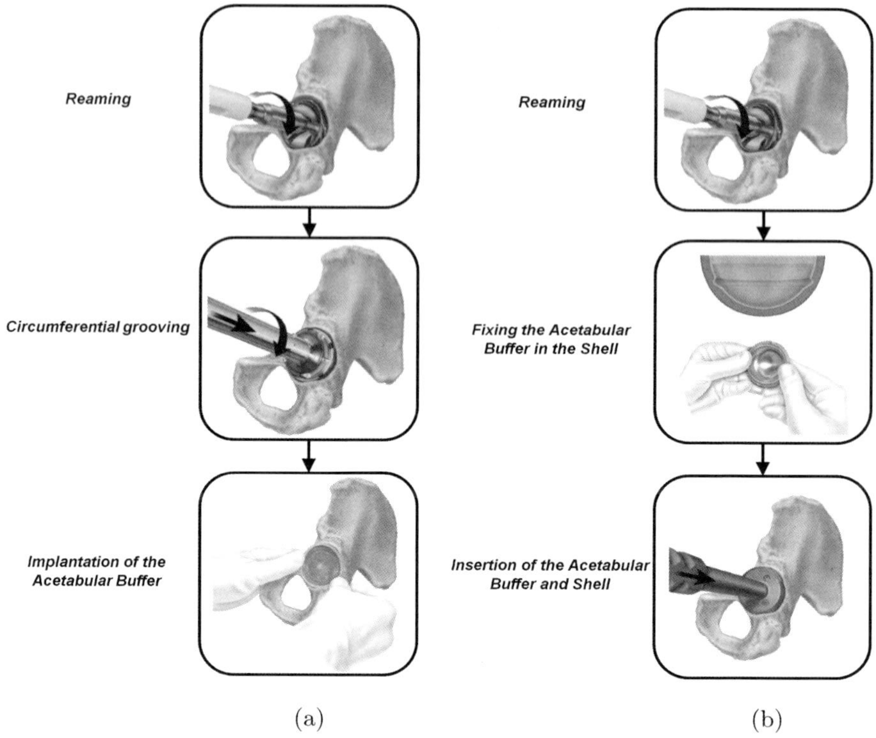

Figure 9-4. An overview of the steps required for preparation and implantation of the Tribofit® PCU Buffer, (a) when implanted directly against bone, and (b) when used as a liner backed by a metal shell.

Implantation with a metal shell component follows the standard surgical technique as with any cementless hemispherical metal shell component. Once proper reaming and sizing is carried out, the buffer implant is snapped into place and can then be inserted as a monoblock acetabular component (Figure 9-4(b), middle). Implantation and component insertion is carried out as with any standard cementless conventional acetabular component (Figure 9-4(b), bottom).

3.1.3. *In vitro evaluation*

Several wear studies were performed in recent years to evaluate the wear-rate of the PCU acetabular buffer. Fisher and Jennings (2002) tested a configuration of the buffer, which simulated implantation directly on bone (without a backside metal shell). The PCU buffers were placed in Sawbone replicas of the acetabulum that were reamed and grooved as mentioned before. The implants were loaded according to ISO standard 14242 for 5 million cycles in a new born calf serum diluted to 25%. The wear-rate gradient was measured between 2 and 5 Mc, after the buffers had reached a steady creep state and wear rate. The average wear rate measured in this interval was 2.8 mm^3/Mc.

St. John and Gupta (2012) compared the wear characteristics of UHMWPE, crosslinked UHMWPE, and PCU buffers of a similar geometry against cobalt alloy femoral components. Over the course of 5 million load cycles, the PCU buffers were seen to have the lowest wear rate, with an average material loss of 19.1 mm^3/Mc. The crosslinked UHMWPE components had a loss rate of 25 mm^3/Mc, while the UHMWPE components had a much higher rate of material loss ~100 mm^3/Mc. The finding of about a 70% reduction in wear due to crosslinking reconfirms the theory that crosslinking of UHMWPE is beneficial in reducing wear, but the material loss for the PCU samples appears to have been at least 24% lower than for the crosslinked UHMWPE.

The longest controlled laboratory wear study of the commercially available PCU buffer was conducted on a buffer implanted against a metal shell (Elsner *et al.*, 2010a, 2011). An ISO-based simulation was performed for a duration of 20 million cycles. Gravimetric and particulate wear analyses by means of filtration and bioferrography were used in this study. The PCU buffer showed excellent wear characteristics in terms of its low and steady volumetric wear rate (5.8–7.7 mm^3/Mc) and low particle generation rate (2–3 $\times$ 10^6 particles/Mc). The latter is 5–6 orders of magnitude lower than that reported for crosslinked UHMWPE and 6–8 orders of magnitude lower than that of metal-on-metal bearings (Figure 9-5). Microscopic analysis (atomic force microscopy, AFM, and profilometry) of the implants' articulating surface after the simulation demonstrated a low damage level even after 20 Mc. Another important finding in this study was that only 3.4% of the PCU wear particles isolated from the

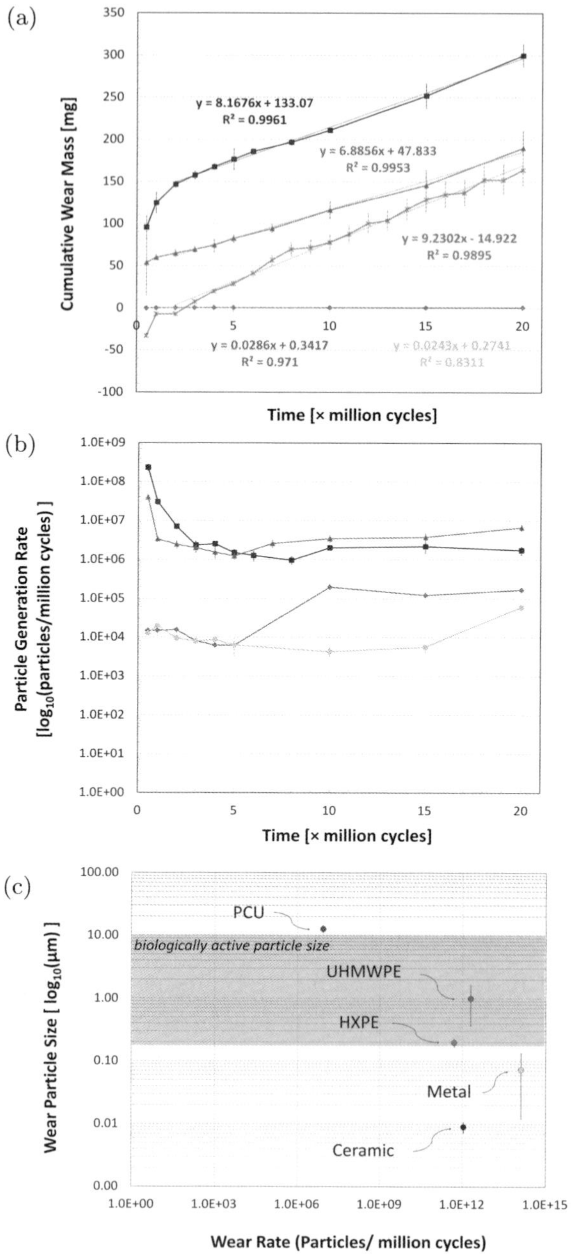
(a)
Cumulative Wear Mass [mg]
y = 8.1676x + 133.07
R² = 0.9961
y = 6.8856x + 47.833
R² = 0.9953
y = 9.2302x - 14.922
R² = 0.9895
y = 0.0286x + 0.3417
R² = 0.971
y = 0.0243x + 0.2741
R² = 0.8311
Time [× million cycles]
(b)
Particle Generation Rate
[log10(particles/million cycles)]
Time [× million cycles]
(c)
Wear Particle Size [log10(μm)]
PCU
biologically active particle size
UHMWPE
HXPE
Metal
Ceramic
Wear Rate (Particles/ million cycles)

←

Figure 9-5. (Figure on facing page) (a) Cumulative mass of worn PCU Buffer material during 20 million loading cycles, as determined by gravimetrical measurements (⟶), analysis of wear particles isolated by filtration (·, articulating surface; •, backside surface), and by Bio-Ferrography (■, articulating surface; ♦, back-side surface). (b) Particle generation rate during 20 Mc. Data are presented as mean ± standard error of the mean. (c) Overview of typical wear particle sizes versus wear rates reported for various acetabular liners used in total hip replacement with respect to the PCU results. Data are presented based on the particle generation wear rate (Elsner *et al.*, 2011).

lubricant lay in the 0.2–10 μm size range, with the majority of particle mass being associated with larger sizes. This particle size range has been shown to stimulate macrophages to produce high levels of the cytokine TNF-α, and the major part of UHMWPE wear particles usually lies in this range (Green *et al.*, 1998). One more potential advantage of PCU in this respect is that, while highly crosslinked UHMWPE and UHMWPE materials share similar values of biological activity (Galvin *et al.*, 2007), a recent study has shown that PCU is less inflammatory to periprosthetic tissue and bone compared to these materials (Smith *et al.*, 2010). Thus, based on the combination of larger wear particles, less reactivity of the material itself, and lower particle generation rate, the authors hypothesized that the osteolytic risk of the PCU buffer may be lower than that of hard bearings.

3.1.4. *Large animal studies*

The *in vivo* biocompatibility and biostability of the TriboFit® Hip System has been tested for a duration of 24 months in a sheep model. Sheep have often been used in studies involving hip arthroplasty, as the bony acetabulum of the sheep is made up of the three bones of the pelvis, as it is in humans, and the anatomy of the soft tissue around the ovine hip is also very similar to that of humans (Timperley *et al.*, 2010). Additionally, instrumented endoprostheses have shown a similar load orientation (Bergmann *et al.*, 1984). However, the walls of the ovine socket are thin, making it very difficult to expose cancellous bone at the rim of the acetabulum. This means that the ovine acetabulum anatomy is an ideal model to test the efficacy of an implant against sclerotic bone at the rim.

Four sheep were implanted with a buffer alone, while four others were implanted with a buffer and hydroxyapatite (HA)-coated shell configuration. One sheep from each study group was euthanized and examined 6 and 12 months after implantation. The remaining sheep in each group were euthanized and examined 24 months after implantation.

Physical examination of the sheep 6, 12, or 24 months post-implantation revealed the animals to be performing well with no gait or functional issues apparent. Specifically, the range of motion appeared unrestricted, and no dislocations or subluxations were noted. At a gross macroscopic level it would appear there are no untoward effects of the componentry.

Evaluations at necropsy 6, 12, and 24 months post-intervention demonstrated that the gentle reaming and removal of articular cartilage followed by grooving of the surface were sufficient to maintain the buffer alone in a good position, and provided rigid fixation of the acetabular component. Similarly, the under-sizing of the reamed acetabulum and impaction of the shell into the acetabulum created a tight interface fixation of the hemispherical HA-coated CoCr shell with the acetabular bone (Figure 9-6). Lucencies visible around the

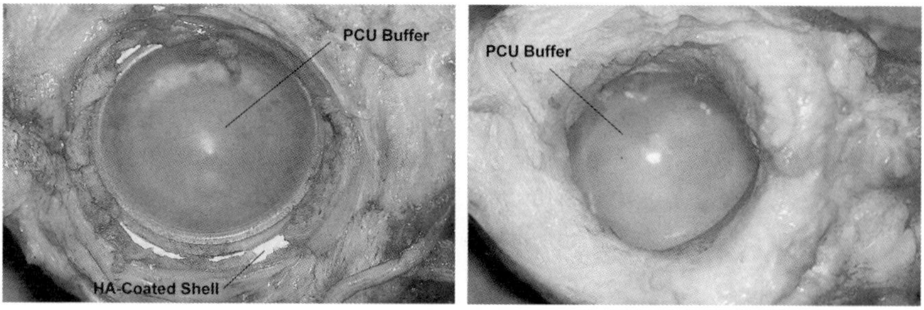

(a) (b)

Figure 9-6. Photographs of explanted PCU buffers which were implanted as a liner with an HA-coated metal shell (a), and directly in the acetabulum (b), 24 months post implantation in sheep.

shell at the time of implantation had filled, presumably with new bone infiltrating the HA surface coating.

The surfaces of the retrieved buffer specimens from both groups appeared intact with no gross evidence of surface abrasion. Some edge wear along the dorsal and cranial aspects of the 24-month explants developed in response to abrasion from the stem during locomotion but this finding was not considered unusual or significant. In one of the buffer-on-bone explants, backside wear was indicated. This appeared to have originated at the interface between the outer buffer surface and the underlying acetabular cartilage/bone in response to load bearing. Further work is needed to evaluate the exact wear mechanism in this case. Nevertheless, the sheep did not show any signs of lameness prior to necropsy and the implant remained in place. Substantial new circumferential bone formation was seen in the acetabulum immediately adjacent to the buffer in both sheep.

Histological examination of the surrounding tissues verified no noticeable untoward biological response to the implant components, and very few traces, if any at all, of wear particles.

3.1.5. *Clinical experience*

The first implantation of the TriboFit® Acetabular Buffer was done in 2006. As of August 2013, the TriboFit® Acetabular Buffer has been implanted in more than 1200 patients, with the longest implantation reaching seven years.

Two case studies describing the early retrieval analysis results of patients, 10.5 and 12 months post-implantation were published by Wippermann *et al.* (2008) and Siebert *et al.* (2008), respectively. Both patients experienced hip pain approximately eight months post-implantation. The retrieved implants were analyzed for wear using SEM and micro-CT technique, and the average wear rate was found to be 1.5 mm^3/year (Wippermann *et al.*, 2008) and 15 mm^3/year (Siebert *et al.*, 2008), respectively. The average particle size was measured in one of the cases (Wippermann *et al.*, 2008) and was found to be 0.9 μm according to laser diffraction analysis and 2.9 μm (range: 0.5–90 μm, plus one at 200 μm) according to SEM analysis. These average particle sizes are lower than that reported in the lab (Elsner *et al.*, 2010). A possible explanation for this discrepancy may be that only particles from the synovial fluid were characterized in the clinical study, and since smaller particle sizes tend to suspend in the fluid better than larger particles, the results could lean towards the lower range of sizes.

In 2011, Giannini *et al.* (2011) reported a prospective controlled randomized study of the buffer, which compared clinical outcomes of 60 osteoporotic patients with femoral neck fracture, treated either with the PCU buffer or bipolar hemiarthroplasy. The Harris Hip Score (HHS) was used to measure subjective outcomes 3 and 12 months post-operatively and adverse events (AEs) were recorded throughout the follow-up period. No statistical difference was found between the groups. The average HHS at 3 and 12 months was 71.6 and 75.5 in the hemiarthroplasy group, and 74.5 and 80.7 in the PCU Buffer group, respectively. In the reported study, no major complications occurred and the authors state that the surgical technique is fast and simple.

In another recent study, serum cobalt (Co) and chromium (Cr) levels were measured in a small group of 15 patients treated with the TriboFit® Buffer (Group A) and in 15 patients treated with metal-on-metal (MoM) total hip arthroplasty (Group B) (Moroni *et al.*, 2012). The metal ions level measured after 18–35 (average 27.3) months was significantly higher in patients treated with MoM implants ($p < 0.05$). Specifically, Co (1.3 μg/L) and Cr (2.9 μg/L) median levels were found to be 5.4 and 4.8 times higher, respectively, from Co (0.24 μg/L) and Cr (0.6 μg/L) levels in patients treated with a PCU buffer. The radiographic results were excellent, and there were no signs of osteolysis or loosening of the buffer. In both groups, the postoperative HHS and Oxford Hip Score (OHS) improved as compared to the pre-operative scores (Table 9-1). Even though patients in Group A showed significantly higher pre-operative scores ($p = 0.014$), at follow-up, neither group showed a statistically significant difference in results (HHS:$p = 0.148$; OHS: $p = 0.683$). Further clinical studies are ongoing.

Table 9-1. Harris Hip Score (HHS) and Oxford Hip Score (OHS) in Group A and B at baseline and at follow-up visit (Moroni *et al.*, 2012).

	Group A 27.8	Group B 26.8	*p*-value
Harris hip score			
Baseline			
Average ± SEM (median)	52.5 ± 4.3 (50.5)	39.3 ± 3.6 (37.8)	0.014
Range, SD	31.8–87.7, 16.1	22.2–71.9, 13.8	
Follow-up			
Average ± SEM (median)	94 ± 2.9 (98)	93.2 ± 1.9 (96.3)	0.148
Range, SD	55.2–100, 11.5	73.8–100, 7.33	
Oxford hip score			
Baseline			
Average ± SEM (median)	25.1 ± 2.4 (22)	15.3 ± 2.7 (13)	0.014
Range, SD	14–41, 9.4	1–35, 10.6	
Follow-up			
Average ± SEM (median)	45.2 ± 1.7 (47)	44.9 ± 1.2 (47)	0.683
Range, SD	23–48, 6.4	34–48, 4.6	

SD: Standard Deviation

3.2. *Meniscus Replacement*

The menisci play an important role in functionality of the knee joint. Clinical studies have shown that the loss of the meniscus leads to degenerative arthritis due to changes in cartilage load distribution (McDermott and Amis, 2006). In these cases, there is clearly a need to protect the articular cartilage by either repairing or replacing the meniscus.

Meniscus replacement still represents an unsolved problem in orthopedics. Meniscal allografts have been shown to heal to the capsule and relieve pain (Verdonk *et al.*, 2005). However, besides problems related to availability, size matching, cost, and risk of disease transmission, allograft menisci undergo remodeling after implantation, causing shrinkage and reduced mechanical strength (Noyes *et al.*, 2004; van Arkel and de Boer 2002). Other substitutes made from synthetic and natural biodegradable polymers have been described (Buma *et al.*, 2007; Chiari *et al.*, 2006; Kobayashi *et al.*,

2003; Tienen *et al.*, 2006). These prostheses form temporary scaffolds that degrade in the body and are replaced gradually by newly formed tissue. Potential shortcomings of this approach include the lack of durability associated with most biodegradable materials under *in vivo* knee loading conditions (Kelly *et al.*, 2007; Kobayashi *et al.*, 2003), as well as the variability in the body response to the implant, limited age of the target population, and the quality of the tissue formed.

Nowadays, conservative care strategies (medication, knee bracing, activity modification, intra-joint injections of hyaluronic acid), and even primary, secondary, or multiple meniscectomies comprise the mainstream treatment for a typical 50-year-old patient with post-meniscectomy pain. At a later age, typically after age 65, clinicians often choose the more invasive treatment options to treat joint pain by performing high tibial osteotomy, unicompartmental, or total knee arthroplasties. Based on the above, there is a clear treatment gap for the middle-aged population, creating a need to accommodate a treatment option which can delay more aggressive treatments by relieving pain associated with meniscal dysfunction and the associated joint overload.

This section will present an overview of a non-anchored PCU medial meniscus implant (NUsurface® Meniscus Implant, Active Implants Corporation, Memphis, TN).

3.2.1. *Design rationale*

The meniscus implant was designed as a composite construct made of PCU, which is reinforced circumferentially with UHMWPE fibers (Figure 9-7(a)). This composite structure aims to reproduce the functional properties and relationship between the structural components of the natural meniscus, which consist of a solid matrix reinforced with a highly orientated collagen fiber network (Adams and Hukins, 1992). Functionally, the pliable matrix material is expected to distribute joint loads and reduce contact pressure by permitting local material deformation, whereas the reinforcement material is designed to restrain matrix flow and bear a high portion of hoop stresses.

In contrast to the acetabular buffer implant, which is used in a total joint arthroplasty, the meniscus implant only consists of one component, and as a hemiarthroplasty implant, it articulates against existing articular surface. A three-dimensional form of the meniscus was developed to match the geometry of existing cartilaginous surfaces (Figure 9-7(b)) and joint tolerances (Elsner *et al.*, 2010b)

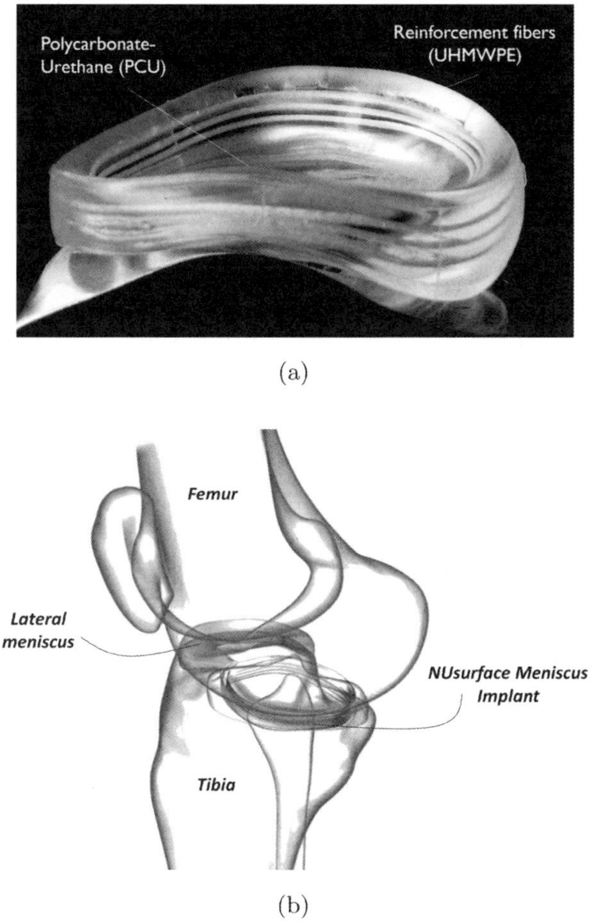

Figure 9-7. (a) A side view of the NUsurface® implant, which consists of PCU, reinforced internally with UHMWPE fibers. The circumferential orientation of the fibers assists in controlling deformation of the PCU material, and improving its pressure distribution performance. (b) An illustration of the knee joint and the location of the meniscus implant (Shemesh *et al.*, 2013).

by using more than 130 human knee MRI scans. Another important design consideration was ease of insertion and leaving all options open for future joint replacement by not drilling into the bone. The semi-lunar geometry of the natural meniscus, which is firmly fixed to the tibia in its horns, was modified into a semi-confined femur-conforming discoid geometry by adding an artificial bridge feature along the lateral side of the implant body. The bridge lies along the gap between the original medial insertion points of the meniscus and is designed to not come into contact with the cruciate ligaments.

3.2.2. *Biomechanics*

The load transfer capability of the implant was evaluated *in vitro* using human cadaveric knees (Linder-Ganz *et al.*, 2010). The implant was inserted into the medial compartment of cadaveric knees following the removal of the natural meniscus, and the knee was loaded under compression representative of the maximum physiological load during gait. The pressure distribution under the implant was measured utilizing flexible sensors (Tekscan Inc., Boston, MA) and compared to that of the natural meniscus prior to meniscectomy (Figure 9-8a). Contact pressure distributions measured on the tibial plateau underneath the PCU implant were found to be in very good agreement with those measured under the intact natural meniscus of the specific knee (Figure 9-8), thus proving that the composite PCU implant fulfills the role of joint load distributor.

Optimization of the implant design, namely determining the ratio of fibers incorporated in the PCU and their configuration, was done by employing a FE model of the medial knee with the PCU implant. The model was developed based on MRI scans of a cadaveric specimen, and analyses were conducted under peak gait loads. Internal strains and stresses which developed in both the PCU matrix and PE fibers were calculated (Elsner *et al.*, 2010c). The tibial plateau contact pressures, measured in cadaveric knees *in vitro* (Linder-Ganz *et al.*, 2010) were used to validate the FE model. The key findings of

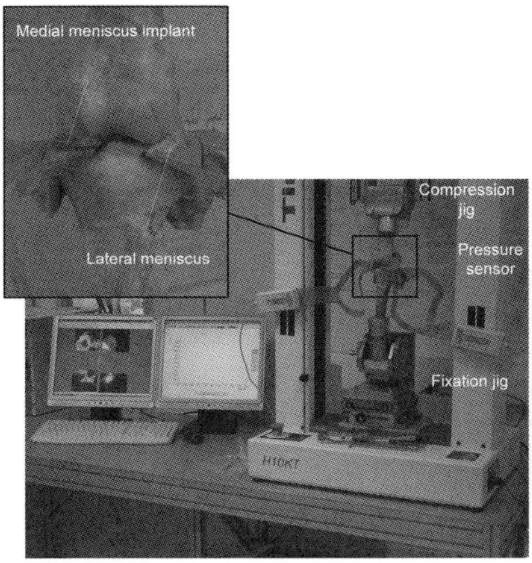

(a)

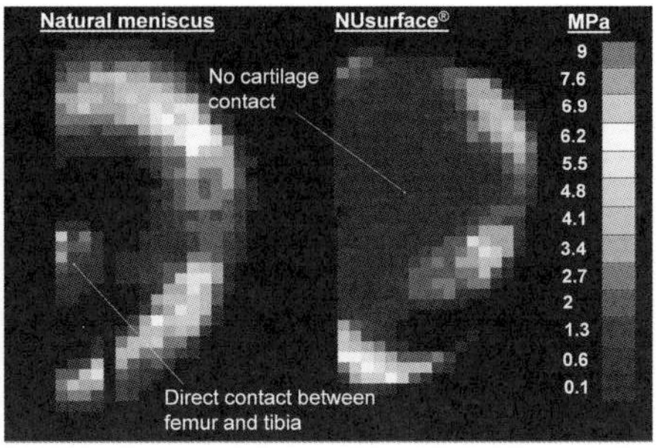

(b)

Figure 9-8. (a) Mechanical compression setup with a representative human cadaveric knee ready to be tested (Linder-Ganz *et al.*, 2010), and (b) a representative pressure distribution under an intact natural meniscus and of the NUsurface® implant, when placed in the same joint following a total meniscectomy.

this study were that peak stresses in the PCU were all lower than the maximal allowed stress for this material (15 MPa). Similarly, the peak tensile stress calculated in the fibers was significantly lower than the material's yield stress (3.1 GPa).

Other biomechanical tests of the implant included strain rate testing, creep, relaxation, and hysteresis measurements of the device under simulated joint conditions (Shemesh *et al.*, 2013). The mechanical properties were measured in a cell containing heated (37° C) simulated physiological fluid (SPF) consisting of bovine serum, which was prepared by diluting the serum 1:4 to approximate protein concentration of 1.6g/100 mL with distilled water, against specially designed PE replicas of tibia and femur. Six months of static soaking in SPF and dynamic fatigue loading for 2 million cycles were used to simulate long-term effects of the physiological environment. As a composite with a unique three-dimensional configuration, the implant's stress-strain response under compression was different from

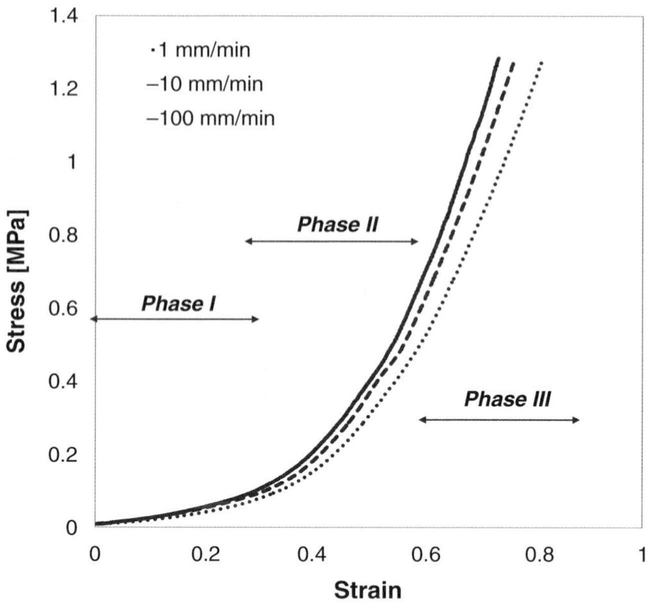

Figure 9-9. Compression stress-strain curves of the meniscus implant at 1, 10, and 100 mm/min strain-rates (Shemesh *et al.*, 2013).

that reported previously for the testing of PCU buttons (Figure 9-2d). It was found to consist of the following three phases (Figure 9-9):

- *Phase I*: A linear phase in which the implant has a relatively low elastic modulus (E∼3 MPa).
- *Phase II*: A non-linear phase of gradual stiffening found to occur between 20–50% strains.
- *Phase III*: A second linear phase in which the implant displays higher resistance to strain (E∼4 MPa), compared to that recorded in phase A (50–80% strain).

Creep and stress relaxation response of the implant were typical of a viscoelastic material. Soaking in SPF and dynamic fatigue simulation were both found to mildly increase the stiffness of the implant. The changes following static soaking stabilized after 28 days, while those measured following fatigue loading became steady after approximately 300,000 load cycles. Preconditioning was found to occur during the first and second loading–unloading cycles in the hysteresis test, but subsequent loading and unloading pathways were found to repeat for the remaining loading cycles (3–10).

In the long term, as seen after 2 million load cycles, the implant's width and length increased slightly (0.9% and 1.1%, respectively) and thickness reduced (−1%) compared to its initial state ($p \leq 0.05$). Moderate creep of the PCU bulk under gait conditions could be considered as an advantage in an implant which is expected to articulate between existing biological surfaces. The implant can adjust itself to variations in the joint morphology of a specific patient, increase conformity, and improve pressure distribution.

The stability of the implant under dynamic loading conditions was investigated in a cadaver-based, robotic knee dynamic simulator (Cleveland Clinic, OH; Elsner *et al.*, 2012). Eight cadaveric knees were placed on a robotic manipulator (Rotopod R2000, Parallel Robotics System, Hampton, NH) in such a way as to retain as much soft tissue as possible. Motion and loading conditions were simulated dynamically by replicating the loads and knee flexion motion for different sizes of the implant and for different surgical conditions or incorrect joint preparation conditions in order to test the sensitivity towards these parameters. In the majority of the cases, the implant was found to be stable. Implantation of an undersized implant and the presence of an anterior cruciate ligament (ACL) tear increased the risk of subluxation/dislocation.

Other dynamic tests of the implant included a mixed-mode wear test, which was conducted according to ISO 14243. Axial load, together with flexion-extension, internal–external, and anterior–posterior movements were applied on the implant, using MRI-based CoCr replicas of the tibia and femur. Five million mixed-mode cycles were applied on each specimen and wear was measured using gravimetry every million cycles. The average wear rate over 5 Mc was found to be less than 20 mg/Mc. The long-term wear rate is even lower, and close to zero since the wear-in rate measured in the first 3 Mc contributed most to the average value (Figure 9-10). This transient wear behavior may be linked to the fact that the meniscus implant articulates against existing joint surfaces, in contrast to a total joint replacement, where tolerances can be tailored in advance

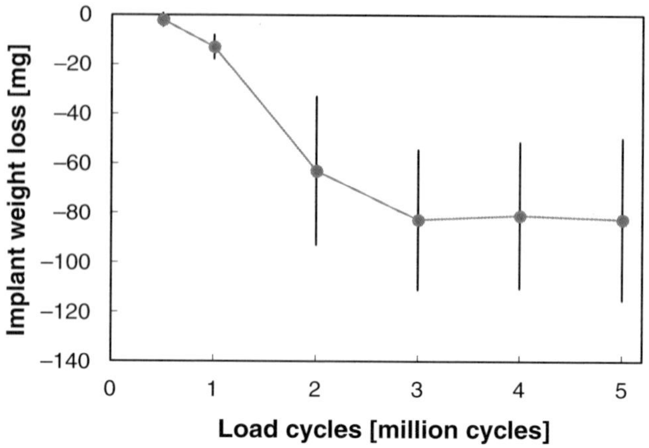

Figure 9-10. Average change in the weight of the NUsurface Meniscus Implants, adjusted by correction against the changes in the weight of the load-soak control (•) (Average ± standard error of the mean).

to assure full film lubrication. Since the meniscus implant is compliant, it undergoes moderate and controlled creep over time (Shemesh *et al.*, 2013), and it is believed that such adaptation to the joint, typically after 2–3 million load cycles, improves the lubrication regime considerably, thus reducing the wear rate. The implant's mechanical properties and functionality remained similar to those measured before the test.

3.2.3. *Large animal study*

A large animal study in sheep was used to evaluate the biological response exerted by the PCU implant when it articulates against cartilage under load. It was hypothesized that the PCU meniscus could provide a protective effect on the underlying cartilage when subjected to repeated loading in the absence of the natural meniscus. The cartilage condition of sheep implanted with a PCU meniscus substitute, following a total meniscectomy, was compared to the cartilage of the intact contralateral joint by using the modified Mankin score (Zur *et al.*, 2011).

Six ewes (1–2 years, weighing 60–80 kg) were implanted with a PCU meniscus substitute following a full meniscectomy of the medial meniscus. Animals were euthanized after three (n = 3) and six (n = 3) months. Cartilage and surrounding soft tissues of both knees were assessed macroscopically and by H&E and Saf-O staining using a semi-quantitative modified Mankin grading scale (Carlson *et al.*, 2002), with the contralateral knee serving as control.

In general, the sheep tolerated the operations well, stood upright immediately and bore weight on their operated hind limbs. Periodic physical examination indicated a full range of motion, no weight loss, and no signs of distress. The PCU implant was durable and remained well secured throughout the trial period. Gross and microscopic examinations of the explanted PCU implant's surfaces did not reveal any changes in their structure. No inflammatory cellular infiltration was observed in the joint. Macroscopically, cartilage in direct contact with the implant was preserved well and did not show significant degeneration (Figure 9-11). In most sheep, the main change in soft tissue was fibrosis of the joint capsule and other regional structures. Histological analysis showed that the total modified Mankin osteoarthritis scores were relatively low in both groups (<45 of 140 possible, Figure 9-12a,b). At both three and six months, there was a trend toward an increase in the total scores, although

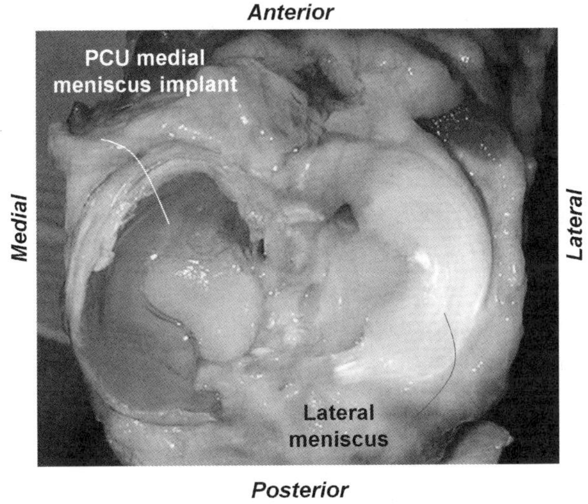

Figure 9-11. A transverse view of a PCU meniscus implant (adapted to the sheep anatomy), in an exposed sheep cadaver joint, six months after implantation (Zur *et al.*, 2011).

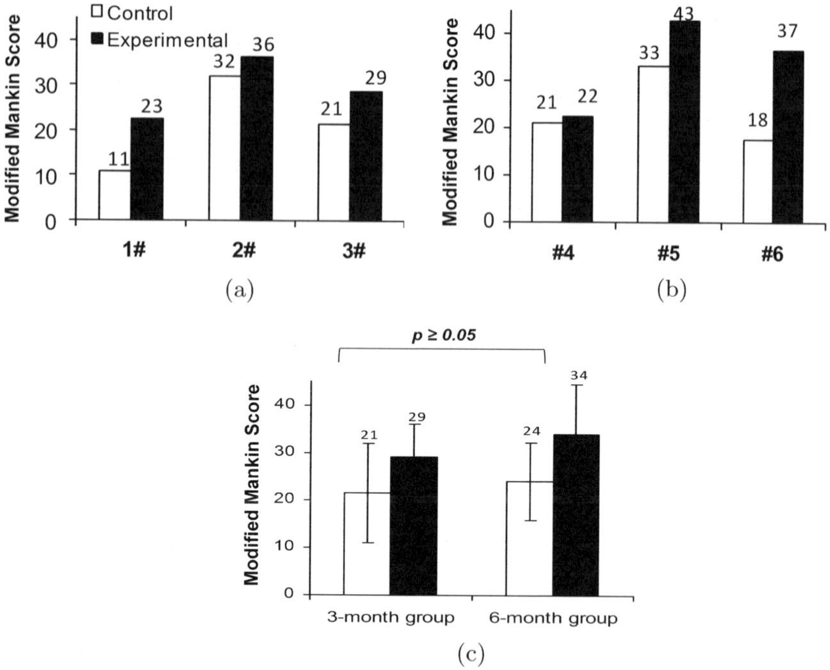

Figure 9-12. Modified Mankin score for cartilage degeneration following implantation of a PCU meniscus for each sheep at three months group (a), six months group (b), and the averaged score of both groups (c).

these differences were not significant (Figure 9-12(c)). Good preservation of articular cartilage was observed generally, particularly on the femoral condyles and tibial plateau. The histological changes observed in this study were generally mild, as previous studies have shown significant loss of cartilage structure and properties following meniscectomy (Appleyard *et al.*, 2003; Little *et al.*, 1997). These findings imply that a compliant PCU implant can delay the progression of degenerative cartilage changes in the short term.

3.2.4. *Clinical experience*

A series of 130 middle-aged patients in Europe and Israel have been treated with the NUsurface® Meniscus Implant for medial knee pain, due to a medial meniscus tear and/or a previous meniscectomy.

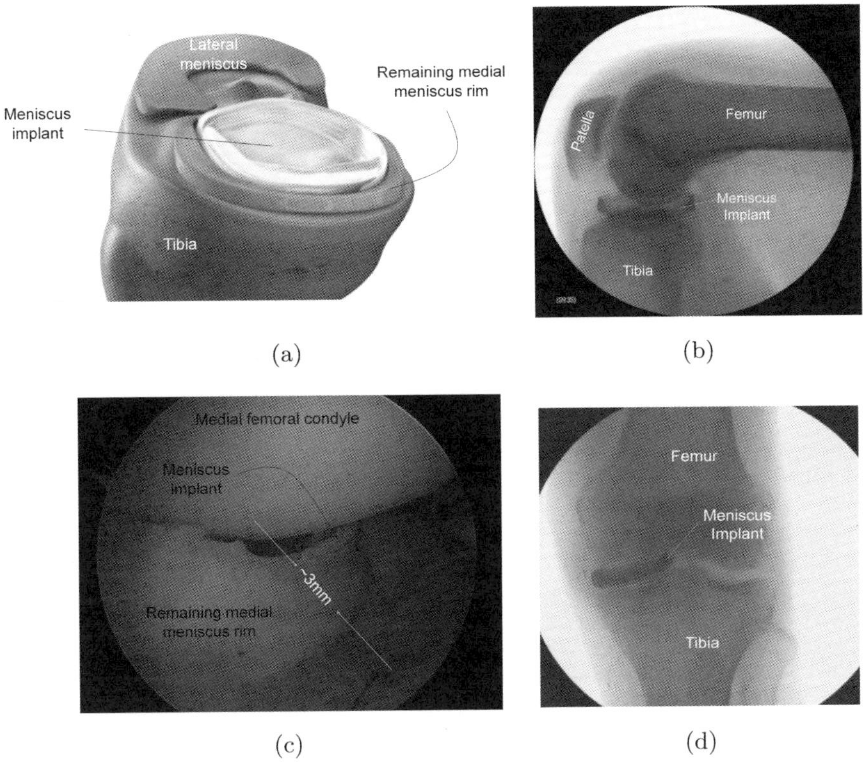

Figure 9-13. (a) An illustration of the positioning of the NUsurface® implant within the remaining rim of the medial meniscus, a postero-medial view of the implant and the remaining medial meniscus rim as seen (b) arthroscopically, (c) sagittal, and (d) coronal fluoroscopic views of a radio-opaque version of the NUsurface® which is used intra-operatively as a trial to select the correct implant size (*Photos courtesy of Dr. Vincenzo Condello*).

Patients with severe cartilage loss (grade IV cartilage loss according to the Outerbridge scale) or knee instability were excluded from the study. The primary clinical outcome was pain relief and improved function as measured by the KOOS scale, with secondary outcomes measured by IKDC and VAS pain scales. MRI scans were conducted periodically as well to evaluate the condition of cartilage over time.

The implantation of the device typically begins with a standard arthroscopic evaluation of the medial compartment, followed by a

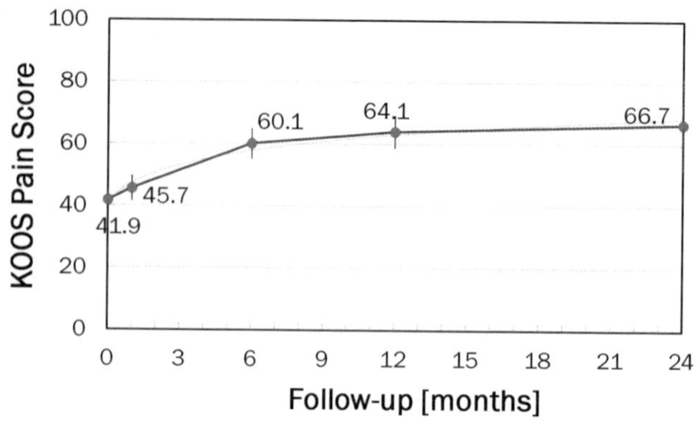

(a)

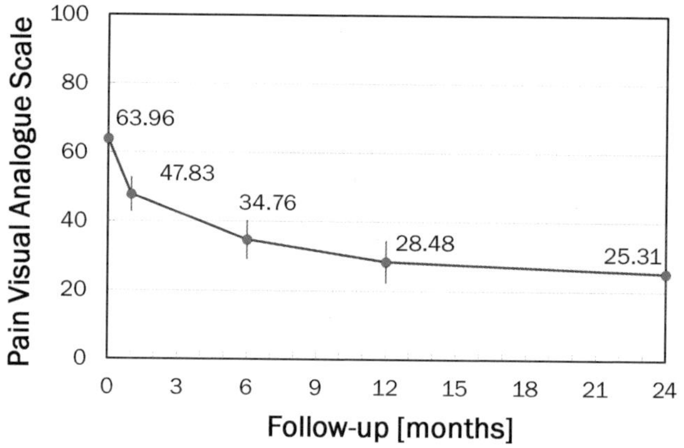

(b)

Figure 9-14. The results of subjective pain questionnaires (a) KOOS (Knee injury and Osteoarthritis Outcome Score), and (b) VAS (Visual Analogue Score), as reported by patients implanted with the NUSurface® meniscus implant over two years, with the following number of patients reaching each time point: $n = 115$ at the baseline, $n = 104$ at 6 weeks, $n = 91$ at 6 months, $n = 61$ at 1 year, and $n = 13$ at 2 years.

sub-total meniscectomy of the non-functional medial meniscus, leaving a thin rim of 2–4 mm, which serves as a pocket for the implant (Figures 9-13(a)–9-13(b)). Next, the implant is inserted through a 4–6 cm incision. Radio-opaque trials are used to determine the final implant size for implantation by allowing the surgeon to evaluate

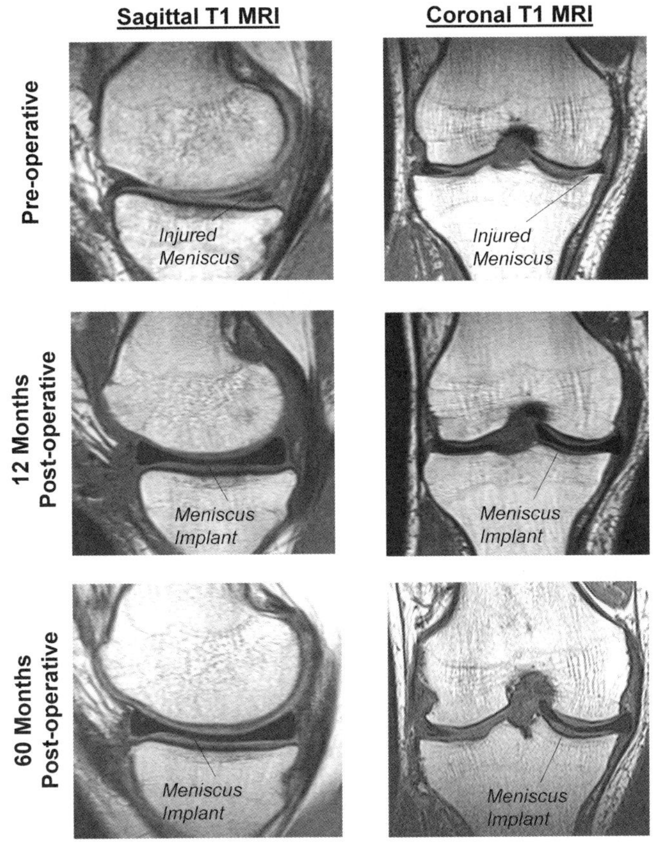

Figure 9-15. Sagittal (left column) and coronal (right column) T1 MRI scans of a patient (60-year-old male) treated with the meniscus implant: Pre-operative, 12 months post-operative, and 60 months post-operative (*Photos, courtesy of Dr. Vincenzo Condello*).

movement of the trial *in vivo* using fluoroscopy (Figures 9-13(c)–9-13(d)).

The patients showed an improvement post-operation. Significant pain relief was indicated by both the KOOS pain subscale (Figure 9-14(a)) and VAS scores (Figure 9-14(b)) after 12 months (Arbel *et al.*, 2013; Verdonk *et al.*, 2013). The first MRI findings showed no signs of further cartilage degradation. Representative coronal and sagittal MRI images of the device, 1.5, 12, and 60 months post-implantation are shown in Figure 9-15. Long-term follow-up is ongoing. While the clinical results in the short term seem to be as promising as the *in vitro* results, long-term results are needed and will be evaluated in years to come.

Acknowledgments

The authors wish to thank Prof. Claudio Zorzi and Dr. Vincenco Condello for providing surgical images and follow-up data, and Mr. Emanuele Nocco for providing the summary of clinical data for the NUsurface® meniscus implant.

References

Adams, M. and Hukins, D. (1992). *The extracellular matrix of the meniscus*, Raven Press, New York.

Appleyard, R.C., Burkhardt, D., Ghosh, P., Read, R., Cake, M., Swain, M.V. *et al.* (2003). Topographical analysis of the structural, biochemical and dynamic biomechanical properties of cartilage in an ovine model of osteoarthritis, *Osteoarthr Cartilage*, **11**, 65–77.

Arbel, R., Israeli, S., Beer, Y., Ben-Haim, Z., Blumberg, N., Shabshin, N. *et al.* (2013). A novel polycarbonate-urethane meniscus implant for the treatment of middle aged patients: First experience from 30 patients, *Int Cartilage Repair Soc (ICRS) Meet 2013*, Izmir.

Auger, D.D., Dowson, D., Fisher, J., and Jin, Z.M. (1993). Friction and lubrication in cushion form bearings for artificial hip joints, *Proc Inst Mech Eng H*, **207**(1), 25–33.

Auger, D.D., Dowson, D. and Fisher, J. (1995a). Cushion form bearings for total knee joint replacement. Part 1: Design, friction and lubrication, *Proc Inst Mech Eng H*, **209**(2), 73–81.

Auger, D.D., Dowson, D. and Fisher J. (1995b). Cushion form bearings for total knee joint replacement. Part 2: Wear and durability, *Proc Inst Mech Eng H*, **209**(2), 83–91.

Bergmann, G., Siraky, J., Rohlmann, A. and Koelbel, R. (1984). A comparison of hip joint forces in sheep, dog and man. *J Biomech*, **17**(12), 907–921.

Buma, P., van Tienen, T. and Veth, R. (2007). The collagen meniscus implant, *Expert Rev Med Devic*, **4**, 507–516.

Carlson, C.S., Guilak, F., Vail, T.P., Gardin, J.F. and Kraus, V.B. (2002). Synovial fluid biomarker levels predict articular cartilage damage following complete medial meniscectomy in the canine knee, *J Orthop Res*, **20**, 92–100.

Chiari, C., Koller, U., Dorotka, R., Eder, C., Plasenzotti, R., Lang, S. *et al.* (2006). A tissue engineering approach to meniscus regeneration in a sheep model, *Osteoarthr Cartilage*, **14**, 1056–1065.

Christenson, E.M., Anderson, J.M. and Hiltner, A. (2007). Biodegradation mechanisms of polyurethane elastomers, *Corr Eng Sci Technol*, **42**(4), 312–323.

Christenson, E.M., Patel, S., Anderson, J.M. and Hiltner, A. (2006). Enzymatic degradation of poly(ether urethane) and poly(carbonate urethane) by cholesterol esterase, *Biomaterials*, **27**(21), 3920–3926.

Dalstra, M. and Huiskes, R. (1995). Load transfer across the pelvic bone, *J Biomech*, **28**, 715–724.

Dowson, D., Fisher, J., Jin, Z.M., Auger, D.D. and Jobbins, B. (1991). Design considerations for cushion form bearings in artificial hip joints, *Proc Inst Mech Eng H*, **205**(2), 59–68.

Elsner, J.J., Portnoy, S., Guilak, F., Shterling, A. and Linder-Ganz, E. (2010b). MRI based characterization of bone anatomy in the human knee for size matching of a medial meniscal implant, *J Biomech Eng*, **132**(10), 101008.

Elsner, J.J., Portnoy, S., Zur, G., Guilak, F., Shterling, A. and Linder-Ganz, E. (2010c). Design of a free-floating polycarbonate-urethane meniscal implant using finite element modeling and experimental validation, *J Biomech Eng*, **132**(9), 095001.

Elsner, J.J., Mezape, Y., Hakshur, K., Shemesh, M., Linder-Ganz, E., Shterling, A. *et al.* (2010a). Wear rate evaluation of a novel polycarbonate-urethane cushion form bearing for artificial hip joints, *Acta Biomater*, **26**(12), 4698–4707.

Elsner, J.J., Shemesh, M., Mezape, Y., Levenshtein, M., Hakshur, K., Shterling, A. *et al* . (2011). Long-term evaluation of a compliant cushion form acetabular bearing for hip joint replacement: A 20 million cycles wear simulation, *J Orthop Res*, **29**(12), 1859–1866.

Elsner, J.J., Bonner, T.F., Greene, A., Gupta, R.R., Butler, R.S., Linder-Ganz, E. *et al.* (2012). *In vitro* stability testing of a non-fixed meniscal implant: The effect of surgical technique and knee condition, *Int Cartilage Repair Soc (ICRS) Meet 2012*, Montreal.

Fisher, J. and Jennings, L. (2002). Investigation of a novel compliant all-polyurethane acetabular resurfacing system, *Int Conf Eng Surg*, London.

Galvin, A.L., Tipper, J.L., Jennings, L.M., Stone, M.H., Jin, Z.M., Ingham, E. *et al.* (2007). Wear and biological activity of highly crosslinked polyethylene in the hip under low serum protein concentrations, *Proc Inst Mech Eng H*, **221**, 1–10.

Giannini, S., Chiarello, E., Cadossi, M., Luciani, D. and Tedesco, G. (2011). Prosthetic surgery in fragility osteopathy, *Aging Clin Exp Res*, **23**(2 Suppl), 40–42.

Green, T.R., Fisher, J., Stone, M., Wroblewski, B.M. and Ingham, E. (1998). Polyethylene particles of a 'critical size' are necessary for the induction of cytokines by macrophages *in vitro*, *Biomaterials*, **19**(24), 2297–2302.

Kelly, B.T., Robertson, W., Potter, H.G., Deng, X.H., Turner, A.S., Lyman, S. *et al.* (2007). Hydrogel meniscal replacement in the sheep knee: Preliminary evaluation of chondroprotective effects, *Am J Sports Med*, **35**, 43–52.

Khan, I., Smith, N., Jones, E., Finch, D.S. and Cameron, R.E. (2005). Analysis and evaluation of a biomedical polycarbonate urethane tested in an *in vitro* study and an ovine arthroplasty model. Part I: Materials selection and evaluation, *Biomaterials*, **26**(6), 621–631.

Khan, I., Smith, N., Jones, E., Finch, D.S. and Cameron, R.E. (2005). Analysis and evaluation of a biomedical polycarbonate urethane tested in an *in vitro* study and an ovine arthroplasty model. Part II: *In vivo* investigation, *Biomaterials*, **26**(6), 633–643.

Kobayashi, M., Toguchida, J. and Oka, M. (2003). Development of an artificial meniscus using polyvinyl alcohol-hydrogel for early return to, and continuance of, athletic life in sportspersons with severe meniscus injury. II: Animal experiments, *Knee*, **10**, 53.

Labow, R., Meek, E., Matheson, L. and Santerre, J. (2002). Human macrophage-mediated biodegradation of polyurethanes: Assessment of candidate enzyme activities, *Biomaterials*, **23**(19), 3969–3975.

Linder-Ganz, E., Elsner, J.J., Danino, A., Guilak, F. and Shterling, A. (2010). A novel quantitative approach for evaluating contact mechanics of meniscal replacements, *J Biomech Eng*, **132**(2), 024501.

Little, C., Smith, S., Ghosh, P. and Bellenger, C. (1997). Histomorphological and immunohistochemical evaluation of joint changes in a model of osteoarthritis induced by lateral meniscectomy in sheep, *J Rheumatol*, **24**(11), 2199–2209.

McDermott, I.D. and Amis, A.A. (2006). The consequences of meniscectomy, *J Bone Joint Surg Br*, **88**(12), 1549–1556.

McTighe, T., Treharne, R. and Greene, A.H. (2009). Design rationale and clinical review of a new compliant bearing material for acetabular reconstruction, *Joint Implant Surgery and Research Foundation*, Ohio. Available at: http://www.jisrf.org/pdfs/joint-implant-surgery-and-research-foundation-chagrin.pdf.

Moroni, A., Nocco, E., Hoque, M., Diremigio, E., Buffoli, D., Cantù, F. *et al.* (2012). Cushion bearings versus large diameter head metal-on-metal bearings in total hip arthroplasty: A short-term metal ion study, *Arch Orthop Trauma Surg*, **132**(1), 123–129.

Noyes, F.R., Barber-Westin, S.D. and Rankin, M. (2004). Meniscal transplantation in symptomatic patients less than fifty years old. *J Bone Joint Surg Am*, **86**, 1392–1404.

Pinchuk, L. (1992). Crack-resistant polycarbonate-urethane polymer prostheses, *US Patent 5,133,742*.

Pinchuk, L. (1993). Crack-resistant polycarbonate-urethane polymer prostheses and the like, *US Patent 5,229,431*.

Pöllänen, R., Tikkanen, A.M., Lammi, M.J. and Lappalainen, R. (2011). The effect of loading and material on the biomechanical properties and vitality of bovine cartilage *in vitro*, *J Appl Biomater Biomech*, **9**(1), 47–53.

Scholes, S.C., Unsworth, A. and Goldsmith, A.A. (2000). A frictional study of total hip joint replacements, *Phys Med Biol*, **45**(12), 3721–3735.

Scholes, S.C., Burgess, I.C., Marsden, H.R., Unsworth, A., Jones, E. and Smith, N. (2006). Compliant layer acetabular cups: Friction testing of a range of materials and designs for a new generation of prosthesis that mimics the natural joint, *Proc Inst Mech Eng H*, **220**(5), 583–596.

Shemesh, M., Asher, R., Zylberberg, E., Guilak, F., Linder-Ganz, E. and Elsner, J.J. (2014). Viscoelastic properties of a synthetic meniscus implant, *J Mech Behav Biomed Mat*, **29**, 42–55.

Shepherd, D.E.T. and Seedhom, B.B. (1999). The 'instantaneous' compressive modulus of human articular cartilage in joints of the lower limb, *Rheumatology*, **38**(2), 124–132.

Siebert, W.E., Mai, S. and Kurtz, S. (2008). Retrieval analysis of a polycarbonate-urethane acetabular cup: A case report, *J Long-Term Eff Med*, **18**(1), 69–74.

Smith, S.L., Ash, H.E. and Unsworth, A. (2000). A tribological study of UHMWPE acetabular cups and polyurethane compliant layer acetabular cups, *J Biomed Mater Res*, **53**(6), 710–716.

Smith, R.A., Maghsoodpour, A. and Hallab, N.J. (2010). *In vivo* response to cross-linked polyethylene and olycarbonateurethane particles, *J Biomed Mater Res A*, **93**, 227–234.

St. John, K. and Gupta, M. (2012). Evaluation of the wear performance of a polycarbonate-urethane acetabular component in a hip joint simulator and comparison with UHMWPE and cross-linked UHMWPE, *J Biomater Appl*, **27**(1), 55–65.

Stokes, K. and Cobian, K. (1982). Polyether polyurethanes for implantable pacemaker leads, *Biomaterials*, **3**(4), 225–231.

Stokes, K., McVenes, R. and Anderson, J.M. (1995). Polyurethane elastomer biostability, *J Biomater Appl*, **9**(4), 321–354.

Tang, Y., Labow, R. and Santerre, J. (2001). Enzyme-induced biodegradation of polycarbonate-polyurethanes: Dependence on hard-segment chemistry, *J Biomed Mater Res*, **57**(4), 597–611.

Tang, Y.W., Labow, R.S., Revenko, I. and Santerre, J.P. (2002). Influence of surface morphology and chemistry on the enzyme catalyzed biodegradation of polycarbonate-urethanes, *J Biomater Sci Polym Ed*, **13**(4), 463–483.

Tienen, T.G., Heijkants, R.G., de Groot, J.H., Pennings, A.J., Schouten, A.J., Veth, R.P. *et al.* (2006). Replacement of the knee meniscus by a porous polymer implant: A study in dogs, *Am J Sports Med*, **34**, 64–71.

Timperley, A.J., Nusem, I., Wilson, K., Whitehouse, S.L., Buma, P. and Crawford, R.W. (2010). A modified cementing technique using BoneSource to augment fixation of the acetabulum in a sheep model, *Acta Orthop*, **81**(4), 503–507.

Unsworth, A. (1991). Tribology of human and artificial joints, *Proc Inst Mech Eng H*, **205**(3), 163–172.

Van Arkel, E.R. and de Boer, H.H. (2002). Survival analysis of human meniscal transplantations, *J Bone Joint Surg Br*, **84**, 222–231.

Verdonk, P., Dhollander, A.A.M. and Verdonk, R. (2013). Treatment of post-meniscectomy syndrome with a free-floating meniscus implant: A prospective, open label, single-arm trial, *Int Cartilage Repair Soc (ICRS) Meet 2013*, Turkey.

Verdonk, P.C., Demurie, A., Almqvist, K.F., Veys, E.M., Verbruggen, G. and Verdonk, R. (2005). Transplantation of viable meniscal allograft. Survivorship analysis and clinical outcome of one hundred cases, *J Bone Joint Surg Am*, **87**, 715–724.

Wiggins, M.J., Wilkoff, B., Anderson, J.M. and Hiltner, A. (2001). Biodegradation of polyether polyurethane inner insulation in bipolar pacemaker leads, *J Biomed Mater Res*, **58**(3), 302–307.

Wippermann, B., Kurtz, S., Hallab, N. and Treharne, R. (2008). Explantation and analysis of the first retrieved human acetabular cup made of polycarbonate urethane: A case report, *J Long Term Eff Med Implants*, **18**(1), 75–83.

Yang, M., Zhang, Z., Hahn, C., King, M.W. and Guidoin, R. (1999). Assessing the resistance to calcification of polyurethane membranes used in the manufacture of ventricles for a totally implantable artificial heart, *J Biomed Mater Res*, **48**(5), 648–659.

Zhao, Q., Agger, M.P., Fitzpatrick, M., Anderson, J.M., Hiltner, A., Stokes, K. *et al.* (1990). Cellular interactions with biomaterials: *In vivo* cracking of pre-stressed Pellethane 2363-80A, *J Biomed Mater Res*, **24**(5), 621–637.

Zur, G., Linder-Ganz, E., Elsner, J.J., Shani, J., Brenner, O., Agar, G. *et al.* (2011). Chondroprotective effects of a polycarbonate-urethane meniscal implant: Histopathological results in a sheep model, *Knee Surg Sport Tr A*, **19**(2), 255–263.

Chapter 10

Hydrogels and Surface Modification

Masayuki Kyomoto[a,b,c] and Kazuhiko Ishihara[a]

[a] *Department of Materials Engineering, Department of Bioengineering, School of Engineering,*

[b] *Division of Science for Joint Reconstruction, School of Medicine, The University of Tokyo, Tokyo, Japan*

[c] *Research Department, KYOCERA Medical Corporation, Osaka, Japan*

1. Articular Cartilage

1.1. *Articular Cartilage as Hydrogel Matrix and its Lubrication Mechanism*

The surface of articular cartilage is made up of a collagen network, hyaluronic acid, and proteoglycan subunits (Mow *et al.*, 1992). The proteoglycan subunits form a gel-like surface layer, owing to hydration, along with the joint synovia. Although the binding that exists between the proteoglycan subunits and the hyaluronic acid can be detected (Buckwalter and Rosenberg, 1983), that between the hyaluronic acid and the collagen network has not yet been confirmed. Obara *et al.* (1997) reported that the friction coefficient of joints increases when the gelled material on the cartilage surface has been removed with gauze. Once the gelled material has been removed, the joint surface is lubricated only by the joint synovia or hyaluronic acid; following the loss of the gel comprising proteoglycan subunits, the friction coefficient of the joints increases and cannot be lowered again. This fact indicates that the proteoglycan aggregates not only bond with the collagen network through physical

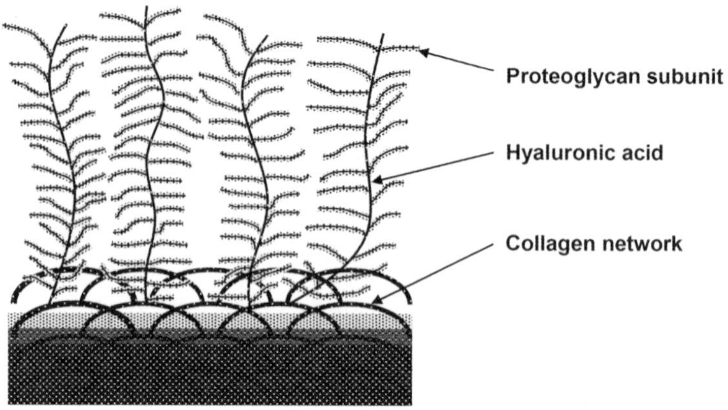

Figure 10-1. Schematic model of the brush-like structure of cartilage surface.

adsorption but also that the hydrophilic macromolecules on the joint surface play an important role in reducing friction. A previous study reported that the hydrophilic macromolecules present on the cartilage surface are likely to have a brush-like structure: A part of this proteoglycan aggregate brush bonds with the collagen network on the cartilage surface (Figure 10-1) (Ishikawa *et al.*, 2006). The rest of the proteoglycan aggregate floats freely in the joint synovia.

Although the lubrication mechanism of human joints has been studied extensively since the 1930s, it is not yet clearly understood. Longfield *et al.* (1969) and Ikeuchi *et al.* (1999) reported that the lubrication of joints is mainly of the hydration lubrication. Hydrophilic macromolecules reduce friction by promoting the formation of a fluid film that is retained by the water molecules' attraction forces, indicating that these attraction forces are critical for realizing low friction for the smooth motion of the joints (Wright and Dowson, 1976). The lubrication of human joints appears to occur by hydration lubrication because the structure of the surface layer of the joints is similar to the gelled material. Sasada *et al.* have proposed a new mechanism, named 'surface gel hydration lubrication', to describe joint lubrication in cases when such hydrophilic macromolecules are involved (Ishikawa *et al.*, 2006).

Water is attracted by the hydrophilic macromolecules in the surface layer and plays an important role in lubrication. As most

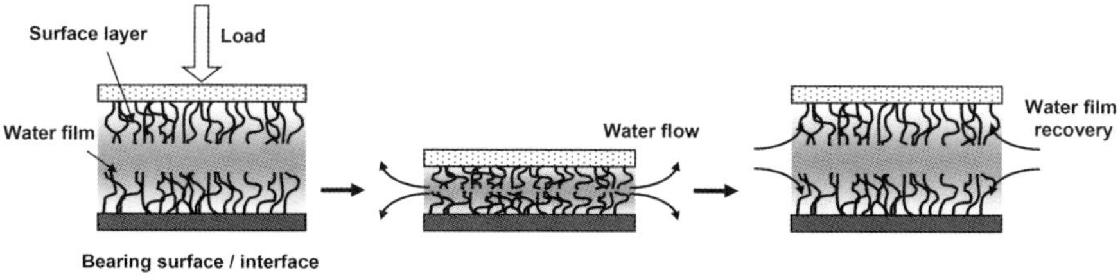

Figure 10-2. Schematic model of hydration lubrication.

macromolecules are flexible, they cannot support a load by themselves. It is thus likely that the water in the surface layer supports most of the load. Frictional forces arise owing to the adhesion of macromolecules to the counter surface. The time-dependent properties of these friction forces can be interpreted as follows (Figure 10-2) (Yoshida *et al.*, 2003). Under a load, water exudes slowly from the surface layer with or without sliding. As the result of water loss, the thickness of the surface layer reduces and the water content of the surface layer decreases. Consequently, the degree of adhesion of the surface to the opposite bearing surface increases and so does the frictional force. Therefore, it may be concluded that the amount of friction essentially depends on the water content of the surface layer. Hydration lubrication can thus be said to lead to low friction and wear.

1.2. *Articular Cartilage and Materials for Designing Artificial Joints*

The lubrication of the artificial hip joint principally occurs through a different mechanism than in the case of natural human joints and is considerably less effective as well. As mentioned above, the most popular artificial hip joint is a bearing couple composed of a cup of a plastic such as crosslinked polyethylene (CLPE) and a head that is made of a metal such a cobalt–chromium–molybdenum (CoCrMo) alloy or ceramics (Figure 10-3). The bearing couple is structurally rigid and made of non-porous materials, which do not allow for the biophysical mechanisms responsible for lubrication in natural joints. The primary advantage of this bearing couple is that it allows for the

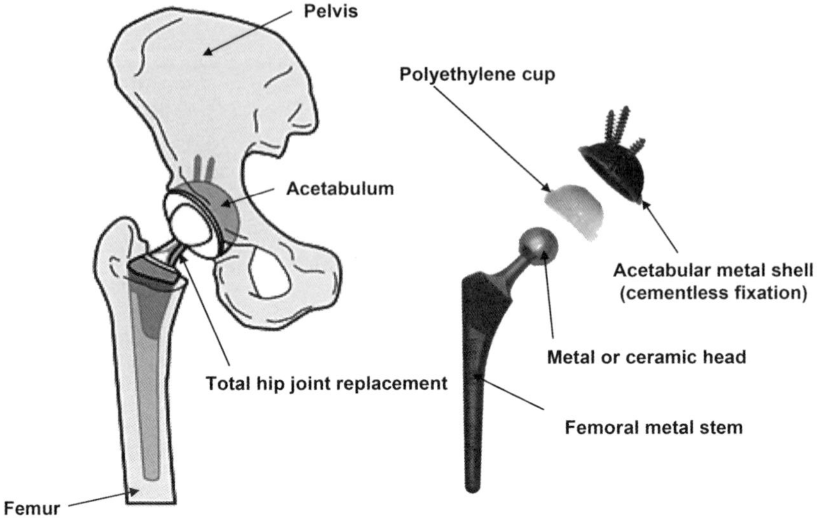

Figure 10-3. Schematic model of total hip joint replacement and typical implant.

design of anatomically accurate hip joints. Therefore, substituting or modifying the bearing surfaces of artificial joints with a hydrogel structure should increase lubrication to levels that match that of articular cartilage under physiological conditions. A bearing surface with a hydrogel structure comprising hydrophilic macromolecules should be very similar to that of articular cartilage. Thus, hydrogel materials that allow for hydration lubrication are well suited for this purpose.

2. Hydrogel Materials and Surface Modification of Orthopedic Implants

2.1. *Hydrogels as Artificial Materials*

Gels consist of a solid three-dimensional (3D) network that spans the volume of a liquid medium and ensnares it through surface tension effects. The internal network structure may result from physical bonds (physical gels) or chemical bonds (chemical gels), as well as owing to crystallites or other junctions that remain intact within the extending fluid. Hydrogels are hydrophilic macromolecule

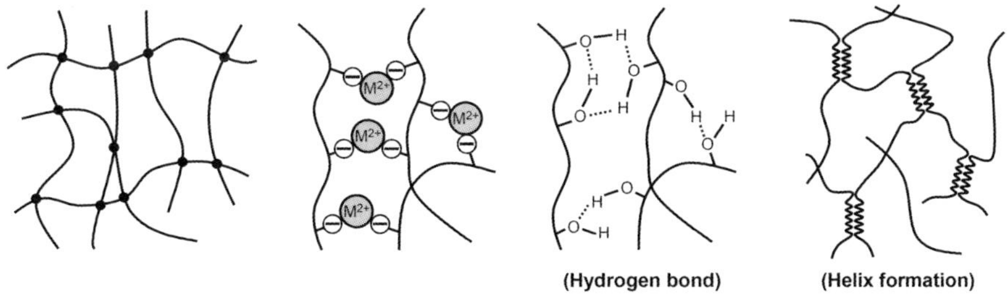

(a) Covalent bond (b) Ionic bond (c) Noncovalent interaction

Figure 10-4. Three-dimensional networks formed by various crosslink structures.

(hydrophilic polymer) based gels and are able to retain large quantities of water within their structure without dissolving. In contrast, organogels swell with organic solvents. Hydrogels have a 3D structure and the crosslinks responsible for this structure can be formed through either covalent or ionic bonds (Figure 10-4). In addition, weaker forces such as van der Waals forces and hydrogen bonds can also serve as crosslinks. Finally, non-crosslinked hydrophilic polymers can also form hydrogels upon swelling because the crystallites present in them are insoluble in water and can act as physical crosslinks.

Hydrogels may be classified in a number of ways, depending on their physical and chemical structures. A common classification scheme that is particularly useful in the case of medical devices is to label hydrogels as being nonionic/neutral, cationic, anionic, or zwitterionic hydrogels, or being based on a swollen interpenetrating polymer networks (IPN). A few typical nonionic hydrophilic polymers and hydrogels are summarized in Table 10-1. Poly(2-hydroxyethyl methacrylate) (PHEMA), its derivatives, and its copolymers with other vinyl monomers have been widely investigated as hydrogel materials. Polyacrylamide (PAAm), poly(N-vinyl-pyrrolidone) (PVPy), poly(vinyl alcohol) (PVA), poly(ethylene glycol) (PEG), poly(oligo[ethylene glycol] methacrylate) (POEGMA), poly(2-[dimethylamino]ethyl methacrylate) (PDMAEMA), poly(2-methacryloyloxyethyl phosphate) (PMPA), and poly(2-methacryloyloxyethyl phosphorylcholine) (PMPC; MPC, 2-methacryloyloxyethyl phosphorylcholine) have also been investigated as hydrogels.

Table 10-1. Chemical structures of monomers used to form hydrophilic polymer and hydrogels.

Electric charge	Hydrophilic group	Typical monomer
Nonion	–OH	Vinyl alcohol (VA)* 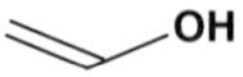 * VA is unstable in normal condition.
	$-C_2H_4OH$	2-Hydroxyethyl methacrylate (HEMA) 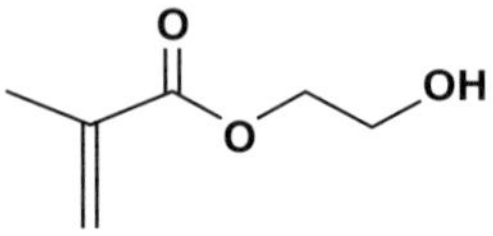
	$-(O-C_2H_4)_nOH$	Oligo(ethylene glycol) methacrylate (OEGMA) 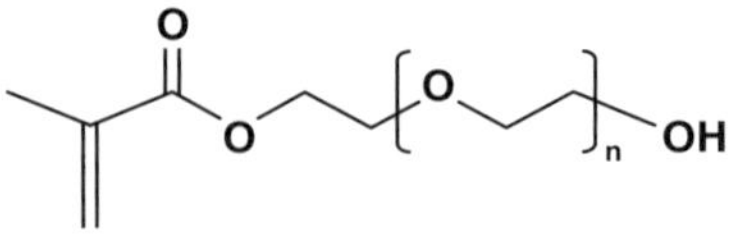
	$-CONH_2$	Acrylamide (AAm) 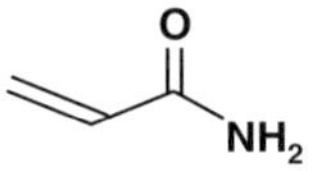
	–CONR–	N-Vinylpyrrolidone (VPy) 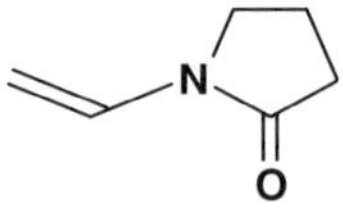
Cation	$-NR_2H^+$	2-(Dimethylamino)ethyl methacrylate (DMAEMA) 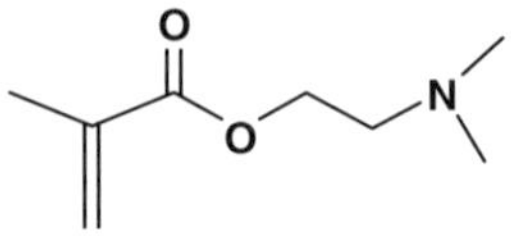
Anion	$-COO^-$	Acrylic acid (AA) 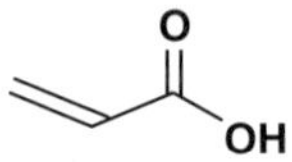

(*Continued*)

Table 10-1. (*Continued*)

Electric charge	Hydrophilic group	Typical monomer
	$-SO_3^-$	2-Acrylamido-2-methylpropane sulfonic acid (AMPS) 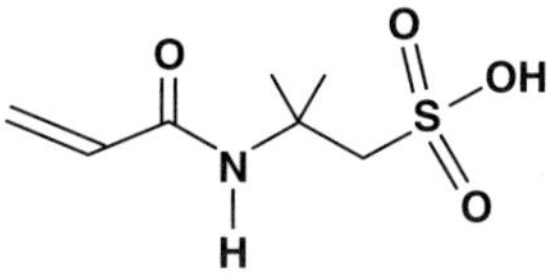
	$-PO_4^{2-}$	2-Methacryloyloxyethyl phosphate (MPA) 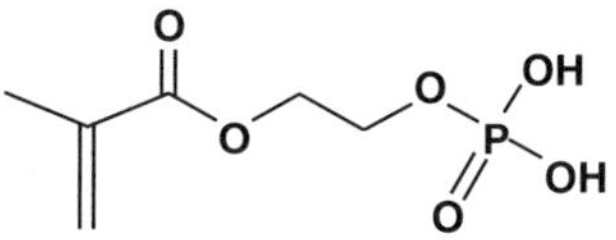
Zwitterion	$-PO_4^-\ (CH_2)_2N^+ \equiv$	2-Methacryloyloxyethyl phosphorylcholine (MPC) 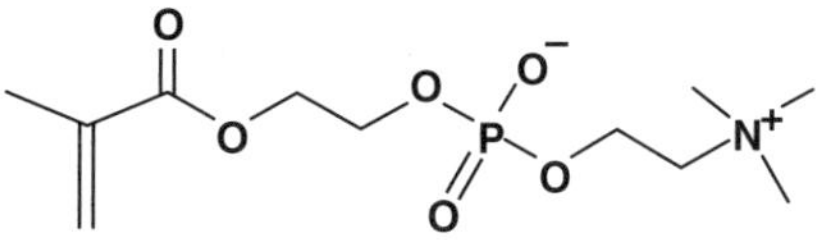

PVA was synthesized in 1924 by Hermann *et al.* for use as a synthetic fiber (Paradossi, 2013). The hydrophilic nature of the polymer, attributable to the hydroxyl groups in its repeating unit, is considered as a key feature. The alcoholic functional groups present in it are also responsible for the unusual chemical versatility of PVA. Bray and Merrill (1973) were the first to report that PVA hydrogels are structurally and functionally similar to cartilage. PVA in aqueous solution form can be crosslinked to produce hydrogels through the formation of acetal linkages by using di-functional crosslinking agents. PVA hydrogels can also be produced via physical crosslinks owing to crystallization induced by annealing, dehydration, freeze-thaw cycling, and phase separation. Hyon *et al.* (1989) developed the low-temperature crystallization technique using water/dimethyl sulfoxide-mixed solvent for the transparent PVA hydrogels with high

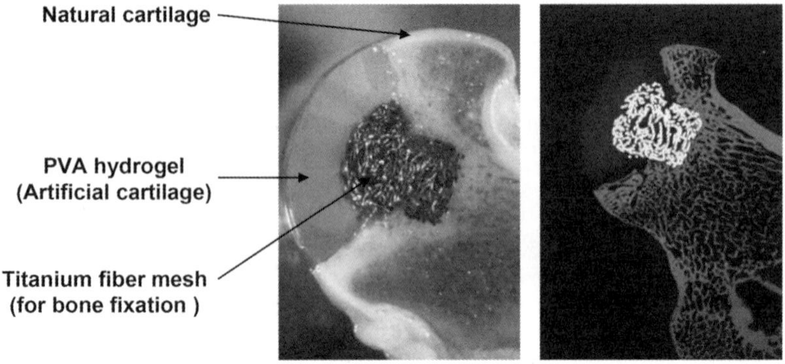

Figure 10-5. Artificial cartilage made of poly(vinyl alcohol).

strength and modulus. It is known that PVA hydrogels are similar to articular cartilage in terms of their mechanical and lubrication properties, directing fluid to the contact surface as per squeeze-film lubrication under low-load conditions and boundary lubrication under high-load ones. On the basis of the fact that PVA hydrogels are effective in producing fluid film lubrication, Ushio *et al.* (2003) used PVA hydrogels with a titanium fiber mesh for bone fixation during hemi-arthroplasty in order to induce a high degree of lubrication in the replacement joint (Figure 10-5). This PVA hydrogel implant for hemi-arthroplasty exhibited lubricity at the PVA hydrogel/natural articular cartilage interface.

Elisseeff *et al.* (1999) prepared hydrogels from PEG by modifying methacrylate groups to allow for photoinduced crosslinking and used them as injectable photoinduced polymerizable hydrogels for repairing cartilage defects. Like PVA hydrogels, PEG hydrogels can also be modified easily and have been useful in studying the effects of hydrogel properties on articular cartilage.

MPC, a methacrylate monomer with a phospholipid polar group in the side chain, was designed and developed by Ishihara *et al.* (1990) and is a novel biomaterial that mimics the neutral phospholipids of cell membranes. MPC polymers are the most biocompatible polymers, as well as the hydrophilic ones, studied thus far and have potential for application in a variety of fields such as biology, biomedical science, and surface chemistry. This is because of their high biocompatibility, high lubricity, low friction, anti-protein adsorptivity, and cell membrane-like surface (Ishihara *et al.*, 1990). Hence, MPC polymers can induce the formation of thin films of free water under physiological conditions. Several medical devices such as intravascular stents (Kuiper and Nordrehaug, 2000), soft contact lenses (Selan *et al.*, 2009), and artificial hearts (Snyder *et al.*, 2007) have been developed using MPC polymers. These devices have been approved by the Ministry of Health, Labour and Welfare (MHLW) of Japan and the Food and Drug Administration (FDA) of the United States. Therefore, the efficacy and safety of MPC polymers as biomaterial is well established (Table 10-2).

Arakaki *et al.* (2010) investigated the *in vivo* effects of a poly (2-acrylamido-2-methylpropane sulfonic acid)/poly(N, N-dimethyl acrylamide) (PAMPS/PDMAAm) IPN hydrogel (i.e. a double-network (DN) hydrogel) on counterface cartilage in rabbit knee joints and its *ex vivo* friction properties with respect to normal cartilage. They found that the PAMPS/PDMAAm DN hydrogel has an extremely low friction coefficient with respect to normal cartilage and that it has no significant detrimental effects on counterface cartilage *in vivo*.

Thus, owing to their superior chemical and physical properties, hydrogels have received much attention for use as biomedical materials.

2.2. *Surface Modification with Hydrogels*

2.2.1. *Polymer surface modification*

Generally, hydrogels have several good characteristics; for instance, they exhibit antibiofouling properties. However, their mechanical strength is not high enough for use as medical devices. Therefore, hydrophilic polymers and hydrogels have to be crosslinked or grafted onto polymeric substrates.

In artificial hip joints, bearing surfaces with a brush-like structure made up of hydrophilic macromolecules can thus be assumed to be similar to that of articular cartilage. The hydration lubrication interface of such joints can also be regarded to mimic natural joint cartilage *in vivo*. The grafting of polymers onto various surfaces has been

Table 10-2. Medical devices with MPC polymer.

Medical device	Product name	Manufacturer	Clinical introduction	Reference
Artificial heart	Evaheart	Sun Medical	2011	Yamada *et al.*, 2012
Artificial joint	Aquala	KYOCERA Medical	2011	Takatori *et al.*, 2013
Artificial lung	Mimesys	Sorin Biomedica	2002	Myers *et al.*, 2005
	Synthesis	Sorin Biomedica	2003	Myers *et al.*, 2003
	Physio	Sorin Italia	2005	—
Catheter	Eliminate	Clinical Supply	—	MHLW approval
Contact lens	Proclear	Cooper Vision	1998	FDA approval
Guide wire	Aqua diver	Clinical Supply	—	MHLW approval
	Inter through	Clinical Supply	—	—
	Hunter	Biocompatible	1997	FDA approval
Micro catheter	Londis	Clinical Supply	2005	MHLW approval
Stent	Endeavor	Medtronic	2008	Gershlick *et al.*, 2007
	Endeavor I	Medtronic	2008	Kandzari and Leon, 2006
	Endeavor II	Medtronic	2008	Fajadet *et al.*, 2006
	Endeavor II CA	Medtronic	2008	Sakurai *et al.*, 2007
	Endeavor III	Medtronic	2008	Kandzari *et al.*, 2006
	TriMaxx	Abbott Laboratories	2005	Abizaid *et al.*, 2007b
	ZoMaxx	Abbott Laboratories	—	Abizaid *et al.*, 2007a
	Biodiv Ysio	Biocompatible	2000	Rodriguez *et al.*, 2005 Han *et al.*, 2006
Tympanostomy tube	—	Gyrus, Grace Medical	2000	FDA approval

studied for over 50 years. This type of grafting plays an important role in many areas of biomaterial science and technology, including in colloidal stabilization, adhesion, lubrication, tribology, and rheology. Recent efforts have focused on the synthesis of polymer brushes, in which the polymer chains stretch out away from the surface of the substrate (Milner, 1991; Nagasaki and Kataoka, 1996). There are three primary methods for modifying a planar substrate with an organic polymer: (a) physical coating, (b) chemical coating or 'grafting to'; and, (c) 'grafting from' (Figure 10-6). Examples of physical coating techniques are spin and dip coating. However, in these techniques, the polymer is merely adsorbed onto the substrate surface and may diffuse away when the substrate is immersed into a solvent in which polymer is soluble. Chemical coating methods involve chemically attaching the functional groups of the polymer to the substrate surface via various techniques. Robust layers can be created by making use of self-assembled monolayers (SAMs) to immobilize a reactive functional group. Thus, the polymer can be attached to the substrate surface provided the preformed polymer possesses a functional group that is capable of bonding with the substrate. For example, a polymer containing a primary amine could form an amide bond with a carboxylic acid-terminated SAM. This approach is known as the 'grafting to' technique and has been considerably successful in the synthesis of robust layers 1–50 nm in thickness. However, the grafting to technique is limited by diffusion barriers, which prevent the preformed polymer from intercalating through the tethered polymer to the reactive substrate. As a result, the grafting to method yields low-density brushes. In contrast, the grafting from approach can be used to synthesize high-density polymer brushes (Edmondson *et al.*, 2004). The conformation of these polymer brushes in solvents can change dramatically with the graft density. At low-graft densities, these brushes will assume a mushroom-like conformation, with the coil dimensions being similar to that of their free chains. With an increase in the graft density, the graft chains are forced to stretch away from the substrate, forming a polymer brush. Such high-density brushes are much thicker and range in size from a few nanometers to several micrometers. This significant increase in thickness

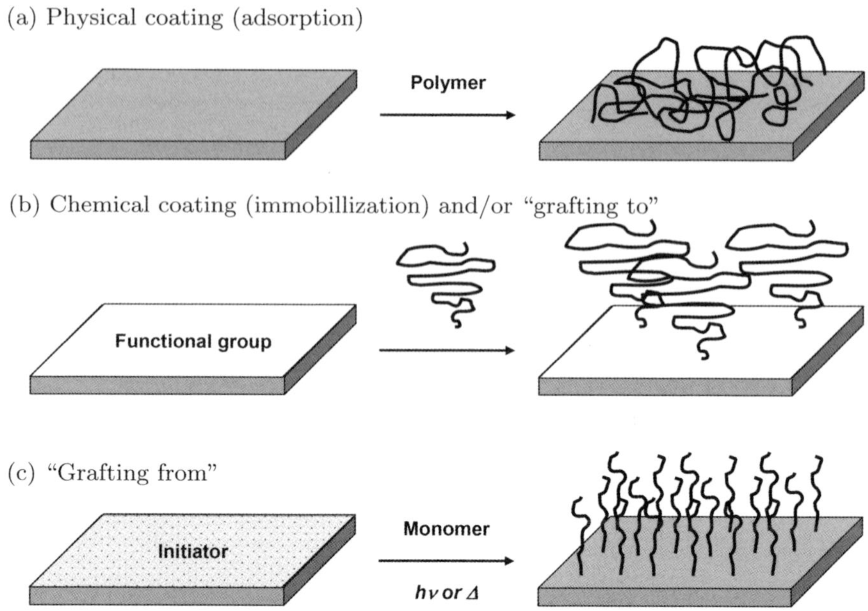

Figure 10-6. Approaches for modifying substrate with polymer: (a) physical coating (adsorption), (b) chemical coating (immobilization) and/or 'grafting to'; and, (c) 'grafting from'.

is attributable to the fact that the grafting-from layers have much higher grafting densities than those of the grafting-to layers.

2.2.2. *Photoinduced surface 'grafting-from' polymerization*

Photochemical initiation has several advantages over thermal initiation. First, certain functional groups are not thermally stable, therefore it is desirable to initiate the polymerization process at room temperature. This also simplifies manufacturing processes. Furthermore, most alkylthiolate SAMs are not stable at temperatures greater than 70°C and may begin to degrade at the temperatures required for thermally initiating the polymerization of most polymers. Second, photoinitiation is generally faster than thermal initiation. Finally, the photoinitiation can be performed at almost any temperature. This allows for great flexibility when controlling the reactivity and processability of a layer. Surface-initiated polymerization can be

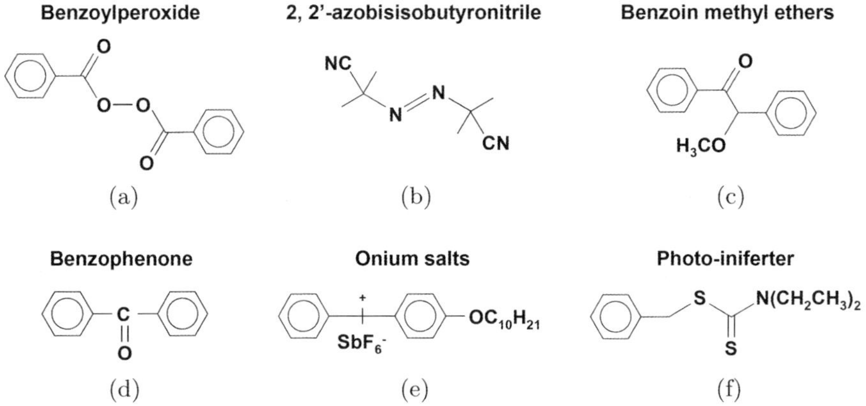

Figure 10-7. Various types of photoinitiators: (a) peroxides, (b) azo compounds based on AIBN, (c) benzoin methyl ethers, (d) triplet photosensitizers, (e) onium salts for cationic polymerization; and, (f) controlled free radical polymerization with photoiniferters.

performed with a variety of initiators; Figure 10-7 shows some of the most commonly used ones (Dyer, 2006). Typically, during surface-initiated polymerization, these initiators are modified and made to covalently bond with the substrate, resulting in 'grafting-from' polymerization. Alternatively, photosensitizers can be added to bulk solutions in order to abstract hydrogen atoms from the substrate. For example, benzophenone (BP) (Figure 10-7(d)) is converted to a reactive triplet state when subjected to ultraviolet (UV) irradiation; this triplet is capable of abstracting hydrogen atoms from various moieties. Tertiary amines or thiol-ene systems can be activated with photosensitizers but have not been used for surface-initiated polymerization until recently. Other photoinitiators include peroxides (Figure 10-7(a)) and benzoin derivatives (Figure 10-7(c)); of the two, only peroxides have been used for surface-initiated polymerization. The most common free radical photoinitiators are derivatives of 2, 2/-azobisisobutyronitrile (AIBN) (Figure 10-7(b)); several research groups have used these for grafting-from polymerizations involving various substrates. Recently, controlled free radical polymerization processes have gained much recognition because the resulting polymers have low polydispersities and living polymerization-like characteristics (Dyer, 2006). Indeed, polymerization techniques that yield living-like polymers have a tremendous advantage with respect to surface-initiated polymerization because they make it possible to grow block copolymers and to terminate the polymerized chain with specific end groups. However, most free-radical polymerization processes yielding living polymers require thermal initiation. For example, atom-transfer radical polymerization may be used to initiate surface polymerization; however, the rate of initiation and propagation is relatively low compared to that of photoinitiated polymerization and typically leads to layers that are less than 50 nm thick. Thus, there exist a number of photopolymerization strategies that may be used in the future, even though few of them have been investigated in detail as of now.

2.2.3. *Surface modification with polyelectrolyte*

2.2.3.1. Surface modification

A nanometer-scaled hydrated polyelectrolyte layer that covers the joint cartilage surface provides hydrophilicity and works as an effective boundary lubricant (Bhosale and Richardson, 2008; Goldberg *et al.*, 2011a, 2011b; Kirk *et al.*, 1993). Hence, grafting a cartilage-like hydrophilic polymer layer onto the bearing surfaces of artificial joints may bestow on them the same hydrophilicity and lubricity as that seen in physiological joint surface (Raviv *et al.*, 2003).

Kyomoto *et al.* (2012) synthesized nanometer-scaled hydrophilic layers having various types of charges (nonionic/neutral, cationic, anionic, or zwitterionic) on CLPE surfaces to increase the lubrication to levels that matched those of articular cartilage under physiological conditions. This type of nanometer-scaled surface modification was performed using a photoinduced radical polymerization technique that was similar to the grafting from method. The approach used renders only the surface of the CLPE substrate susceptible to modification and does not affect its bulk properties (Kyomoto *et al.*, 2007a, 2011). As can be seen from the cross-sectional transmission electron microscope (TEM) images in Figure 10-8, the graft polymerization processes resulted in the formation of uniform polyelectrolyte layers on the CLPE surface; the thicknesses of the layers

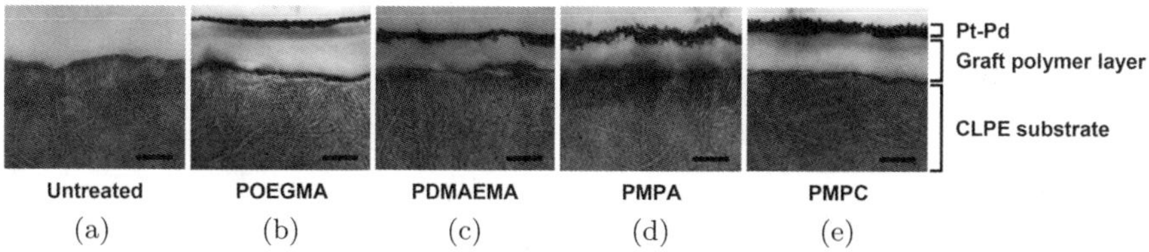

Figure 10-8. Cross-sectional TEM images of untreated CLPE and various polyelectrolyte-grafted CLPE. Bar: 100 nm.

were 100–150 nm. The hydrophilicity of the polyelectrolyte-grafted CLPE surfaces increased gradually with the photoirradiation time (Figure 10-9) (Kyomoto *et al.*, 2011). Thus, it was evident that the photoirradiation time affects the hydration kinetics of the polyelectrolyte graft chains. In contrast, the static-water contact angle of the polyelectrolyte-grafted CLPE surfaces differed significantly, with the lowest values ranging from 20° to 60°.

2.2.3.2. Wettability and lubricity in several lubricant conditions

It can be seen from Figure 10-10c that the coefficients of dynamic friction for the polyelectrolyte-grafted CLPE samples ranged from 0.01 to 0.05 in water, representing a 40–85% reduction compared to those of untreated CLPE. A calcified, mineralized morphology was observed on the surface of the PMPA-grafted CLPE samples after they had been pre-soaked in acellular simulated body fluid (SBF) for 24 h before the friction test; the inorganic ion concentrations of the SBF were analogous to those of human extracellular fluid. The coefficients of dynamic friction of the POEGMA- and PMPC-grafted CLPE surfaces with respect to different lubricants did not differ significantly. For all lubricants, the coefficient of dynamic friction of the PMPC-grafted CLPE sample was significantly lower than that of the POEGMA-grafted CLPE sample; a similar relation was noticed for the values of the static-water contact angles of the two types of polyelectrolyte-grafted CLPE surfaces. In contrast, the coefficients of dynamic friction of the PDMAEMA- and PMPA-grafted CLPE surfaces increased drastically in SBF and

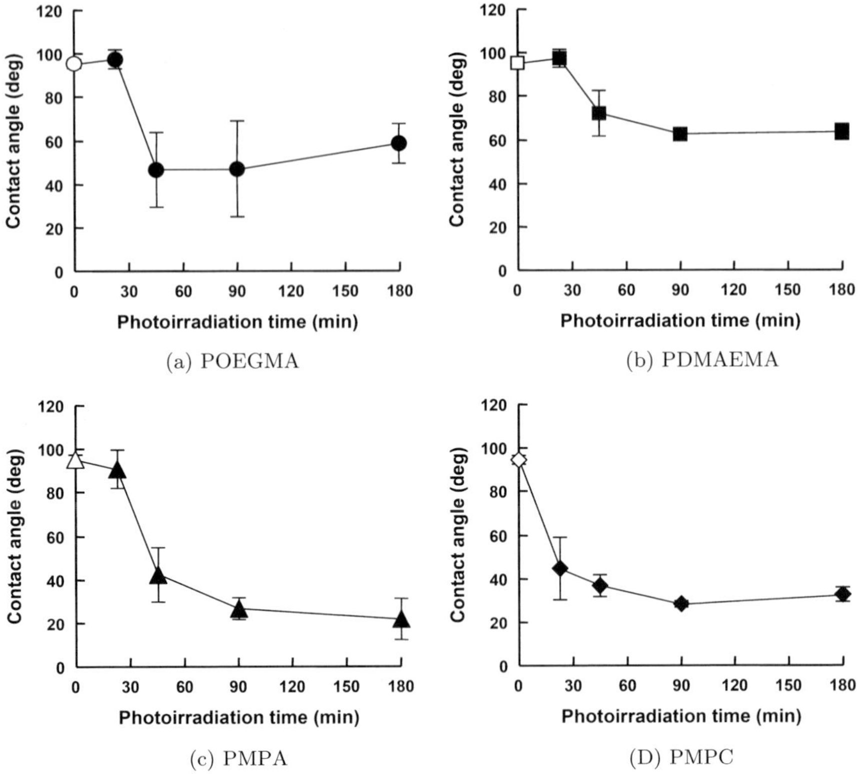

Figure 10-9. Static-water contact angles of various polyelectrolyte-grafted CLPE surfaces as functions of photoirradiation time. (a) POEGMA-grafted, (b) PDMAEMA-grafted, (c) PMPA-grafted, and (d) PMPC-grafted CLPE. Data are expressed as mean ± standard deviation.

bovine serum, respectively. In addition, the untreated CLPE sample also exhibited increased friction in bovine serum (BS) lubricant compared with that in water. As can be seen in the figure, the surface zeta potentials of the untreated CLPE and the POEGMA- and PMPC-grafted CLPE surfaces with nonionic and zwitterionic grafted polymer layers were almost zero (Figure 10-10a). In contrast, that of the PDMAEMA-grafted CLPE sample with cationic grafted polymer layers was strongly positive, and that of the PMPA-grafted CLPE sample with anionic grafted polymer layers was strongly negative. The amounts of BSA adsorbed on the surface

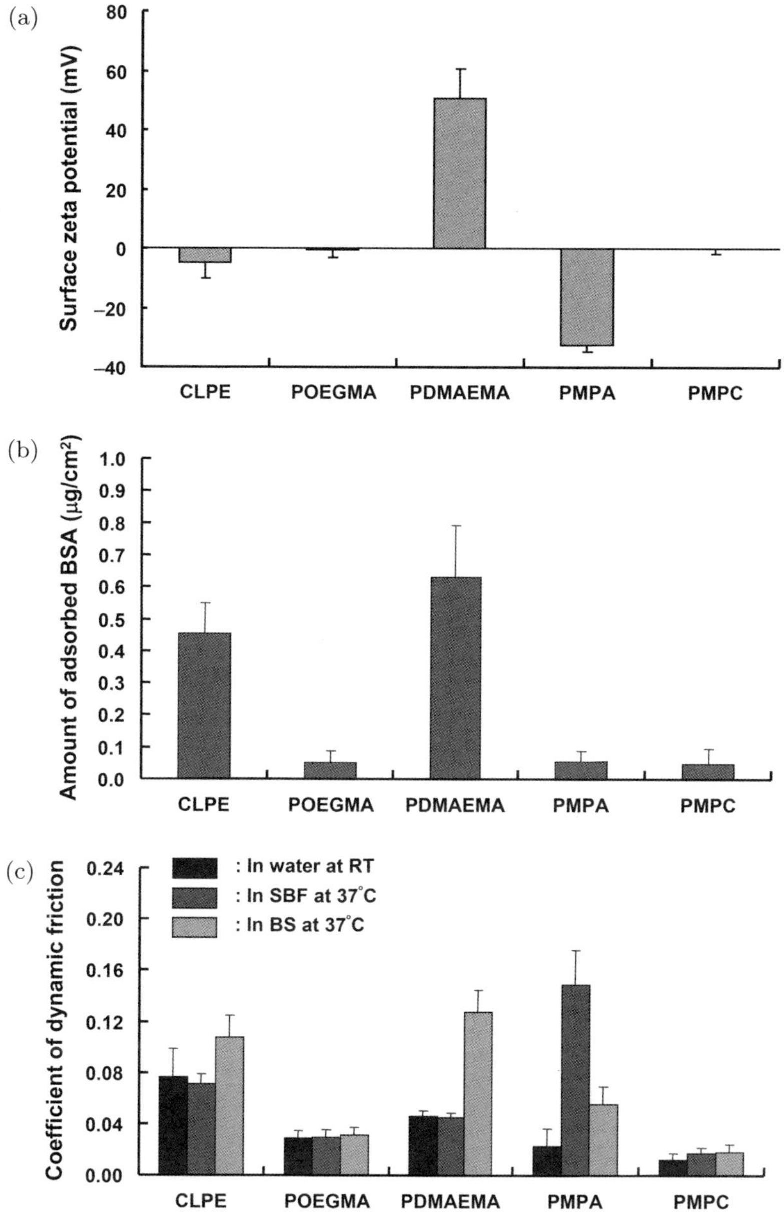

Figure 10-10. (a) Surface zeta potentials, (b) amounts of adsorbed BSA, and (c) coefficients of dynamic friction in the ball-on-plate friction test under various lubrication conditions for untreated CLPE and various polyelectrolyte-grafted CLPE samples. Data are expressed as mean ± standard deviation.

of the POEGMA-, PMPA-, and PMPC-grafted CLPE samples with nonionic, anionic, and zwitterionic polymer layers grafted on the were significantly lower (Figure 10-10b). In contrast, that in the case of the PDMAEMA-grafted CLPE sample with a grafted cationic polymer layer was higher. These findings show that the type of charge (nonionic, cationic, anionic, or zwitterionic) of the graft layer affects the hydration and friction kinetics of the CLPE bearing surface. The coefficient of dynamic friction during the ball-on-plate friction test using water as lubricant depends on the hydrophilicity of the surface (i.e. on the static-water contact angles), as shown in Figures 10-9 and 10-10c. The surfaces of all the polyelectrolyte-grafted CLPE samples exhibited considerably higher lubricity than did the surface of the untreated CLPE sample when water was used as a lubricant. This is because the water molecules in the hydration layers of the hydrophilic polymer or polyelectrolytes act as highly efficient lubricants (Kyomoto *et al.*, 2012; Raviv *et al.*, 2003). However, when other lubricants were used, the surface of the polyelectrolyte-grafted CLPE samples with cationic and anionic polymer layers exhibited characteristics that were significantly different from those of the hydrophilic polymer- and zwitterionic polyelectrolyte-grafted CLPE samples, even though all the surfaces were highly hydrophilic. The PDMAEMA-grafted CLPE samples exhibited a higher coefficient of dynamic friction in BS, which contained proteins such as albumin and globulin, than in water or SBF during the ball-on-plate friction test (Kobayashi and Takahara, 2010). PDMAEMA contains a positively charged $-NH^+(CH_3)_2$ group at neutral pH; this group, in turn, attracts negatively charged molecules. For example, albumin molecules have a negatively charge at neutral pH (Figure 10-10). This implies that the presence of protein molecules at the bearing interface increases the resistance to sliding motion. Because proteins are adsorbed on the CoCrMo alloy counterface (Crockett *et al.*, 2009; Serro *et al.*, 2006), the high resistance to sliding motion can be attributed to being the result of stronger adhesive interaction or the interpenetration of the adsorbed protein films formed on both the PDMAEMA-grafted CLPE and the CoCrMo alloy surfaces. However, the PDMAEMA-grafted CLPE cups exhibited high wear resistance at high loads during the hip simulator test despite the fact that they exhibited a high coefficient of dynamic friction in BS during the ball-on-plate friction test. This may be because the protein film adsorbed from the BS is squeezed out of the bearing interface at high loads (Fang *et al.*, 2009). In contrast, the surface of the PMPA-grafted CLPE samples exhibited considerably lower lubricity in SBF during the ball-on-plate friction test. The chemical structure of the negatively charged PMPA is characterized by the presence of a large number of trap sites for positively charged inorganic ions. Hence, the poor lubricity of the surface of the PMPA-grafted CLPE samples can be attributed to the shrinkage or bridging of the negatively charged polyelectrolyte chains; this reduces the mobility of the chains in solutions containing positively charged inorganic ions (Kobayashi and Takahara, 2010; Kyomoto *et al.*, 2012; Raviv *et al.*, 2003). Kato *et al.* (1996) reported that PMPA-grafted poly(ethylene terephtalate) surfaces induce hydroxyl apatite deposition in SBF, mimicking biological mineralization. A similar phenomenon was observed, in that PMPA-grafted CLPE surfaces exhibited calcification-like mineralization after being pre-soaked in SBF for 24 h before the friction test. The BS sample used as lubricant during the hip simulator test contained not only protein molecules but also inorganic ions. Further, the test cups were soaked in BS for over 30 days during the hip simulator test. Therefore, it can be assumed that the negatively charged PMPA attracts only positively charged inorganic ions and repels the negatively charged molecules. Finally, the PMPA-grafted CLPE cups exhibited higher wear than did the other polyelectrolyte-grafted CLPE cups; this was owing to the abrasive wear by the mineralized, hardened surface layer (Tretinnikov *et al.*, 1994).

2.2.3.3. Wear resistance

The POEGMA- and PMPC-grafted CLPE cups exhibited high wear resistance during the hip simulator tests (Figure 10-11) as well as low coefficients of dynamic friction during the ball-on-plate friction tests (Figure 10-10c). In particular, the highly hydrated surface layer of the PMPC-grafted CLPE sample provided extremely efficient lubrication under all conditions. Moreover, the zeta potential

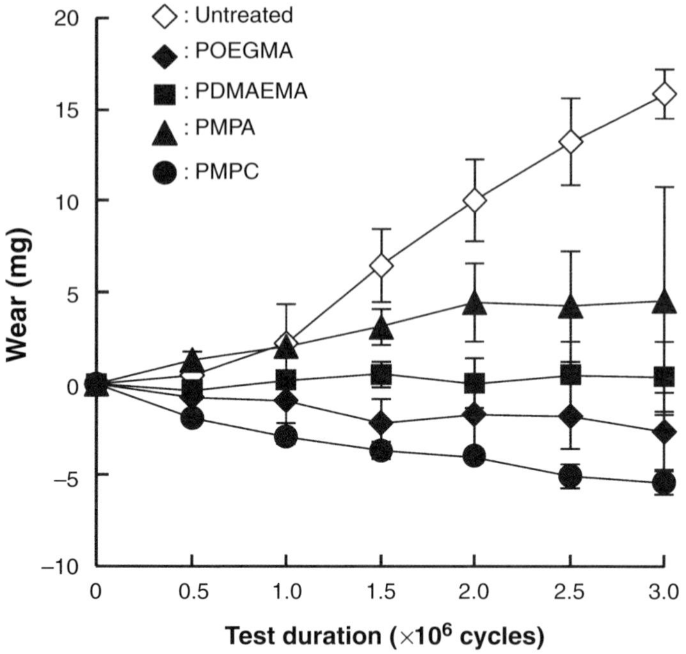

Figure 10-11. Time course of gravimetric wear of various polyelectrolyte-grafted CLPE cups during hip simulator test. A CoCrMo alloy ball with a diameter of 26 mm was used as the femoral head. Data are expressed as means ± standard deviations.

of the surface of the PMPC-grafted CLPE sample was close to zero because the ionic group in the MPC unit forms an inner salt and the electrostatic effects are diminished. Therefore, the zwitterionic grafted polymer layers attract only water molecules, repel protein molecules (Figure 10-10b), and positively charged inorganic ions. This characteristic is similar to that of the nonionic-grafted polymer layers. Chen *et al.* (2009) reported that the water molecules adsorbed on the surfaces of highly hydrophilic polyzwitterionic (i.e. PMPC) brushes act as lubricants to reduce the friction between the brushes and the counter surface. Recent efforts to identify hydrophilic polymers or polyelectrolytes have focused on nanotribological studies of surface-attached molecules, seeking to emulate those found at the cartilage surface (Briscoe *et al.*, 2006; Kitano *et al.*, 2009; Raviv *et al.*, 2003). However, the results obtained for the PDMAEMA- and PMPA-grafted CLPE samples during the hip joint simulator tests demonstrate that the mechanism of action of the polyelectrolyte-grafted layer cannot be explained merely in terms of fluid-film lubrication. Therefore, it is assumed that the primary factor responsible for the low friction and the high wear resistance is the high level of hydration of the polyelectrolyte layer, such as the case for the zwitterionic PMPC-grafted layer; water molecules in the hydration layers act as highly efficient lubricants (Kitano *et al.*, 2009; Kobayashi *et al.*, 2007; Raviv *et al.*, 2003). Another factor is the repulsion of protein molecules by the positively charged inorganic ions of the polyelectrolyte layer in the synovial fluid; this may weaken the adhesive interaction or reduce interpenetration between the opposing femoral head surfaces of CoCrMo alloy implants or the protein films adsorbed on the femoral head surfaces (Chen *et al.*, 2009; Kyomoto *et al.*, 2010a).

After the hip simulator test, the POEGMA-, PDMAEMA-, and PMPC-grafted CLPE cups exhibited a greater than 97% reduction in the steady wear rate compared with the untreated CLPE sample (Figure 10-11). This suggests the current approach may be promising for extending the longevity of total hip arthroplasty (THA) prosthetics (Moro *et al.*, 2006). Kyomoto *et al.* (2011) assumed that the hydrated bearing surfaces of artificial joints modified with PMPC exhibited fluid-film lubrication (i.e. hydration lubrication (Ishikawa *et al.*, 2006; Raviv and Klein, 2002)) and suggested that such artificial hips mimic cartilage or the surface-active phospholipid layer (SAPL) on the cartilage in natural joints. Although the PMPC layer has no direct analog to cartilage surface, which contains an SAPL, the findings underline the fact that highly hydrated macromolecules on such surfaces play a role in chondroprotection and lubrication. Finally, a nanometer-scaled hydrophilic polymer or polyelectrolyte layer on a CLPE surface can confer high durability on the acetabular cup bearings used in THA. These findings may have implications for future studies on surface modification using cartilage-like or SAPL layer-like layers, which are of great importance in the design of lubricated surfaces for artificial joints.

2.2.4. *PMPC-grafted polyethylene*

2.2.4.1. Surface modification

Moro *et al.* have fabricated an artificial hip joint based on the concept of hydration lubrication by grafting PMPC onto the surface of CLPE (PMPC-grafted CLPE). This device was designed to reduce wear and suppress bone resorption (Moro *et al.*, 2004, 2006, 2009). A previous study has reported that hydrogel cartilage surfaces can be assumed to have a brush-like structure: A part of the proteoglycan aggregate brush is bonded with the collagen network on the cartilage surface (Ishikawa *et al.*, 2006). Therefore, in artificial hip joints, the bearing surface with PMPC is assumed to have a brush-like structure similar to that of articular cartilage (Figure 10-12). The hydration lubrication interface can therefore be considered to mimic natural joint cartilage *in vivo*.

The grafting of biocompatible and hydrophilic PMPC onto CLPE was performed using a photoinitiated grafting-from polymerization process. The photoinitiated graft polymerization reaction, which used a typical BP photoinitiator, is shown in Figure 10-13. First, the physically coated layer of BP on the CLPE surface is excited by UV irradiation. As a result, the BP is excited to its triplet state and extracts a hydrogen atom from the $-CH_2-$ group, generating a radical that is capable of initiating the graft polymerization of MPC. This technique has several important benefits. These include the direct grafting of PMPC on CLPE, resulting in the formation of C–C covalent bonds between the PMPC and the CLPE substrate; high mobility of the PMPC chains; high density; and the ability to control the length of the introduced PMPC.

Figure 10-14 shows cross-sectional TEM images of the PMPC-grafted CLPE samples fabricated by polymerization using different photoirradiation times (Kyomoto *et al.*, 2007b). For photoirradiation times greater than 45 min, a 100–200-nm thick grafted layer of PMPC was clearly observed on the surface of the CLPE substrate. The MPC-covered region was coexistent with uncovered regions when the photoirradiation time was 23 min, although the thickness of the covered region on the PMPC layer remained the same (100–200 nm).

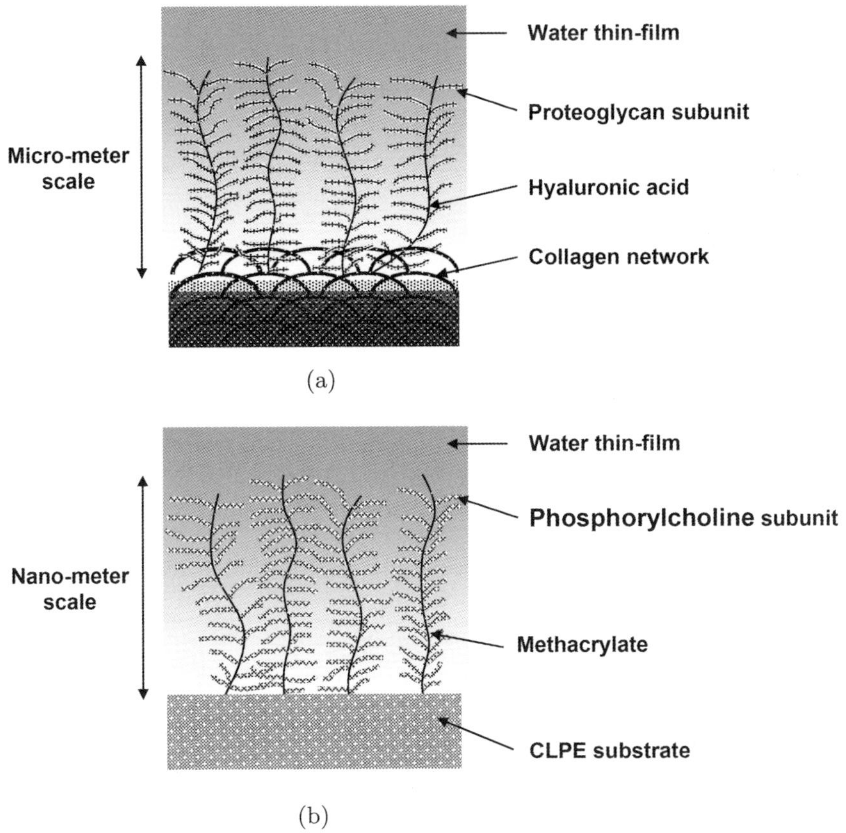

Figure 10-12. Schematic model of PMPC-grafted CLPE surface mimicking cartilage. (a) Cartilage; (b) PMPC-grafted CLPE.

These results indicate that the extent of PMPC grafting can be controlled by the polymerization time. This is attributable to the fact that the number of polymer chains produced during a radical polymerization reaction is generally correlated to the photoirradiation time.

2.2.4.2. Lubricity and wear resistances

Figure 10-15 shows the static-water contact angle of the PMPC-grafted CLPE sample as a function of the photoirradiation time used for polymerization (Kyomoto *et al.*, 2007b). The static water contact

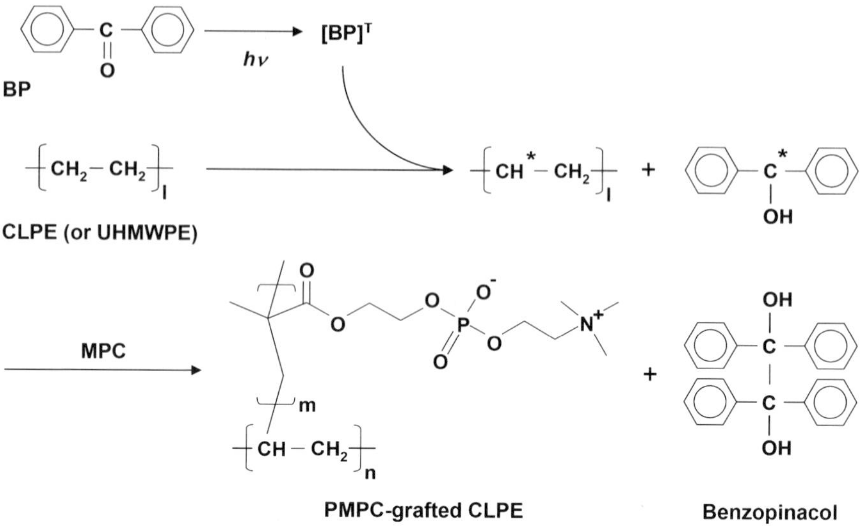

Figure 10-13. Schematic illustration of MPC graft polymerization using BP system.

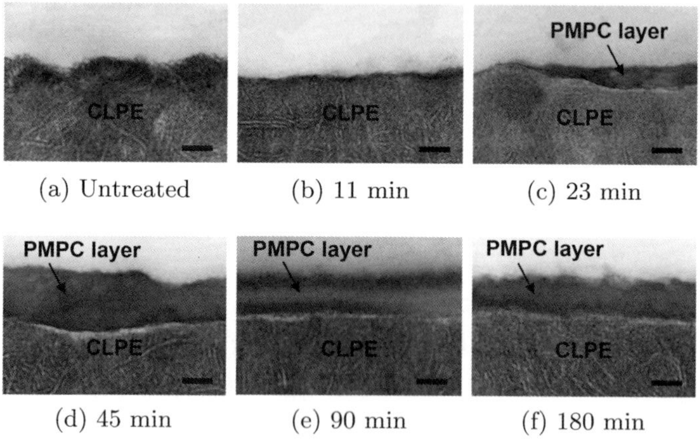

Figure 10-14. Cross-sectional TEM images of PMPC-grafted CLPE samples obtained for various photoirradiation times. Bar: 100 nm.

angle of untreated CLPE was 90° and decreased markedly with an increase in the photoirradiation time. Figure 10-16, meanwhile, shows the relationship between the coefficient of dynamic friction and the contact angle (Kyomoto *et al.*, 2008). The coefficient of dynamic

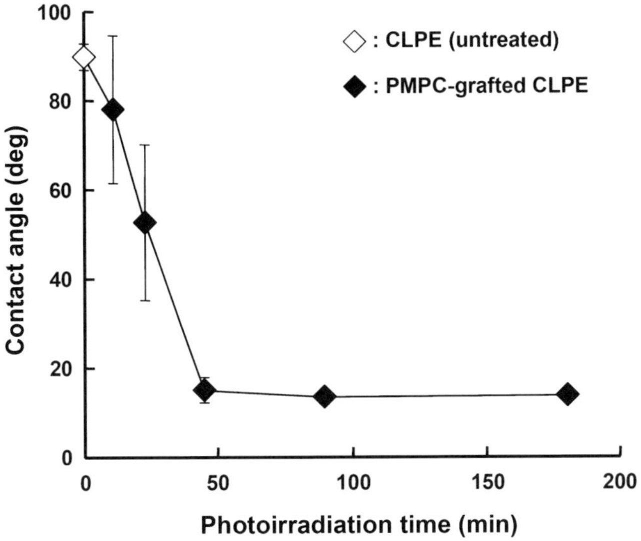

Figure 10-15. Static water contact angle of PMPC-grafted CLPE sample as a function of photo-irradiation time. Data are expressed as means ± standard deviations.

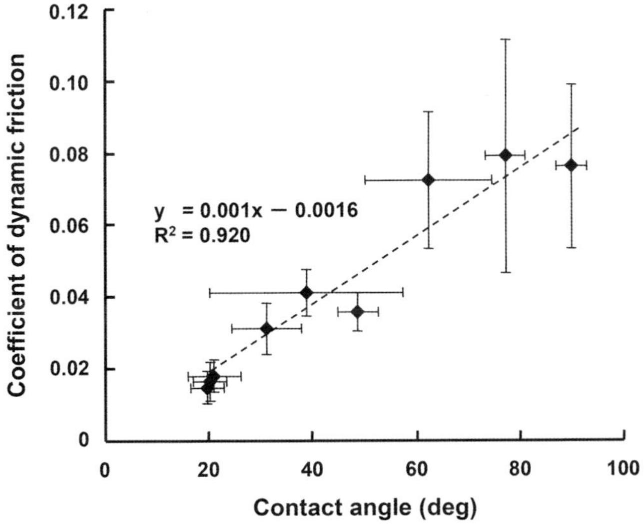

Figure 10-16. Relationship between coefficient of dynamic friction and contact angle of PMPC-grafted CLPE surface. Data are expressed as means ± standard deviations.

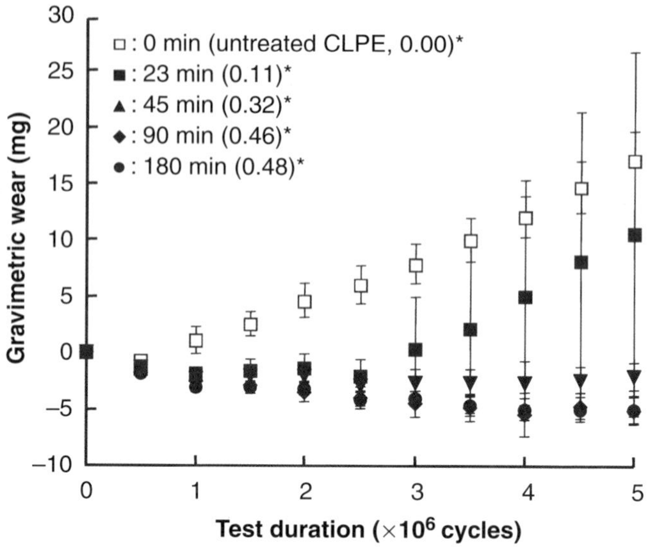

Figure 10-17. Weight change (gravimetric wear) of PMPC-grafted CLPE cups for a MPC concentration of 0.5 mol/L and various photoirradiation times during hip joint simulator wear test. A CoCrMo alloy ball with a diameter of 26 mm was used as the femoral head. Data are expressed as means ± standard deviations. *P–O group indexes are in parentheses.

friction tended to increase with the contact angle. This increase was linear to a degree of accuracy, and the coefficient of determination was 0.920.

After the hip simulator test, it was confirmed that the PMPC-grafted CLPE cups with a high P–O group index exhibited a relatively low steady wear rate (Figure 10-17). The PMPC-grafted CLPE cups with a P–O group index greater than 0.32 exhibited a greater than 90% reduction in their steady wear rate as compared to untreated CLPE as well as the PMPC-grafted CLPE cups having a low P–O group index and a low density of PMPC graft chains. This effect was independent of whether or not the CLPE substrate was crosslinked, as well as of the material used for the femoral heads (Moro *et al.*, 2009). The steady wear rate of the PMPC-grafted CLPE cups subjected to photoirradiation for 23 min and that of the untreated CLPE were almost the same. This result indicates that when the PMPC-graft layer is removed from the CLPE substrate, only the surface of the substrate is exposed. In a previous study, Moro *et al.* (2014) subjected hip joints to long-term wear tests and found that the PMPC-grafted liners exhibited almost no wear even after 7×10^7 cycles. The PMPC-grafted CLPE cups showed a slight increase in weight. This was partially attributable to the fluid absorption in the tested cups being higher than that in the load-soak controls, which was in keeping with the standard ISO14242. When using the gravimetric method, the weight loss in the tested cups was corrected by subtracting the weight gain in the case of the load-soak controls; however, this correction could not be made perfectly because only the tested cups were continuously subjected to motion and load. Usually, the fluid absorption in the tested cups is slightly higher than that in the load-soak controls. Consequently, correcting the amount of fluid absorbed by using the load-soak data as the correction factor leads to a slight underestimation of the actual weight loss, in addition to resulting in the use of large femoral heads or in metal-shell fixation. The advantage of using photoinduced graft polymerization stems from the fact that the grafted PMPC increases the high lubricity of only the surface of the CLPE substrate and has no effect on its bulk properties. In the case of the PMPC-grafted CLPE cups, the number of wear-generated particles isolated from the lubricants decreased. However, because the wear-generated particles were produced in extremely small amounts, they could not be classified according to size. The majority of the wear-generated particles from the untreated CLPE surfaces were 0.1 to 1.0 μm in size. In addition to enhancing the wear resistance of the cups, reducing the bone resorptive responses to the wear-generated particles is also important for preventing periprosthetic osteolysis. Such responses are dependent not only on the total number of wear-generated particles, but also on the proportion of particles that are within the most biologically active size range. Moro *et al.* (2004) have shown that polymer particles (most of the particles were approximately 0.5 μm in size) covered with PMPC are biologically inert with respect to phagocytosis by macrophages and subsequent bone resorptive.

2.2.4.3. Clinical applications

Desirable results of *in vitro* studies do not automatically imply clinical success. Takatori *et al.* (2013) conducted multicenter clinical trials of the PMPC-grafted CLPE cups in 80 patients between 2007 and 2009 at the University of Tokyo and various hospitals in Japan. Close monitoring of the clinical performance of the cups and accurate quantification of their wear rates were essential for the early recognition of unforeseen problems. On the basis of other related evidence and the results of the clinical trials, the Japanese government (Ministry of Health, Labour, and Welfare) approved the clinical use of PMPC-grafted CLPE acetabular liners (Aquala® liner; KYOCERA Medical Corp.) in artificial hip joints in April 2011. Osteolysis was not observed and neither was revision surgery necessary for up to six years post-surgery. Regarding the efficacy of PMPC grafting in reducing wear, Moro *et al.* (2013) reported that the steady-state wear rate of PMPC-grafted CLPE acetabular liners was 0.002 mm/year. However, further studies, including long-term follow-ups, are needed to confirm whether this preliminary observation is valid.

2.2.5. *PMPC-grafted poly-ether–ether–ketone*

Recently, poly-ether–ether–ketone (PEEK) has emerged as the leading high-performance super-engineering plastic candidate for replacing metal implant components, especially in the field of orthopedics and spinal surgery (Kurtz and Devine, 2007). However, conventional single-component PEEK cannot satisfy the requirements (antibiofouling nature, wear resistance, and the ability to fix to bone) for use as material for fabricating artificial joints or intervertebral body fusion cages (Kurtz and Devine, 2007). In order to improve the further applicability of PEEK as an implant biomaterial, a number of studies have focused on improving the lubricating and antibiofouling nature of the polymer, either via reinforcing agents or through surface modifications (Fan *et al.*, 2004; Yu *et al.*, 2005). Therefore, a number of multicomponent polymer systems have been designed in order to synthesize new multifunctional biomaterials. In order to use PEEK and its related composites (including carbon fiber-reinforced

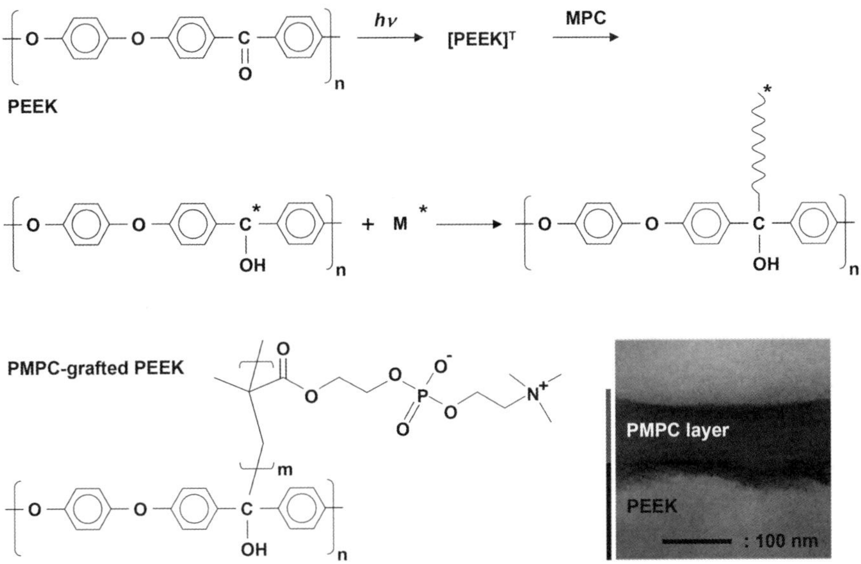

Figure 10-18. Schematic illustration for the fabrication of PMPC-grafted PEEK and cross-sectional TEM image of fabricated sample.

PEEK (CFR-PEEK)) as implant materials, they have to be engineered to exhibit a wide range of physical, mechanical, and surface properties.

2.2.5.1. Surface modification

It is well known that when BP is exposed to radiation such as UV rays, a pinacolization reaction is induced; this results in the formation of semi-benzopinacol radicals (i.e. ketyl radicals) that act as photoinitiators. Kyomoto and coworkers focused on a BP unit in PEEK and formulated a novel self-initiated surface-graft polymerization method that utilizes the BP unit in grafting-from polymerization (Figure 10-18) (Kyomoto and Ishihara, 2009; Kyomoto *et al.*, 2010b). This polymerization reaction (involving free radicals) is photoinduced by UV irradiation. Under UV irradiation, a BP unit in PEEK can undergo the following reactions in monomeric aqueous solutions (Cole and Casella, 1992; Giancaterina *et al.*, 2000; Nguyen and Ishida, 1986; Qiu and Si, 1996; Qiu *et al.*, 2007; Wang *et al.*, 2007;

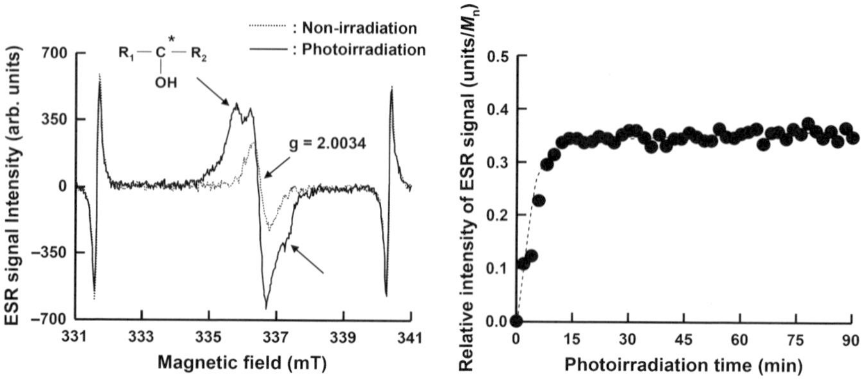

Figure 10-19. Free radical production in PEEK under photoirradiation. (a) ESR spectra of PEEK before and after photoirradiation (90 min), (b) time course of the relative intensity of ESR signal of PEEK during UV irradiation.

Yang and Rånby, 1999). The pinacolization reaction (photoreduction by the H-abstraction of a BP unit in PEEK) results in the formation of a semi-benzopinacol radical, which can initiate the grafting-from polymerization of the feed monomer (this is the main reaction). In addition, grafting-to polymerization, during which the radical chain end of the active-polymer couples with the semi-benzopinacol radical of the PEEK surface, also takes place as a sub-reaction. In addition, another sub-reaction, a photoscission reaction, occurs; this reaction may not require a hydrogen (H)-donor. The cleavage reaction induces recombination and grafting-from polymerization. When water-based polymerization is performed in the presence of an H-donor, a phenol unit may be subsequently formed owing to H-abstraction. Figure 10-19 shows that the UV irradiation produced ketyl radicals within the molecular structure of PEEK. It is assumed that the ketyl radicals were produced by the pinacolization reaction under UV irradiation. The number of free radicals produced (as determined by the relative intensity of electron spin resonance (ESR) signal) initially increased rapidly and then became almost constant during the irradiation process. It is assumed that this phenomenon should allow the graft polymerization process to be controlled. Kyomoto and coworkers were actually able to control the grafting of the PMPC layer by controlling the number of the ketyl radicals produced by the BP units in PEEK. It is likely that the produced ketyl radicals undergo pinacolization in monomer aqueous solutions under UV irradiation (Kyomoto and Ishihara, 2009; Kyomoto *et al.*, 2010b, 2013). This results in the formation of ketyl radicals that can initiate the grafting-from polymerization of the feed monomer as the main reaction, and the grafting-to polymerization (the radical chain end of the active polymer couples with the ketyl radical on the PEEK surface) as a sub-reaction. The reaction enables the direct grafting of the functional polymer (PMPC in this study) onto the PEEK surface in the absence of a photoinitiator, resulting in the formation of a C–C covalent bond between the functional polymer and the PEEK substrate.

2.2.5.2. Surface properties

It is important to control the properties of the graft layers on both PEEK and CFR-PEEK surfaces in order to optimize their lubrication and resistance to wear. Kyomoto *et al.* (2013) demonstrated that the extent of grafting of both the PMPC-grafted PEEK and CFR-PEEK surfaces increases gradually with the photoirradiation time, suggesting that the graft chain propagates steadily with irradiation (Figure 10-20). Therefore, to control the extent of grafting, the irradiation time must be controlled. Moreover, it was observed that, for a particular irradiation time, the higher the monomer concentration, the greater was the extent of grafting. Thus, the extent of the PMPC graft should increase with the photoirradiation time and the monomer concentration (Kyomoto *et al.*, 2013).

Interestingly, the rate at which the extent of the PMPC graft increased was low in the case of CFR-PEEK. The self-initiated surface graft polymerization process is photoinduced by the UV irradiation of the BP units on the PEEK surface. When PAN-based carbon fibers were used in an amount of 30 mass %, the self-initiated surface graft polymerization between the radicals on the PEEK surface and the MPC monomer occurred gradually, resulting in the formation of comparatively small graft chains on the surface. It is therefore assumed that the rate of increase of the extent of the PMPC graft

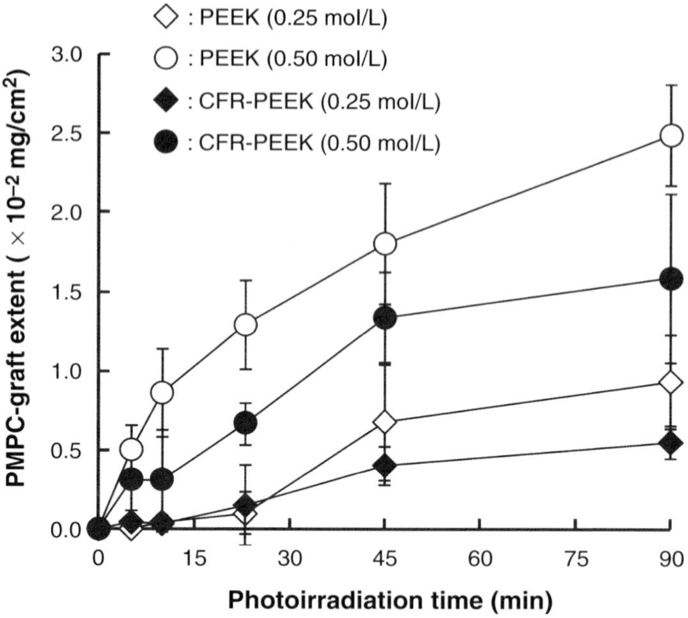

Figure 10-20. Extent of the PMPC grafts on PEEK and CFR-PEEK surfaces as a function of photoirradiation time. Data are expressed as means ± standard deviations.

depends only on the number of free radicals produced from the PEEK matrix. Hence, the production of free radicals on the PEEK surface would be affected by the presence of the blended carbon fiber because the latter would occupy some of the surface. For a photoirradiation time of 90 min, the extents of the PMPC graft on CFR-PEEK for MPC concentrations of 0.25 and 0.50 mol/L were 0.55×10^{-2} and 1.59×10^{-2} mg/cm^2, respectively. These were respectively 40.9% and 36.1% lower than those on PEEK. As can be observed, the differences are close to the carbon fiber content. However, neither cracks nor delamination was observed at the interface between the grafted PMPC layer and the carbon fibers. A detailed study of the effects of the carbon fiber is thus underway. This includes an investigation of the effects of different types and content ratios of carbon fibers and/or PEEK resins.

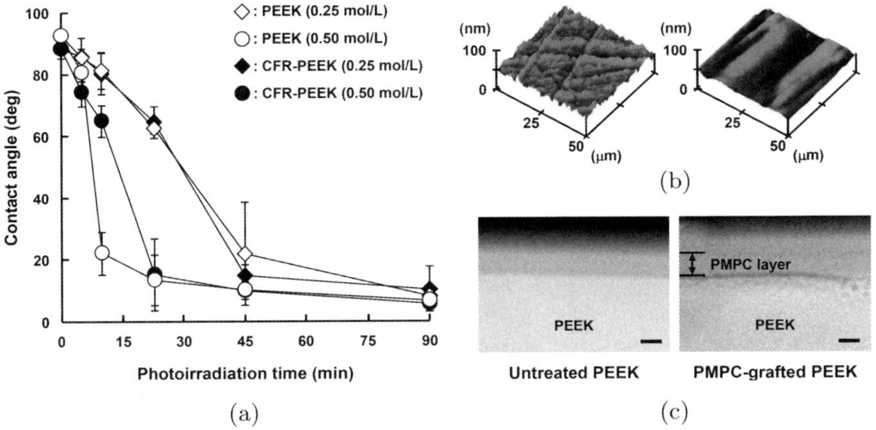

Figure 10-21. (a) Static-water contact angles of PMPC-grafted PEEK and CFR-PEEK surfaces as a function of photoirradiation time. Data are expressed as means ± standard deviations. (b) AFM and (c) cross-sectional TEM images of untreated and PMPC-grafted PEEK samples fabricated using an MPC concentration of 0.5 mol/L and 90 min of photoirradiation. Scale bar indicates 100 nm.

2.2.5.3. Wear resistance

The water wettabilities of the PMPC-grafted PEEK and CFR-PEEK surfaces were considerably greater than those of the untreated PEEK and CFR-PEEK surfaces (Figure 10-21). This was because of the presence of a nanometer-scaled smooth PMPC layer on the former surfaces. As mentioned above, MPC is a highly hydrophilic compound; this makes PMPC water-soluble. The coefficients of dynamic friction of the PMPC-grafted PEEK and CFR-PEEK surfaces were significantly lower than those of the untreated PEEK and CFR-PEEK surfaces. This observation is related to the significant reduction of the static-water contact angles in the case of the PMPC-grafted surfaces. That the friction in the case of the untreated PEEK and CFR-PEEK surfaces is higher is one of their chief disadvantages because it results in greater wear as well as the seizure (melting) of bearing couples. The higher friction in the case of the untreated PEEK and CFR-PEEK surfaces actually affected their wear properties, as determined by the results of the hip simulator wear test.

The wear properties of PEEK and CFR-PEEK when used as bearing materials in hip joint articulations have been investigated in previous studies (Brockett *et al.*, 2012; Scholes *et al.*, 2008; Wang *et al.*, 1998, 2012). During the hip simulator wear tests performed on the PMPC-grafted PEEK and CFR-PEEK cups, the significant improvements in the water wettabilities, frictional properties, and/or carbon fiber-reinforced properties of the PMPC-grafted PEEK and CFR-PEEK cups resulted in substantial improvements in their wear resistances (Figure 10-22). The wear rate of the PMPC-grafted CFR-PEEK cups was almost zero, even when they were articulated to CoCrMo alloy femoral heads. Though the concentration of the PAN-based carbon fibers in the composite must be sufficiently high to achieve both high gravimetric and volumetric wear resistance, this can also cause scratches on the CoCrMo alloy femoral heads (Wang *et al.*, 1998). In contrast, the surfaces of the femoral heads were smooth when used against the PMPC-grafted CFR-PEEK cups. It is assumed that the fluid film and/or the hydrated layer produced by the PMPC graft suppress direct contact between the counter-bearing

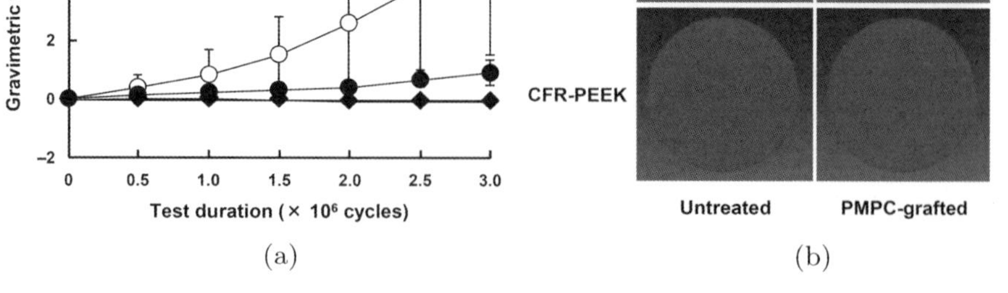

Figure 10-22. (a) Time course of gravimetric wear of PMPC-grafted PEEK and CFR-PEEK cups. A CoCrMo alloy ball with a diameter of 26 mm was used as the femoral head. Data are expressed as mean ± standard deviation. (b) Three-dimensional coordinate measurements of PMPC-grafted PEEK and CFR-PEEK cups after hip simulator test.

face and the hard carbon fibers of the CFR-PEEK substrate. This prevents the metal counter surface from being damaged, regardless of the carbon fiber content of the CFR-PEEK substrate.

Moreover, because the number of wear-generated particles produced by the PMPC-grafted PEEK and CFR-PEEK cups was extremely small, it was not possible to separate them from those produced by the PEEK matrix and the blended carbon fibers. Keeping these results in mind, the authors expect the biological response of the PMPC-grafted PEEK and CFR-PEEK cups *in vivo* to be comparable with those of PE or CLPE (Utzschneider *et al.*, 2010). This assumption is supported by the results of cell culture experiments performed by Howling *et al.* (2003), who reported that CFR-PEEK wear particles had no cytotoxic effects and could not possibly cause adverse tissue reactions *in vivo*. However, no *in vivo* biocompatibility studies using an appropriate animal model have yet been published.

3. Future Perspectives

THA is one of the most successfully performed joint surgeries today. Owing to the increase in the aging global population, the number of primary and revised THA procedures performed annually is increasing significantly (Bozic *et al.*, 2009; Kurtz *et al.*, 2005). As a result, the quality of the implanted artificial joints is becoming increasingly important, necessitating functional, durable, and natural joint-like artificial implants. The authors believe that an important research goal for the future is the creation of an artificial joint interface that mimics the natural joint cartilage. In this chapter, the authors proposed a way of achieving this goal, which is to use PMPC-grafted CLPE liners. Data corresponding to 20,000 instances of the clinical use of PMPC-grafted CLPE liners (March 2015) indicated that the liners exhibited neither wear nor any complications during the follow-up assessment periods, which spanned a minimum of five years and a maximum of seven years. Considering that PMPC-grafted CLPE liners show better lubrication, one can expect improved long-term clinical results from their use. Additionally, a functional, durable, and natural surface would find wide application not only in medical devices such as artificial joints but would also be important to biomaterial and bioengineering sciences. For example, it is well known that the surface of articular cartilage consists of a collagen network, hyaluronic acid, and proteoglycan subunits. However, the functions of the articular cartilage surface have not yet been fully elucidated. The authors consider that a bioengineered surface based on a new hydrogel-like biomaterial would help in this regard. Biotribological studies should also help elucidate the functions of articular cartilage surface. Moreover, none of the recent studies investigated the complete range of loading- and motion-related conditions corresponding to the *in vivo* environment. That is to say, these studies did not explore all the positions possible during the hip joint simulator wear test, variations in the magnitude of loading, or the subjects' daily routines. Advanced simulation technologies that can completely capture these physiological conditions would be highly desirable. The authors believe that such hydrogel biomaterials and bioengineering surfaces can act as key technologies for joint arthroplasty and that this issue will be addressed in the future by scientists working on hydrogel biomaterials and in biotribological science.

Acknowledgments

Part of this research was supported by the Japan Science and Technology Agency (JST), the S-Innovation program, and the Health and Welfare Research Grants for Research on Medical Devices for Improving Impaired QOL (H20-004) and Research on Publicly Essential Drugs and Medical Devices (H23-007) from the Japanese Ministry of Health, Labour and Welfare. We further express our gratitude to Dr. Toru Moro and Dr. Yoshio Takatori of the University of Tokyo for the valuable suggestions that they offered.

References

Abizaid, A., Lansky, A.J., Fitzgerald, P.J., Tanajura, L.F., Feres, F., Staico, R. *et al.* (2007a). Percutaneous coronary revascularization using a trilayer metal phosphorylcholine-coated zotarolimus-eluting stent, *Am J Cardiol*, **99**, 1403–1408.

Abizaid, A., Popma, J.J., Tanajura, L.F., Hattori, K., Solberg, B., Larracas, C. *et al.* (2007B). Clinical and angiographic results of percutaneous coronary revascularization using a trilayer stainless steel-tantalum-stainless steel phosphorylcholine-coated stent: The TriMaxx trial, *Catheter Cardio Inte*, **70**, 914–919.

Arakaki, K., Kitamura, N., Fujiki, H., Kurokawa, T., Iwamoto, M., Ueno, M. *et al.* (2010). Artificial cartilage made from a novel double-network hydrogel: In vivo effects on the normal cartilage and ex vivo evaluation of the friction property, *J Biomed Mater Res A*, **93**, 1160–1168.

Bhosale, A.M. and Richardson, J.B. (2008). Articular cartilage: Structure, injuries and review of management, *Br Med Bull*, **87**, 77–95.

Bozic, K.J., Kurtz, S.M., Lau, E., Ong, K., Vail, T.P. and Berry, D.J. (2009). The epidemiology of revision total hip arthroplasty in the United States, *J Bone Joint Surg Am*, **91**, 128–133.

Bray, J.C. and Merrill, E.W. (1973). Poly(vinyl alcohol) hydrogels for synthetic articular cartilage material, *J Biomed Mater Res*, **7**, 431–443.

Briscoe, W.H., Titmuss, S., Tiberg, F., Thomas, R.K., McGillivray, D.J. and Klein, J. (2006). Boundary lubrication under water, *Nature*, **444**, 191–194.

Brockett, C.L., John, G., Williams, S., Jin, Z., Isaac, G.H. and Fisher, J. (2012). Wear of ceramic-on-carbon fiber-reinforced poly-ether ether ketone hip replacements, *J Biomed Mater Res B Appl Biomater*, **100**, 1459–1465.

Buckwalter, J.A. and Rosenberg, L. (1983). Structural changes during development in bovine fetal epiphyseal cartilage, *Coll Relat Res*, **3**, 489–504.

Chen, M., Briscoe, W.H., Armes, S.P. and Klein, J. (2009). Lubrication at physiological pressures by polyzwitterionic brushes, *Science*, **323**, 1698–1701.

Cole, K.C. and Casella, I.G. (1992). Fourier transform infrared spectroscopic study of thermal degradation in films of poly(etheretherketone), *Thermochim Acta*, **211**, 209–228.

Crockett, R., Roba, M., Naka, M., Gasser, B., Delfosse, D., Frauchiger, V. *et al.* (2009). Friction, lubrication, and polymer transfer between UHMWPE and CoCrMo hip-implant materials: A fluorescence microscopy study, *J Biomed Mater Res A*, **89**, 1011–1018.

Dyer, D.J. (2006). Photoinitiated synthesis of grafted polymers, in Abe, A., Albertsson, A.C., Coates, G.W., Genzer, J., Kobayashi, S., Lee, K.S. *et al.* (eds.), *Advances in Polymer Science*, Springer, Berlin, 47–65.

Edmondson, S., Osborne, V.L. and Huck, W.T.S. (2004). Polymer brushes via surface-initiated polymerizations, *Chem Soc Rev*, **33**, 14–22.

Elisseeff, J., Anseth, K., Sims, D., McIntosh, W., Randolph, M., Yaremchuk, M. *et al.* (1999). Transdermal photopolymerization of poly(ethylene oxide)-based injectable hydrogels for tissue-engineered cartilage, *Plast Reconstr Surg*, **104**, 1014–1022.

Fajadet, J., Wijns, W., Laarman, G.J., Kuck, K.H., Ormiston, J., Münzel, T. *et al.* (2006). Randomized, double-blind, multicenter study of the Endeavor zotarolimus-eluting phosphorylcholine-encapsulated stent for treatment of native coronary artery lesions: Clinical and angiographic results of the ENDEAVOR II trial, *Circulation*, **114**, 798–806.

Fang, H.W., Hsieh, M.C., Huang, H.T., Tsai, C.Y. and Chang, M.H. (2009). Conformational and adsorptive characteristics of albumin affect interfacial protein boundary lubrication: From experimental to molecular dynamics simulation approaches, *Colloids Surf B Biointerfaces*, **68**, 171–177.

Fan, J.P., Tsui, C.P., Tang, C.Y. and Chow, C.L. (2004). Influence of interphase layer on the overall elasto-plastic behaviors of HA/PEEK biocomposite, *Biomaterials*, **25**, 5363–5373.

Gershlick, A., Kandzari, D.E., Leon, M.B., Wijns, W., Meredith, I.T., Fajadet, J. *et al.* (2007). Zotarolimus-eluting stents in patients with native coronary artery disease: Clinical and angiographic outcomes in 1,317 patients, *Am J Cardiol*, **100**, 45M–55M.

Giancaterina, S., Rossi, A., Rivaton, A. and Gardette, J.L. (2000). Photochemical evolution of poly(ether ether ketone), *Polym Degrad Stab*, **68**, 133–144.

Goldberg, R., Schroeder, A., Barenholz, Y. and Klein, J. (2011a). Interactions between adsorbed hydrogenated soy phosphatidylcholine (HSPC) vesicles at physiologically high pressures and salt concentrations, *Biophys J*, **100**, 2403–2411.

Goldberg, R., Schroeder, A., Silbert, G., Turjeman, K., Barenholz, Y. and Klein, J. (2011b). Boundary lubricants with exceptionally low friction coefficients based on 2D close-packed phosphatidylcholine liposomes, *Adv Mater*, **23**, 3517–3521.

Han, S.H., Ahn, T.H., Kang, W.C., Oh, K.J., Chung, W.J., Shin, M.S. *et al.* (2006). The favorable clinical and angiographic outcomes of a high-dose dexamethasone-eluting stent: Randomized controlled prospective study, *Am Heart J*, **152**, 887.e1–e7.

Hyon, S.H., Cha, W.I. and Ikada, Y. (1989). Preparation of transparent poly(vinyl alcohol) hydrogel, *Polym Bull*, **22**, 119–122.

Howling, G.I., Sakoda, H., Antonarulrajah, A., Marrs, H., Stewart, T.D., Appleyard, S. *et al.* (2003). Biological response to wear debris generated in carbon based composites as potential bearing surfaces for artificial hip joints, *J Biomed Mater Res B Appl Biomater*, **67**, 758–764.

Ikeuchi, K., Kusaka, J., Yamane, D. and Fujita, S. (1999). Time-dependent wear process between lubricated soft materials, *Wear*, **229**, 656–659.

Ishikawa, Y., Hiratsuka, K. and Sasada, T. (2006). Role of water in the lubrication of hydrogel, *Wear*, **261**, 500–504.

Ishihara, K., Ueda, T. and Nakabayashi, N. (1990). Preparation of phospholipid polymers and their properties as polymer hydrogel membranes, *Polym J*, **22**, 355–360.

Kandzari, D.E. and Leon, M.B. (2006). Overview of pharmacology and clinical trials program with the zotarolimus-eluting endeavor stent, *J Interv Cardiol*, **19**, 405–413.

Kandzari, D.E., Leon, M.B., Popma, J.J., Fitzgerald, P.J., O'Shaughnessy, C., Ball, M.W. *et al.* (2006). Comparison of zotarolimus-eluting and sirolimus-eluting stents in patients with native coronary artery disease: A randomized controlled trial, *J Am Coll Cardiol*, **48**, 2440–2447.

Kato, K., Eika, Y. and Ikada, Y. (1996). Deposition of a hydroxyapatite thin layer onto a polymer surface carrying grafted phosphate polymer chains, *J Biomed Mater Res*, **32**, 687–691.

Kirk, T.B., Wilson, A.S. and Stachowiak, G.W. (1993). The morphology and composition of the superficial zone of mammalian articular cartilage, *J Orthop Rheumatol*, **6**, 21–28.

Kitano, K., Inoue, Y., Matsuno, R., Takai, M. and Ishihara, K. (2009). Nanoscale evaluation of lubricity on well-defined polymer brush surfaces using QCM-D and AFM, *Colloids Surf B Biointerfaces*, **74**, 350–357.

Kobayashi, M. and Takahara, A. (2010). Tribological properties of hydrophilic polymer brushes under wet conditions, *Chem Rec*, **10**, 208–216.

Kobayashi, M., Terayama, Y., Hosaka, N., Kaido, M., Suzuki, A., Yamada, N. *et al.* (2007). Friction behavior of high-density poly(2-methacryloyloxyethyl phosphorylcholine) brush in aqueous media. *Soft Matter*, **2**, 740–746.

Kuiper, K.K. and Nordrehaug, J.E. (2000). Early mobilization after protamine reversal of heparin following implantation of phosphorylcholine-coated stents in totally occluded coronary arteries, *Am J Cardiol*, **85**, 698–702.

Kurtz, S.M. and Devine, J.N. (2007). PEEK biomaterials in trauma, orthopedic, and spinal implants. *Biomaterials*, **28**, 4845–4869.

Kurtz, S., Mowat, F., Ong, K., Chan, N., Lau, E. and Halpern, M. (2005). Prevalence of primary and revision total hip and knee arthroplasty in the United States from 1990 through 2002, *J Bone Joint Surg Am*, **87**, 1487–1497.

Kyomoto, M. and Ishihara, K. (2009). Self-initiated surface graft polymerization of 2-methacryloyloxyethyl phosphorylcholine on poly(ether-ether-ketone) by photo-irradiation, *ACS Appl Mater Interfaces*, **1**, 537–542.

Kyomoto, M., Moro, T., Takatori, Y., Kawaguchi, H. and Ishihara, K. (2011). Cartilage-mimicking, high-density brush structure improves wear resistance of crosslinked polyethylene: A pilot study, *Clin Orthop Relat R*, **469**, 2327–2336.

Kyomoto, M., Moro, T., Konno, T., Takadama, H., Kawaguchi, H., Takatori, Y. *et al.* (2007a). Effects of photo-induced graft polymerization of 2-methacryloyloxyethyl phosphorylcholine on physical properties of cross-linked polyethylene in artificial hip joints, *J Mater Sci Mater Med*, **18**, 1809–1815.

Kyomoto, M., Moro, T., Konno, T., Takadama, H., Yamawaki, N., Kawaguchi, H. *et al.* (2007b). Enhanced wear resistance of modified cross-linked polyethylene by grafting with poly(2-methacryloyloxyethyl phosphorylcholine), *J Biomed Mater Res A*, **82**, 10–17.

Kyomoto, M., Moro, T., Miyaji, F., Hashimoto, M., Kawaguchi, H., Takatori, Y. *et al.* (2008). Effect of 2-methacryloyloxyethyl phosphorylcholine concentration on photo-induced graft polymerization of polyethylene in reducing the wear of orthopaedic bearing surface, *J Biomed Mater Res A*, **86**, 439–447.

Kyomoto, M., Moro, T., Saiga, K., Hashimoto, M., Ito, H., Kawaguchi, H. *et al.* (2012). Biomimetic hydration lubrication with various polyelectrolyte layers on cross-linked polyethylene orthopedic bearing materials, *Biomaterials*, **33**, 4451–4459.

Kyomoto, M., Moro, T., Saiga, K., Miyaji, F., Kawaguchi, H., Takatori, Y. *et al.* (2010a). Lubricity and stability of poly(2-methacryloyloxyethyl phosphorylcholine) polymer layer on Co–Cr–Mo surface for hemi-arthroplasty to prevent degeneration of articular cartilage, *Biomaterials*, **31**, 658–668.

Kyomoto, M., Moro, T., Takatori, Y., Kawaguchi, H., Nakamura, K. and Ishihara, K. (2010b). Self-initiated surface grafting with poly(2-methacryloyloxyethyl phosphorylcholine) on poly(ether-ether-ketone), *Biomaterials*, **31**, 1017–1024.

Kyomoto, M., Moro, T., Yamane, S., Hashimoto, M., Takatori, Y. and Ishihara, K. (2013). Poly(ether-ether-ketone) orthopedic bearing surface modified by self-initiated surface grafting of poly(2-methacryloyloxyethyl phosphorylcholine), *Biomaterials*, **34**, 7829–7839.

Longfield, M.D., Dowson, D., Walker, P.S. and Wright, V. (1969). "Boosted lubrication" of human joints by fluid enrichment and entrapment, *Biomed Eng*, **4**, 517–522.

Milner, S.T. (1991). Polymer brushes, *Science*, **251**, 905–914.

Moro, T., Takatori, Y., Ishihara, K., Nakamura, K. and Kawaguchi, H. (2006). Grafting of biocompatible polymer for longevity of artificial hip joints, *Clin Orthop Relat R*, **453**, 58–63.

Moro, T., Kawaguchi, H., Ishihara, K., Kyomoto, M., Karita, T., Ito, H. *et al.* (2009). Wear resistance of artificial hip joints with poly(2-methacryloyloxyethyl phosphorylcholine) grafted polyethylene: Comparisons with the effect of polyethylene cross-linking and ceramic femoral heads, *Biomaterials*, **30**, 2995–3001.

Moro, T., Takatori, Y., Ishihara, K., Konno, T., Takigawa, Y., Matsushita, T. *et al.* (2004). Surface grafting of artificial joints with a biocompatible polymer for preventing periprosthetic osteolysis, *Nature Mater*, **3**, 829–837.

Moro, T., Takatori, Y., Kyomoto, M., Ishihara, K., Hashimoto, M., Ito, H. *et al.* (2014). Long-term hip simulator testing of the artificial hip joint bearing surface grafted with biocompatible phospholipid polymer, *J Orthop Res*, **32**, 369–376.

Moro, T., Takatori, Y., Kyomoto, M., Kamogawa, M., Oda, H., Morimoto, S. *et al.* (2013). Clinical results of PMPC-grafted polyethylene acetabular liners. *Trans Orthop Res Soc*, **38**, 1071.

Mow, V.C., Ratcliffe, A. and Poole, A.R. (1992). Cartilage and diarthrodial joints as paradigms for hierarchical materials and structures, *Biomaterials*, **13**, 67–97.

Myers, G.J., Gardiner, K., Ditmore, S.N., Swyer, W.J., Squires, C., Johnstone, D.R. *et al.* (2005). Clinical evaluation of the Sorin Synthesis oxygenator with integrated arterial filter, *J Extra-Corp Technol*, **37**, 201–206.

Myers, G.J., Johnstone, D.R., Swyer, W.J., McTeer, S., Maxwell, S.L., Squires, C. *et al.* (2003). Evaluation of Mimesys phosphorylcholine (PC)-coated oxygenators during cardiopulmonary bypass in adults, *J Extra-Corp Technol*, **35**, 6–12.

Nagasaki, Y. and Kataoka, K. (1996). An intelligent polymer brush, *Trends Polym Sci*, **4**, 59–64.

Nguyen, H.X. and Ishida, H. (1986). Molecular analysis of the melting behaviour of poly(aryl–ether–ether–ketone), *Polymer*, **27**, 1400–1405.

Obara, T., Mabuchi, K., Iso, T. and Yamaguchi, T. (1997). Increased friction of animal joints by experimental degeneration and recovery by addition of hyaluronic acid, *Clin Biomech*, **12**, 246–252.

Paradossi, G. (2013). Hydrogels formed by cross-linked poly(vinyl alcohol), in Dumitriu, S. and Popa, V. (eds.), *Polymeric Biomaterials*, CRC press, Boca Raton, 37–56.

Qiu, C., Nguyen, Q.T. and Ping, Z. (2007). Surface modification of cardo polyetherketone ultrafiltration membrane by photo-grafted copolymers to obtain nanofiltration membranes, *J Membrane Sci*, **295**, 88–94.

Qiu, K.Y. and Si, K. (1996). Grafting reaction of macromolecules with pendant amino groups via photoinitiation with benzophenone, *Macromol Chem Phys*, **197**, 2403–2413.

Raviv, U., Giasson, S., Kampf, N., Gohy, J.F., Jérôme, R. and Klein, J. (2003). Lubrication by charged polymers, *Nature*, **425**, 163–165.

Raviv, U. and Klein, J. (2002). Fluidity of bound hydration layers, *Science*, **297**, 1540–1543.

Rodriguez, A., Rodríguez Alemparte, M., Fernández Pereira, C., Sampaolesi, A., da Rocha Loures Bueno, R. *et al.* (2005). Latin American randomized trial of balloon angioplasty vs coronary stenting for small vessels (LASMAL): Immediate and long-term results, *Am J Med*, **118**, 743–751.

Sakurai, R., Hongo, Y., Yamasaki, M., Honda, Y., Bonneau, H.N., Yock, P.G. *et al.* (2007). Detailed intravascular ultrasound analysis of Zotarolimus-eluting phosphorylcholine-coated cobalt–chromium alloy stent in de novo coronary lesions (results from the ENDEAVOR II trial), *Am J Cardiol*, **100**, 818–823.

Scholes, S.C., Inman, I.A., Unsworth, A. and Jones, E. (2008). Tribological assessment of a flexible carbon-fibre-reinforced poly(ether–ether–ketone) acetabular cup articulating against an alumina femoral head, *Proc Inst Mech Eng H*, **222**, 273–283.

Selan, L., Palma, S., Scoarughi, G.L., Papa, R., Veeh, R., Di Clemente, D. *et al.* (2009). Phosphorylcholine impairs susceptibility to biofilm formation of hydrogel contact lenses, *Am J Ophthalmol*, **147**, 134–139.

Serro, A.P., Gispert, M.P., Martins, M.C., Brogueira, P., Colaço, R. and Saramago, B. (2006). Adsorption of albumin on prosthetic materials: Implication for tribological behavior, *J Biomed Mater Res A*, **78**, 581–589.

Snyder, T.A., Tsukui, H., Kihara, S., Akimoto, T., Litwak, K.N., Kameneva, M.V. *et al.* (2007). Preclinical biocompatibility assessment of the EVAHEART ventricular assist device: Coating comparison and platelet activation, *J Biomed Mater Res A*, **81**, 85–92.

Takatori, Y., Moro, T., Kamogawa, M., Oda, H., Morimoto, S., Umeyama, T. *et al.* (2013). Poly(2-methacryloyloxyethyl phosphorylcholine)-grafted highly cross-linked polyethylene liner in primary total hip replacement: One-year results of a prospective cohort study, *J Artif Organs*, **16**, 170–175.

Tretinnikov, O.N., Kato, K. and Ikada, Y. (1994). *In vitro* hydroxyapatite deposition onto a film surface-grated with organophosphate polymer, *J Biomed Mater Res*, **28**, 1365–1373.

Ushio, K., Oka, M., Hyon, S.H., Yura, S., Toguchida, J. and Nakamura, T. (2003). Partial hemiarthroplasty for the treatment of osteonecrosis of the femoral head. An experimental study in the dog, *J Bone Joint Surg Br*, **85**, 922–930.

Utzschneider, S., Becker, F., Grupp, T.M., Sievers, B., Paulus, A., Gottschalk, O. *et al.* (2010). Inflammatory response against different carbon fiber-reinforced PEEK wear particles compared with UHMWPE in vivo, *Acta Biomater*, **6**, 4296–4304.

Wang, H., Brown, H.R. and Li, Z. (2007). Aliphatic ketones/water/alcohol as a new photoinitiating system for the photografting of methacrylic acid onto high-density polyethylene, *Polymer*, **48**, 939–948.

Wang, A., Lin, R., Polineni, V.K., Essner, A., Stark, C. and Dumbleton, J.H. (1998). Carbon fiber reinforced polyether ether ketone composite as a bearing surface for total hip replacement, *Tribol Int*, **31**, 661–667.

Wang, Q.Q., Wu, J.J., Unsworth, A., Briscoe, A., Jarman-Smith, M., Lowry, C. *et al.* (2012). Biotribological study of large diameter ceramic-on-CFR-PEEK hip joint including fluid uptake, wear and frictional heating, *J Mater Sci Mater Med*, **23**, 1533–1542.

Wright, V. and Dowson, D. (1976). Lubrication and cartilage, *J Anat*, **121**, 107–118.

Yamada, Y., Saito, S., Nishinaka, T. and Yamazaki, K. (2012). Myocardial size and fibrosis changes during left ventricular assist device support, *ASAIO J*, **58**, 402–406.

Yang, W. and Rånby, B. (1999). Photoinitiation performance of some ketones in the LDPE–acrylic acid surface photografting system, *Eur Polym J*, **35**, 1557–1568.

Yoshida, H., Morita, Y. and Ikeuchi, K. (2003). Biological lubrication of hydrated surface layer in small intestine, in Dowson D. (ed.), *Tribological research and design for engineering systems*, Elsevier, Amsterdam, 425–428.

Yu, S., Hariram, K.P., Kumar, R., Cheang, P. and Aik, K.K. (2005). *In vitro* apatite formation and its growth kinetics on hydroxyapatite/polyetheretherketone biocomposites, *Biomaterials*, **26**, 2343–2352.

Chapter 11

Surface-Oxidized Zirconium

Shantanu Patil and Darryl D. D'Lima
Shiley Center for Orthopaedic Research & Education, Scripps Health, La Jolla, USA

Cobalt chrome alloys articulating against ultra-high molecular weight polyethylene are currently the most popular bearing surfaces for total joint arthroplasty. Ceramic materials wear less due to their greater hardness but carry a risk of implant fracture. Zirconium with an oxidized surface layer has the dual advantage of toughness comparable to metal components and surface hardness comparable to ceramic components. This chapter reviews the performance of oxidized zirconium as an alternative bearing surface for hip and knee arthroplasty. Results integrating *in vitro* and clinical studies as well as retrievals are presented. *In vitro* studies have reported increased surface hardness, reduced polyethylene wear, and low cytotoxicity of particles generated from oxidized zirconium. Oxidized zirconium has not been associated with significant material-related adverse events supporting the high safety of this bearing material. However, clinical studies have not yet supported the promise of better clinical performance or longer survival, in part because of the lack of long-term follow-up investigations and in part because of the high survival rates of current-generation cobalt chrome alloy femoral head designs.

1. Background

Ceramic oxides such as alumina and zirconia have greater wear performance compared to metals and have attributed to higher hardness and enhanced wettability. Niobium (2.5%) when alloyed with zirconium generates a two-phase microstructure that provides the mechanical strength necessary for joint replacement implants. Zirconium and niobium have excellent biocompatibility, which is

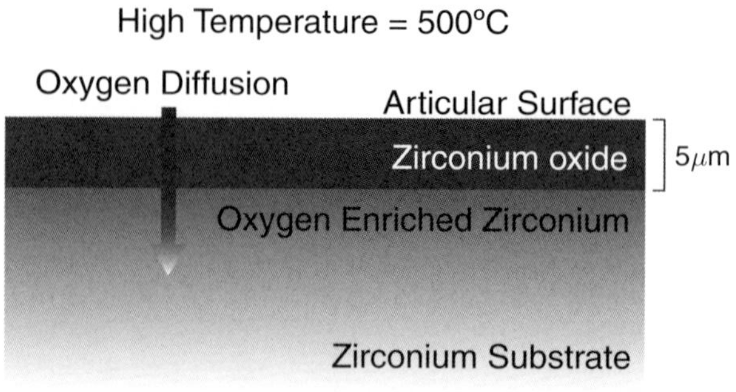

Figure 11-1. Schematic of the process of oxidizing zirconium.

comparable to that of titanium and cobalt–chromium alloys (Rose *et al.*, 2012). Wrought zirconium–niobium alloy is then oxidized by thermal diffusion in heated air (500°C) to generate a nominally 5 μm thick surface of zirconia (ZrO2) (Hobbs *et al.*, 2005). Below the oxide layer is a 1.5–2 μm thick oxygen-rich transition zone called the diffusion-hardened zone (DHZ) (Figure 11-1) (Pawar *et al.*, 2011). More recently a two-step heat treatment process has been described, which increases the thickness of the DHZ tenfold (although implants with this treatment are not yet available) (Pawar *et al.*, 2011). The diffusion process can oxidize complex surface geometries making it highly attractive for joint arthroplasty components. In contrast to a surface coating, surface oxidization transforms the original metal surface into a ceramic layer, and the oxygen gradient results in a more gradual transition between ceramic and metal layers. The advantage is the absence of a coating–metal interface that can be susceptible to debonding. For total knee arthroplasty (TKA) femoral components, the back surface is typically grit blasted since cement does not adhere to the smooth oxide layer.

The nanohardness of the oxidized zirconia (12.1 GPa) is about 80% that of zirconia and more than twice the hardness of cobalt-chromium (5.4 GPa) or titanium (5.6 GPa) alloys (Pawar *et al.*, 2011). The fatigue strength is greater than 450 MPa for 10 million cycles, supporting the claims of increased toughness (Tsai *et al.*, 2001). However, the bulk hardness of oxidized zirconium has been reported to be lower than that of cobalt chrome due to the softer zirconium metal underlying the oxidized layer (Kop *et al.*, 2007).

2. Total Knee Arthroplasty

2.1. *Wear Resistance*

Major factors influencing the wear of polyethylene articulating with metal surfaces are lubrication, bearing hardness, surface roughness, and third-body debris. From a materials perspective, oxidized zirconium combines the toughness of metal with the surface hardness of ceramic, which makes it an attractive alternative as a bearing surface. The free energy of oxidized zirconium surfaces is low and decreases adhesion to polyethylene (Galetz *et al.*, 2010). To document the effect on wear performance, several studies have been conducted *in vitro* under ISO standards (ISO 14243-1:2009) as well as under adverse conditions replicating surface roughening, third-body wear, aggressive kinematics, and loading. Under test conditions simulating normal walking in displacement-controlled knee wear simulators, ultra-high molecular weight polyethylene (UHMWPE) wear rates against oxidized zirconium femoral components were 42–89% lower than those against cobalt chrome femoral components with the same design (Ezzet *et al.*, 2004; Spector *et al.*, 2001) (Figure 11-2). Testing in a force-controlled wear simulator also found a similar (82%) reduction in polyethylene wear rates (DesJardins *et al.*, 2008) (Figure 11-3).

To simulate scratching of femoral components during implantation or *in vivo*, oxidized zirconium and cobalt chrome components were roughened by tumbling in alumina powder (Ries *et al.*, 2002). Tumbling increased the surface roughness of cobalt chrome femoral components to a significantly greater degree than that of oxidized zirconium femoral components. Consequently, UHMWPE wear rates against roughened oxidized zirconium femoral components were 89% lower than those against roughened cobalt chrome femoral components.

One displacement-controlled wear simulator study simulated athletically active patients with varus malalignment and reported 55%

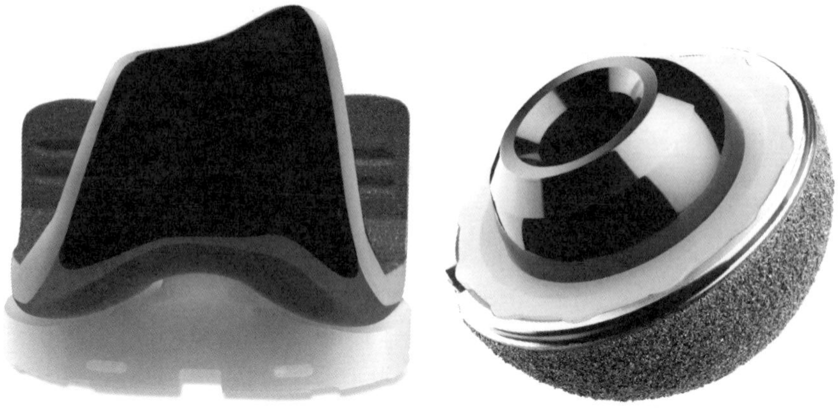

(a) (b)

Figure 11-2. Oxidized zirconium femoral component for knee arthroplasty (a) and femoral head for hip arthroplasty (b).

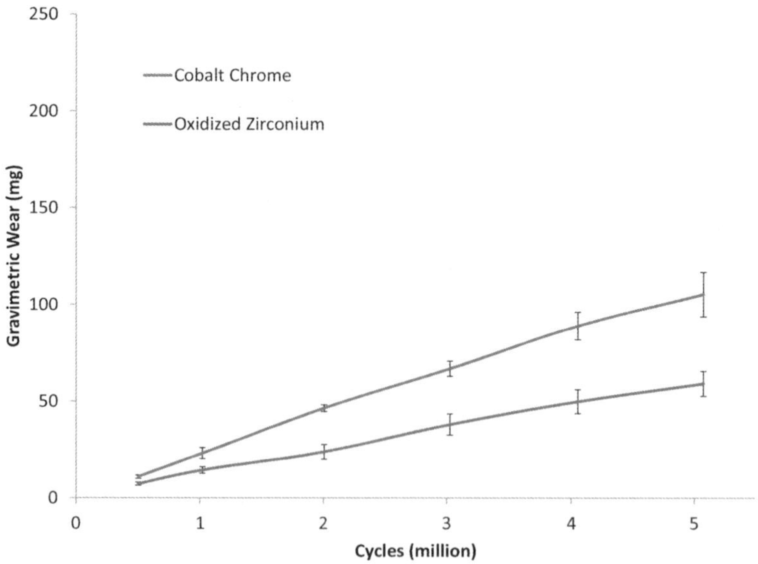

Figure 11-3. Comparison between polyethylene wear against cobalt chrome and oxidized zirconium femoral components in an AMTI knee wear simulator. (Reprinted from Ezzet *et al.* (2004), with permission from Wolters Kluwer Health.)

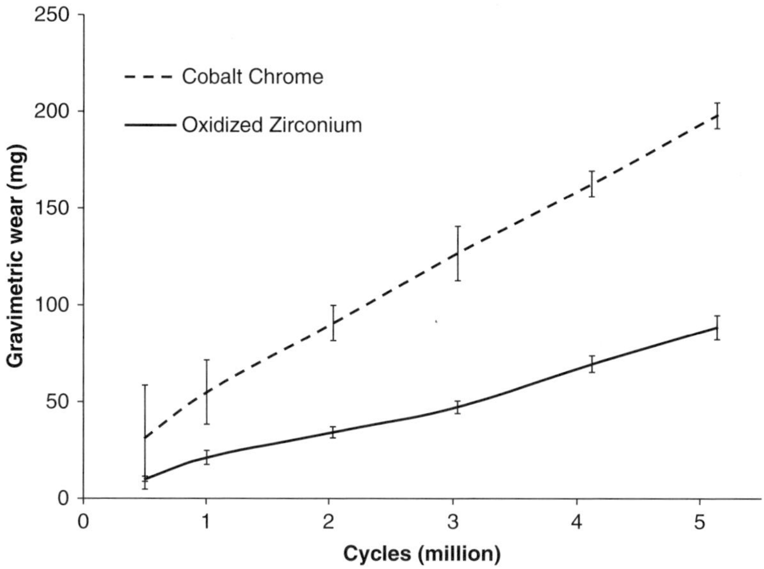

Figure 11-4. Polyethylene wear was lower against oxidized zirconium components tested even when under aggressive test conditions. (Reprinted from Ezzet *et al.* (2012), with permission from Elsevier.)

lower polyethylene wear in the oxidized zirconium group (Ezzet *et al.*, 2012) (Figure 11-4). In a force-controlled wear simulator, increasing shear force and internal–external rotation torque resulted in greater increase in the surface roughness of cobalt chrome femoral components compared to oxidized zirconium femoral components, and a 78% reduction in wear in polyethylene inserts articulating against oxidized zirconium femoral components (Lee *et al.*, 2009).

In bilateral randomized TKA studies of the oxidized zirconium or cobalt chrome Genesis II design (Smith & Nephew, Memphis, TN), no differences were found in weight, size, aspect ratio, or roundness of polyethylene wear particles aspirated from the knees of 100 patients at the 5- to 6-year follow-up or 120 patients at the 6- to 8-year follow-up (Kim *et al.*, 2010; Kim *et al.*, 2012). A smaller study (N = 6) also reported no difference in particle number and morphology (Minoda *et al.*, 2013). In addition, cytotoxicity to wear particles from oxidized zirconium appears to be low: Comparable to Ti_6Al_4V alloy and lower than particles from cobalt or cobalt-chrome alloy (Rose *et al.*, 2012).

2.2. *Retrievals and Damage*

Two retrieval studies of oxidized zirconium femoral components matched with cobalt chrome alloy femoral components for body mass index, insert type (cruciate-retaining or cruciate-substituting), and implantation duration revealed higher surface roughness and grooving damage in the cobalt chrome alloy components but higher gouging damage in the oxidized zirconium components (Brandt *et al.*, 2013; Heyse *et al.*, 2011). The high nanohardness of the oxidized zirconium surface layer likely contributes to the resistance to abrasion but the lower bulk hardness can make it susceptible to damage such as that occurring during contact with the posterior aspect of the tibial tray (Burnell *et al.*, 2011; Kop *et al.*, 2007).

2.3. *Clinical Outcomes*

Randomized studies comparing oxidized zirconium to cobalt chrome femoral components did not find significant differences in clinical outcome scores (e.g. the Knee Society Score) but one study did report a more rapid improvement in flexion and gain of functional milestones that led to early discharge from hospital (Kim *et al.*, 2012; Laskin, 2003). No failure due to wear or aseptic loosening was reported at up to seven years of the retrospective follow-up (Innocenti *et al.*, 2010). A study of bilateral TKAs (N = 40) of the Genesis II design, randomized to an oxidized zirconium femoral component in one knee and a cobalt chrome femoral component in the contralateral knee, did not find any difference in function or revision rates (Hui *et al.*, 2011). However, a greater number of patients preferred the knee with the cobalt chrome femoral component. Polyethylene tibial components retrieved during insert exchange (at the time of subsequent patellar resurfacing in 4 knees at 52 months post-operative) did not reveal any differences in patterns of wear between oxidized zirconium or cobalt chrome designs. A larger randomized bilateral TKA study of the same implant design (N = 331) also reported a similar lack of difference in clinical outcomes between oxidized zirconium and cobalt chrome femoral components, despite no failures at six- to eight-year follow-up (Kim *et al.*, 2012). A large community registry report did not find increased survival in rates in so-called 'premium' TKA designs, which included oxidized zirconium femoral components (Gioe *et al.*, 2011). An analysis of the Kaiser Permanente National Joint Registry reported a slightly higher rate of revision due to tibial insert wear in oxidized zirconium TKAs (N = 1066) with conventional polyethylene inserts compared to cobalt chrome femoral components with highly crosslinked polyethylene inserts (N = 7618) (Inacio *et al.*, 2013). Note that earlier oxidized zirconium TKA designs were implanted with non-crosslinked polyethylene inserts. In 2008, crosslinked polyethylene inserts were made available with oxidized zirconium femoral components.

2.4. *Metal Sensitivity*

Sensitivity to metallic implant components is a poorly understood, difficult to predict, and relatively rare complication of joint arthroplasty (Granchi *et al.*, 2008; Hallab *et al.*, 2001; Merritt and Rodrigo, 1996). Sensitivity to nickel and cobalt, and even chromium has been reported. Since oxidized zirconium femoral components do not contain these metals, the risk of adverse reactions is greatly reduced. There is anecdotal evidence of case reports of resolution of skin reactions and local synovitis and other symptoms of sensitivity after revision to oxidized zirconium femoral components and titanium tibial trays (Gao *et al.*, 2011; Post *et al.*, 2013; Thakur *et al.*, 2013).

3. Total Hip Arthroplasty

3.1. *Wear*

Oxidized zirconium heads generated lower wear rates in non-crosslinked polyethylene liners compared to cobalt chrome heads (Good *et al.*, 2003). The relative reduction in the wear rate against oxidized zirconium heads was maintained even when the femoral heads were roughened. Wear in highly crosslinked polyethylene was undetectable against smooth cobalt chrome or oxidized zirconium heads. On the other hand, wear in highly crosslinked polyethylene increased when cobalt chrome heads were roughened but not when oxidized zirconium heads were roughened.

Results of low wear *in vitro* were supported by radiographic and radiostereometric measurements of head penetration. Penetration rates of oxidized zirconium heads in highly crosslinked polyethylene liners at two-year follow-up were low but not substantially different from those reported for cobalt chrome heads against highly crosslinked (Garvin *et al.*, 2009; Kadar *et al.*, 2011, 2012).

3.2. *Retrievals and Damage*

Case reports of heads retrieved after dislocation have raised concerns over increased damage to oxidized zirconium heads induced during the dislocation event or during the attempts at closed reduction (Evangelista *et al.*, 2007; Jaffe *et al.*, 2009; Kop *et al.*, 2007; Mai *et al.*, 2010; McCalden *et al.*, 2011) (Figure 11-5). The damage reported included loss of the surface layer of oxidized zirconium and transfer of metal from acetabular shells to the femoral head. One study that simulated dislocation damage *in vitro* in oxidized zirconium heads reported no increase in subsequent wear rates *in vitro* in conventional polyethylene liners when compared to undamaged cobalt chrome heads, and very low wear in crosslinked polyethylene liners (Bourne *et al.*, 2005). Other studies have shown that damaged

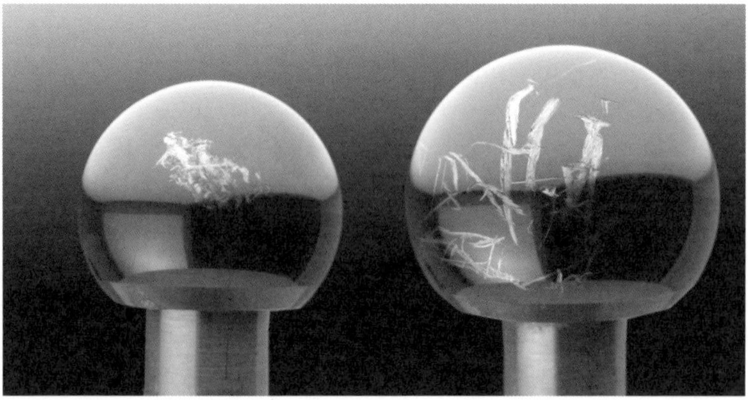

Figure 11-5. Recurrent hip dislocations can scratch the surfaces of oxidized zirconium femoral heads. (Permission pending.)

oxidized zirconium heads, whether obtained from retrievals or damaged *in vitro*, generated higher wear rates in crosslinked polyethylene liners (Jaffe *et al.*, 2009; Lee *et al.*, 2009). Case reports of atypical damage have included third-body damage (due to a trochanteric fixation wire) (Gibon *et al.*, 2013) or polyethylene liner failure leading to direct articulation of an oxidized zirconium head with the titanium acetabular shell (Tribe *et al.*, 2013).

3.3. *Clinical Outcomes*

No difference in clinical outcomes between oxidized zirconium and cobalt chrome femoral heads have been reported at two-year follow-up (Lewis *et al.*, 2008). A large community registry report also did not find increased survival rates in so-called 'premium' total hip arthroplasty (THA) designs (N = 1311), which included oxidized zirconium femoral heads over standard THA designs (N = 868) (Gioe *et al.*, 2011). On the other hand, oxidized zirconium articulating against crosslinked polyethylene has yielded more promising early outcomes. The Australian Registry reported that the cumulative revision rate at five years was the lowest for ceramicized metal femoral heads coupled with crosslinked polyethylene (2%) compared to metal-on = crosslinked polyethylene (2.9%), ceramic-on-ceramic (3.3%), and ceramic-on-crosslinked polyethylene (3.0%) (AOANJR, 2013). Note that the sample size for ceramicized metal-on-crosslinked polyethylene was low compared to the other groups.

4. Summary

Overall, oxidized zirconium has not been associated with significant material-related adverse events, supporting the high safety levels of this bearing material. *In vitro* studies have indicated increased surface hardness, reduced polyethylene wear, and low cytotoxicity of oxidized zirconium particles. Clinical studies have not supported the promise of better clinical performance or longer survival, in part because of the lack of long-term follow-up, and in part because of the high survival rates of current-generation cobalt chrome alloy femoral knee component and head designs. Anecdotal evidence indicates that oxidized zirconium components may be useful in patients with metal sensitivity.

References

AOANJR. (2013). Australian Orthopaedic Association National Joint Replacement Registry. Annual Report 2013, Adelaide.

Bourne, R.B., Barrack, R., Rorabeck, C.H., Salehi, A. and Good, V. (2005). Arthroplasty options for the young patient: Oxinium on cross-linked polyethylene, *Clin Orthop Relat Res*, **441**, 159–167.

Brandt, J.M., Guenther, L., O'Brien, S., Vecherya, A., Turgeon, T.R. and Bohm, E.R. (2013). Performance assessment of femoral knee components made from cobalt-chromium alloy and oxidized zirconium, *Knee*, **20**, 388–396.

Burnell, C.D., Brandt, J.M., Petrak, M.J. and Bourne, R.B. (2011). Posterior condyle surface damage on retrieved femoral knee components, *J Arthroplasty*, **26**, 1460–1467.

DesJardins, J., Burnikel, B. and LaBerge, M. (2008). UHMWPE wear against roughened oxidized zirconium and CoCr femoral knee components during force-controlled simulation, *Wear*, **264**, 245–256.

Evangelista, G.T., Fulkerson, E., Kummer, F. and Di Cesare, P.E. (2007). Surface damage to an Oxinium femoral head prosthesis after dislocation, *J Bone Joint Surg Br*, **89**, 535–537.

Ezzet, K.A., Hermida, J.C., Colwell Jr., C.W. and D'Lima, D.D. (2004). Oxidized zirconium femoral components reduce polyethylene wear in a knee wear simulator, *Clin Orthop Relat R*, **428**, 120–124.

Ezzet, K.A., Hermida, J.C., Steklov, N. and D'Lima, D.D. (2012). Wear of polyethylene against oxidized zirconium femoral components effect of aggressive kinematic conditions and malalignment in total knee arthroplasty, *J Arthroplasty*, **27**, 116–121.

Galetz, M.C., Fleischmann, E.W., Konrad, C.H., Schuetz, A. and Glatzel, U. (2010). Abrasion resistance of oxidized zirconium in comparison with CoCrMo and titanium nitride coatings for artificial knee joints, *J Biomed Mater Res B Appl Biomater*, **93**, 244–251.

Gao, X., He, R.X., Yan, S.G. and Wu, L.D. (2011). Dermatitis associated with chromium following total knee arthroplasty, *J Arthroplasty*, **26**, 665.e13–665.e16.

Garvin, K.L., Hartman, C.W., Mangla, J., Murdoch, N. and Martell, J.M. (2009). Wear analysis in THA utilizing oxidized zirconium and crosslinked polyethylene, *Clin Orthop Relat R*, **467**, 141–145.

Gibon, E., Scemama, C., David, B. and Hamadouche, M. (2013). Oxinium femoral head damage generated by a metallic foreign body within the polyethylene cup following recurrent dislocation episodes, *Orthop Traumatol Surg Res*, **99**, 865–869.

Gioe, T.J., Sharma, A., Tatman, P. and Mehle, S. (2011). Do "premium" joint implants add value?: Analysis of high cost joint implants in a community registry, *Clin Orthop Relat R*, **469**, 48–54.

Good, V., Ries, M., Barrack, R.L., Widding, K., Hunter, G. and Heuer, D. (2003). Reduced wear with oxidized zirconium femoral heads, *J Bone Joint Surg Am*, **85**(Suppl 4), 105–110.

Granchi, D., Cenni, E., Tigani, D., Trisolino, G., Baldini, N. and Giunti, A. (2008). Sensitivity to implant materials in patients with total knee arthroplasties, *Biomaterials*, **29**, 1494–1500.

Hallab, N., Merritt, K. and Jacobs, J.J. (2001). Metal sensitivity in patients with orthopaedic implants, *J Bone Joint Surg Am*, **83**, 428–436.

Heyse, T.J., Chen, D.X., Kelly, N., Boettner, F., Wright, T.M. and Haas, S.B. (2011). Matched-pair total knee arthroplasty retrieval analysis: Oxidized zirconium vs. CoCrMo, *Knee*, **18**, 448–452.

Hobbs, L.W., Rosen, V.B., Mangin, S.P., Treska, M. and Hunter, G. (2005). Oxidation microstructures and interfaces in the oxidized zirconium knee, *Int J Appl Ceram*, **2**, 221–256.

Hui, C., Salmon, L., Maeno, S., Roe, J., Walsh, W. and Pinczewski, L. (2011). Five-year comparison of oxidized zirconium and cobalt–chromium femoral components in total knee arthroplasty: A randomized controlled trial, *J Bone Joint Surg Am*, **93**, 624–630.

Inacio, M.C., Cafri, G., Paxton, E.W., Kurtz, S.M. and Namba, R.S. (2013). Alternative bearings in total knee arthroplasty: Risk of early revision compared to traditional bearings: An analysis of 62,177 primary cases, *Acta Orthop*, **84**, 145–152.

Innocenti, M., Civinini, R., Carulli, C., Matassi, F. and Villano, M. (2010). The 5-year results of an oxidized zirconium femoral component for TKA, *Clin Orthop Relat R*, **468**, 1258–1263.

Jaffe, W.L., Strauss, E.J., Cardinale, M., Herrera, L. and Kummer, F.J. (2009). Surface oxidized zirconium total hip arthroplasty head damage due to closed reduction effects on polyethylene wear, *J Arthroplasty*, **24**, 898–902.

Kadar, T., Hallan, G., Aamodt, A., Indrekvam, K., Badawy, M., Skredderstuen, A. *et al.* (2011). Wear and migration of highly cross-linked and conventional cemented polyethylene cups with cobalt chrome or Oxinium femoral heads: A randomized radiostereometric study of 150 patients, *J Orthop Res*, **29**, 1222–1229.

Kadar, T., Furnes, O., Aamodt, A., Indrekvam, K., Havelin, L.I., Haugan, K. *et al.* (2012). The influence of acetabular inclination angle on the penetration of polyethylene and migration of the acetabular component: A prospective, radiostereometric study on cemented acetabular components, *J Bone Joint Surg Br*, **94**, 302–307.

Kim, Y.H., Kim, J.S., Huh, W. and Lee, K.H. (2010). Weight of polyethylene wear particles is similar in TKAs with oxidized zirconium and cobalt–chrome prostheses, *Clin Orthop Relat R*, **468**, 1296–1304.

Kim, Y.H., Park, J.W. and Kim, J.S. (2012). Comparison of the Genesis II total knee replacement with oxidised zirconium and cobalt-chromium femoral components in the same patients: A prospective, double-blind, randomised controlled study, *J Bone Joint Surg Br*, **94**, 1221–1227.

Kop, A.M., Whitewood, C. and Johnston, D.J. (2007). Damage of Oxinium femoral heads subsequent to hip arthroplasty dislocation three retrieval case studies, *J Arthroplasty*, **22**, 775–779.

Laskin, R.S. (2003). An oxidized Zr ceramic surfaced femoral component for total knee arthroplasty, *Clin Orthop Relat R*, **416**, 191–196.

Lee, J.K., Maruthainar, K., Wardle, N., Haddad, F. and Blunn, G.W. (2009). Increased force simulator wear testing of a zirconium oxide total knee arthroplasty, *Knee*, **16**, 269–274.

Lee, R., Essner, A., Wang, A. and Jaffe, W.L. (2009). Scratch and wear performance of prosthetic femoral head components against crosslinked UHMWPE sockets, *Wear*, **267**, 1915–1921.

Lewis, P.M., Moore, C.A., Olsen, M., Schemitsch, E.H. and Waddell, J.P. (2008). Comparison of mid-term clinical outcomes after primary total hip arthroplasty with Oxinium vs cobalt chrome femoral heads, *Orthopedics*, **31**, 109–112.

Mai, K.T., Verioti, C., D'Lima, D., Colwell Jr., C.W. and Ezzet Jr., K.A. (2010). Surface roughness of femoral head prostheses after dislocation, *Am J Orthop* (*Belle Mead NJ*), **39**, 495–500.

McCalden, R.W., Charron, K.D., Davidson, R.D., Teeter, M.G. and Holdsworth, D.W. (2011). Damage of an Oxinium femoral head and polyethylene liner following 'routine' total hip replacement, *J Bone Joint Surg Br*, **93**, 409–413.

Merritt, K. and Rodrigo, J.J. (1996). Immune response to synthetic materials. Sensitization of patients receiving orthopaedic implants, *Clin Orthop Relat R*, **326**, 71–79.

Minoda, Y., Hata, K., Iwaki, H., Ikebuchi, M., Hashimoto, Y., Inori, F. *et al.* (2013). No difference in *in vivo* polyethylene wear particles between oxidized zirconium and cobalt–chromium femoral component in total knee arthroplasty, *Knee Surg Sports Traumatol Arthrosc*, **22**, 680–686.

Pawar, V., Weaver, C. and Jani, S. (2011). Physical characterization of a new composition of oxidized zirconium-2.5 wt% niobium produced using a two step process of biomedical applications, *Appl Surf Sci*, **257**, 6118–6124.

Post, Z.D., Orozco, F.R. and Ong, A.C. (2013). Metal sensitivity after TKA presenting with systemic dermatitis and hair loss, *Orthopedics*, **36**, e525–e528.

Ries, M.D., Salehi, A., Widding, K. and Hunter, G. (2002). Polyethylene wear performance of oxidized zirconium and cobalt-chromium knee components under abrasive conditions, *J Bone Joint Surg Am*, **84**(Suppl 2), 129–135.

Rose, S.F., Weaver, C.L., Fenwick, S.A., Horner, A. and Pawar, V.D. (2012). The effect of diffusion hardened oxidized zirconium wear debris on cell viability and inflammation — An *in vitro* study, *J Biomed Mater Res B Appl Biomater*, **100**, 1359–1368.

Spector, B.M., Ries, M.D., Bourne, R.B., Sauer, W.S., Long, M. and Hunter, G. (2001). Wear performance of ultra-high molecular weight polyethylene on oxidized zirconium total knee femoral components, *J Bone Joint Surg Am*, **83** (Suppl 2), 80–86.

Thakur, R.R., Ast, M.P., McGraw, M., Bostrom, M.P., Rodriguez, J.A. and Parks, M.L. (2013). Severe persistent synovitis after cobalt–chromium total knee arthroplasty requiring revision, *Orthopedics*, **36**, e520–e524.

Tribe, H., Malek, S., Stammers, J., Ranawat, V. and Skinner, J.A. (2013). Advanced wear of an Oxinium femoral head implant following polyethylene liner dislocation, *Ann R Coll Surg Engl*, **95**, e133–e135.

Tsai, S., Sprague, J., Hunter, G., Thomas, R. and Salehi, A. (2001). Mechanical testing and finite element analysis of oxidized zirconium femoral components, *Trans Soc Biomater*, **24**, 163.

Chapter 12

Oxidized Titanium

Hasan Güleryüz[a], Faiz Muhaffel[b] and Hüseyin Çimenoğlu[b]

[a]*Department of Metallurgical and Materials Engineering, Sinop University, Sinop, Turkey*

[b]*Department of Metallurgical and Materials Engineering, Istanbul Technical University, Istanbul, Turkey*

1. Introduction

Medical devices such as dental and orthopedic implants always require utilization of metallic materials possessing high strength (static/dynamic) and corrosion resistance as well as good biological compatibility. Early biomedical applications of titanium relied on its two principal properties: High strength that can be tailored by alloying and/or heat treatment, and good corrosion resistance. Also, the low density (providing high strength to weight ratio) and low elastic modulus (leading to a reduction in stress shielding effect) of titanium alloys appeared to be additional advantages over other competing metallic materials, including stainless steels and cobalt-chromium alloys (Boyer *et al.*, 1994; Donachie, 1989). The practical use of titanium implants started in the 1960s with the first studies published in 1969, and later on their usage in dentistry and orthopedics rapidly increased to the level we find in the present day (Brunette *et al.*, 2001).

The commercially pure (Cp) titanium grades and Ti_6Al_4V alloy were the first titanium materials introduced to implantable components and devices, but new alloy systems and improved versions of older alloys were produced to obtain better performance (Brunette *et al.*, 2001; Imam and Fraker, 1996). Cp-titanium, which is available in four grades (Grades 1 to 4) with tensile strength levels of 240–740 MPa, is generally preferred for dental implants (Muddugangadhar*et al.*, 2011). Owing to its higher strength, Ti_6Al_4V alloy is mostly used in manufacturing of load bearing orthopedic implants. After the toxicity of Ti_6Al_4V alloy was discovered as the result of *in vivo* release of vanadium in the late 1980s, Ti_6Al_7Nb alloy became an alternative load bearing implant material (Dearnley, 2005; Geetha *et al.*, 2009; Leyens and Peters, 2003).

Due to the fact that titanium is very reactive with oxygen at ambient conditions, it is usually protected by a very stable self-healing passive oxide film consisted of mainly TiO_2. This passive oxide film, which easily forms in any oxidizing media, is responsible for providing corrosion resistance to titanium and its alloys in many aqueous media, and ensures their biocompatibility (Dong and Bell, 2000; Komotori *et al.*, 2001; Long and Rack, 1998). Nevertheless, surface treatments may be applied to titanium and its alloys for the following purposes:

i. Optimizing the surface topography to provide better integration of bone cells onto the surface of the implant.
ii. Enhancing hardness of the surface to increase the wear resistance.
iii. Inducing passivity of the surface in order to increase corrosion resistance against body fluids.
iv. Increasing fatigue strength (e.g. shot peening).

Various techniques that aim to enhance functionality of the surface of the titanium-based implants were utilized. These techniques are mainly based on physical (sol-gel, vapor deposition, thermal spraying, thermal oxidation), mechanical (grinding, sand blasting), chemical (etching with acidic or alkali solutions), and electrochemical (electrolytic polishing, anodic oxidation, micro arc oxidation) modifications (Brunette *et al.*, 2001).

2. Tribology of Titanium and its Alloys

In contrast to the superior combination of mechanical and corrosion properties, titanium alloys suffer from poor tribological performance, with issues including high and unstable friction coefficients, severe adhesive wear, and susceptibility to fretting (Dong and Bell, 2000; Long and Rack, 1998). The poor tribological behavior of titanium and its alloys is due to the inherent characteristics of titanium and mainly related to its electron configuration, crystal structure, and inefficient lubrication (Boettcher *et al.*, 2002; Qi *et al.*, 2002). It has been reported that there is a strong correlation between friction and chemical reactivity of the transition metals (Buckley and Miyoshi, 1984). The relative chemical reactivity of the transition metals (metals with partially filled d-shells) can be determined from their percentage of d-bond character. The greater the percentage of the d-bond character, the less reactive the metal, and the lower the friction. The electron configuration of titanium possesses a low value of d-bond character, which leads to the extreme reactivity of the titanium surface (Bhushan, 2013; Buckley, 1981). Pure titanium and the majority of the titanium alloys have a hexagonal close packed (HCP) structure at low temperatures. At high temperatures, the HCP structure transforms to the body centered cubic (BCC) structure (at 885°C in pure titanium), which is stable up to melting temperature. The HCP and BCC structures of titanium are named α-titanium and β-titanium phases, respectively. The structure of α-titanium is distinguished from other HCP metals by a low axial ratio (c/a ratio) of 1.588, which is a less than ideal close packed structure with an axial ratio of 1.633. Most of the metals with HCP structure exhibit good frictional properties; however, titanium is different. The low axial ratio allows prismatic and pyramidal slip planes to operate in addition to the slip occurring on the basal planes (Donachie, 1989; Leyens and Peters, 2003). The increased number of operational slip systems and possible mechanical twinning enhances ductility and promotes plastic deformation at the asperity junctions, leading to higher friction during sliding contact. Another factor that affects the frictional properties of titanium is the poor response to lubrication. It has been reported that all conventional lubricants (mineral oils and greases), which are successfully and widely used for most metals, have been shown to be ineffective when applied to titanium alloys. The difficulty with titanium is that no strong natural bonding or reaction between the lubricant and the titanium surface takes place (Rabinowicz, 1955; Shapiro and Gisser, 1963). Additionally, sluggish heat conduction in titanium causes copious frictional heating and adds to the inefficiency of lubrication problem.

The blend of material properties mentioned above render titanium and its alloys very susceptible to adhesive and abrasive wear. The high reactivity of the surface and extensive deformation of the subsurface regions cause severe damage while making a large contribution to the friction of titanium mating either with itself or another material (Long and Rack, 1998). The ductility and chemical reactivity of titanium alloys enhance plastic deformation and adhesion at the asperity junctions. The adhesion strength of junctions may be much higher than the strength of titanium alloy. Such junctions eventually rupture within titanium asperities and create many craters on the worn surface. Ruptured particles may transfer to the counter material or form small wear debris. Long and Rack (2001) studied the reciprocating sliding wear of several titanium alloys against steel. The worn surfaces of the titanium alloys showed shear delaminating and smearing accompanied by heavy transfer to the steel surface and mechanical alloying with the steel. After multiple contacts between the coupled surfaces, work hardening of wear debris or transferred titanium developed and resulted in severe abrasive damage to the titanium surface (Long and Rack, 2001). A typical worn surface exhibits grooves aligned with the sliding direction, indicating plastic deformation as well as microplowing and microcracking perpendicular to the sliding direction (Dearnley *et al.*, 2004).

In general, the availability of oxygen in the environment radically changes the friction and wear behavior of metals and alloys. Frictional heating increases the temperature of the contacting surfaces and enhances the oxidation of titanium. Formation of a durable lubricating oxide film inhibits wear; however, regular formation and destruction of a weak oxide film increases wear rate (Stachowiak and

Bachelor, 2001). Molinari *et al.* (1997) investigated the dry sliding wear mechanism of a Ti_6Al_4V alloy mating with itself. Microscopic examinations revealed drastic plastic deformation of the worn surfaces even under low contact pressure. The wear mechanism was described as oxidative wear of a plastically strained surface. Insufficient protection of the oxide film was due to the mechanical instability of the surface, which led to generation of oxide wear debris and a high wear rate. Fracture of the oxide film created the potential for abrasive wear because hard oxide debris acted as third-body abrasive components (Molinari *et al.*, 1997). Dong and Bell (1999) investigated the wear of a Ti_6Al_4V alloy sliding against Al_2O_3 balls. Wear debris analysis indicated some tribochemical reactions developing as a result of the high reactivity and low thermal conductivity of the titanium alloy. Ti_6Al_4V alloy was considered to have poor oxidative wear resistance because of the tribochemical reactions concentrating at the overheated contact area (Dong and Bell, 1999).

For the determination of tribological properties in aqueous media, the combined action of corrosion and wear (i.e. corrosion-wear) should be accounted for (Dearnley, 1999; Dearnley *et al.*, 2004; Komotori *et al.*, 2001). As a matter of fact, a synergy that may arise between corrosion and wear tends to accelerate the degradation of the naturally formed thin oxide film. (Dearnley, 1999; Komotori *et al.*, 2001). Continuous removal of the oxide film due to sustained wear action threatens the long-term corrosion resistance of titanium surfaces. Galliano *et al.* (2001) investigated the simultaneous effects of corrosion and wear by conducting sliding wear tests in 0.9% NaCl solution. The experimental setup allowed monitoring of electrochemical parameters during wear tests. They reported that initiation of wear led to a sharp increase in anodic current and the formation of a galvanic couple between the wear track (anode) and the remaining surface (cathode). Ongoing wear action decreased the corrosion potential and increased corrosion rate (Galliano *et al.*, 2001). Komotori *et al.* (2001) studied the effects of prior abrasion on corrosion of titanium alloys. They observed that dissolution of the alloys was enhanced with increasing abrasion damage (Komotori *et al.*, 2001).

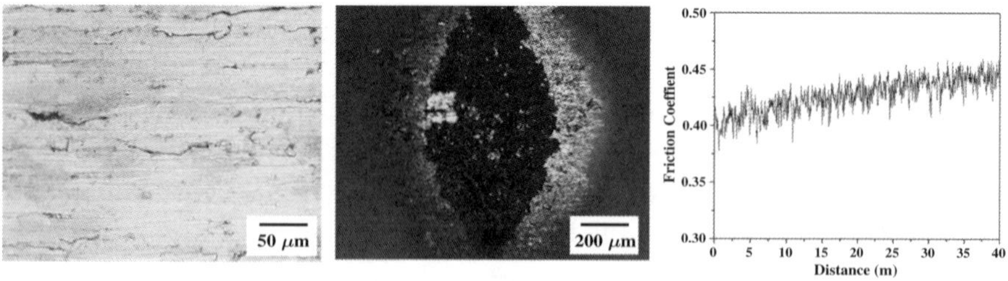

(a) (b) (c)

Figure 12-1. Contact surfaces of (a) Cp-Ti and (b) alumina ball tribocouple after sliding wear test conducted in SBF at 37°C and (c) friction trace recorded during the same wear test (Muhaffel *et al.*, 2014).

Micrographs of contact surfaces and friction trace of Cp-Ti/alumina ball tribocouple subjected to a sliding wear test in simulated body fluid (SBF) at 37°C are presented in Figure 12-1 (Muhaffel *et al.*, 2014). While severe wear was developed by the adhesion mechanism, the friction coefficient increased gradually from 0.40 to 0.45 with oscillations on the friction trace owing to the stick-slip phenomenon at the interface. Transfer of the material removed from titanium to the counterface caused darkening at the contact surface of the alumina ball. Furthermore, removal of the native oxide layer during wear tests enhances the release of alloying elements. Atar (2013) examined the wear performance of a Ti_6Al_4V alloy against an alumina ball under different contact loads in SBF. Characterization studies and spectroscopic analysis of SBF indicated generation of wear debris and release of metallic ions. When the weight ratios of the main alloying elements (Ti, Al, and V) are considered, selective dissolution of V was more prominent as compared to Ti and Al (Atar, 2013).

3. Oxidation Treatments of Titanium and its Alloys

Analysis of retrieved titanium implants and the surrounding tissue indicated formation of wear debris and release of metal ions, which gradually caused adverse tissue reactions and implant loosening, leading to inevitable revision surgery (Dearnley, 1999). Therefore, the need for better biological response of titanium-based implants eventually stimulated research aiming to enhance their corrosion-wear properties.

The poor corrosion-wear resistance of titanium alloys requires utilization of surface engineering methods to minimize generation of wear debris. Since increased surface hardness alleviates friction and develops resistance to adhesive and abrasive wear, various methods including deposition of hard coatings, ion implantation, thermochemical diffusion and oxidation treatments may be considered (Boyer *et al.*, 1994; Donachie, 1989). Hard coatings with a thickness of 3–5 μm can be coated on titanium and titanium alloys by means of chemical and physical vapor deposition processes. However, there are several limiting factors for the use of such coatings in practice. Coating may fail because of insufficient substrate adhesion and localized corrosion (Dearnley, 2005). Ion implantation of titanium by nitrogen and oxygen forms solid solutions of these elements with titanium and changes the chemical composition and properties of the surface. Despite the fact that the concentration of the implanted elements is quite low, a notable increase in surface hardness is possible. However, the hardened surface layer is relatively shallow compared to other surface modification techniques (Boyer *et al.*, 1994).

Thermochemical treatments offer the advantage of producing deeper hardened surface layers owing to thermally induced diffusion of species like carbon, nitrogen, and boron forming solid solutions at elevated temperatures. These treatments are high temperature processes that cause irreversible grain growth, resulting in low mechanical properties and are usually conducted in hydrogen-containing atmospheres. It is a matter of fact that the mechanical properties of titanium alloys are highly dependent on hydrogen contamination (Boyer *et al.*, 1994). Oxidation treatments produce mechanically stable, hard surface layers with good substrate adhesion. Oxide layers, which can be produced by means of thermal or electrolyic methods, significantly alter the surface nature and behavior of titanium. Thereby, they may provide substantial improvement in corrosion-wear performance and/or biocompatibility of titanium and its alloys.

Oxidation of metals is defined as a chemical reaction of metal with oxygen to form an oxide. In general, this reaction occurs naturally; however, it can be initiated and sustained by providing external energy which can be supplied thermally or by creating an electric field. Thermal and electrolytic oxidation treatments of titanium and its alloys produce oxide layers with very distinct characteristics which will be discussed in the following sections.

3.1. *Thermal Oxidation*

Thermal oxidation is a promising surface treatment for titanium and its alloys because of processing simplicity and enhanced resistance to wear and corrosion (Bloyce *et al.*, 1998; Boettcher *et al.*, 2002; Borgioli *et al.*, 2001; Dearnley *et al.*, 2004; Dong *et al.*, 1999; Dong and Bell, 2000; Garcia-Alonso *et al.*, 2003; Komotori *et al.*, 2001; Lopez *et al.*, 2003; Qi *et al.*, 2002; Wiklund and Hutchings, 2001). Depending on the holding time and ambient conditions, thermal oxidation carried out between the temperatures 400°C and 700°C produces a relatively thick and adherent oxide layer with an oxygen-rich diffusion zone beneath it, as presented in Figure 12-2. Diffusion of oxygen atoms

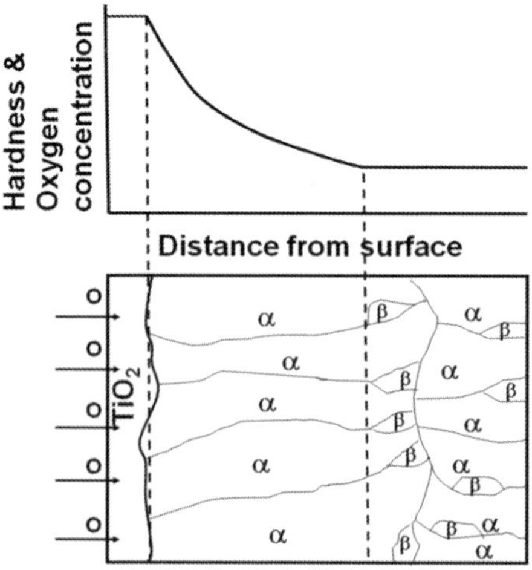

Figure 12-2. Schematic depiction showing hardness and oxygen concentration vs. depth profile and cross-sectional microstructural appearance of a titanium alloy after thermal oxidation.

beneath the oxide layer results in interstitial solid solution formation and stabilization of the α-Ti. The hardness gradually decreases from the surface to the inner regions of the metal as a result of decreasing oxygen concentration. This treatment is also named 'oxygen diffusion hardening of titanium' after innovative studies carried out at the University of Birmingham and SULZER (Dong and Bell, 2000; Dong and Li, 2000; Semlitsch *et al.*, 1992; Streicher *et al.*, 1991). It should be noted that oxidation conditions should be optimized to produce the most corrosion- and wear-resistant surface by elaborating the kinetics of oxidation and oxygen diffusion in titanium.

3.1.1. *Oxidation kinetics of titanium and its alloys*

In order to clarify the oxidation mechanism of titanium and its alloys over broad temperature range, an understanding of oxidation kinetics is required. Oxidation mechanisms of titanium alloys change both with time and temperature, and obey different kinetic rate laws (Bertrand *et al.*, 1983; Kofstad, 1988), as follows:

Logarithmic oxidation: Oxidation is initially rapid and then slows down and becomes negligible.

$$X = k\log(t + t_o). \tag{12.1}$$

Parabolic oxidation: Oxidation rate decreases with time.

$$X^2 = kt. \tag{12.2}$$

Linear oxidation: Oxidation rate is constant with time.

$$X = kt. \tag{12.3}$$

In the equations given above, X is the measured quantity during oxidation; k is rate constant of oxidation, and t is oxidation time. The logarithmic oxidation involves formation of oxide nuclei which grow together to make a continuous thin titanium oxide film below 400°C. Above 600°C simultaneous oxygen dissolution and thick oxide layer formation lead to parabolic oxidation. Between 400°C and 600°C a transition occurs between logarithmic and parabolic oxidation, where dissolution of oxygen becomes more prominent with increasing temperature. It is suggested that the parabolic oxidation of titanium is governed by the diffusion of oxygen in both the oxide and the metal core. Oxygen diffuses inwards through the compact oxide and is consumed by oxide growth and oxygen dissolution at the metal/oxide interface (Kofstad, 1988). Above 800°C, linear oxidation reflects the increased rate of oxide formation, while oxygen dissolution continues at a rate determined by the oxygen gradient and the diffusion coefficient of oxygen in the metal (Kofstad, 1988). This penetration is a result of the relative ease of interstitial diffusion (Shamblen and Redden, 1968). Diffusion of oxygen, like other interstitial solute atoms N and C, takes place by the interstitial mechanism where the solute atoms successively jump from one interstitial site to another. Experimental studies carried out by measuring weight gain during oxidation provide information for overall oxidation (oxide formation and oxygen diffusion) kinetics of titanium alloys. It has been reported that according to weight gain measurements, total oxidation kinetics obey the parabolic rate law between the temperatures 600°C and 800°C (Du *et al.*, 1994; Frangini *et al.*, 1994). In fact, oxide scale TiO_{2-y} has a very small oxygen solubility range and the value of y is approximately 0.01–0.02. On the other hand, it has been shown that the oxygen solid solution zone exhibits a steep concentration gradient which governs the parabolic oxidation kinetics of titanium (Unnam *et al.*, 1986).

Temperature dependence of oxidation rate constant (k) can be quantified by the Arrhenius equation (Kofstad, 1988):

$$k = A \exp\left(\frac{-Q_o}{RT}\right), \tag{12.4}$$

where A is the frequency factor, Q_o is the activation energy of oxidation, R is the gas constant (8.3143 J/mol), and T is the absolute oxidation temperature. Du *et al.* (1994) studied the air oxidation behavior of Ti_6Al_4V alloy in the temperature range 650–850°C by using the weight gain method and calculated Q_o as 267 kJ/mol. Also, Guleryuz and Cimenoglu (2009) utilized the weight gain method to investigate the oxidation behavior of Ti_6Al_4V alloy in air between 600°C and 700°C and reported Q_o as 276 kJ/mol. However, by using the weight gain method, Frangini *et al.* (1994) reported Q_o of Ti_6Al_4V alloy as 192 kJ/mol between 600°C and 700°C. They also determined the activation energy for oxide layer growth by measuring oxide thickness and quantified it as 147 kJ/mol (Frangini *et al.*, 1994). Unnam *et al.* (1986) investigated the oxidation of commercially pure titanium in the temperature range 593–760°C and they reported activation energy for oxide layer growth as 114 kJ/mol.

3.1.2. *Kinetics of oxygen diffusion in titanium and its alloys*

The large oxygen solubility range in the oxygen solid solution zone necessitates the utilization of an analytical solution of Fick's second law (Unnam *et al.*, 1986):

$$\frac{C - C_s}{C_o - C_s} = erf\left(\frac{z}{2\sqrt{Dt}}\right), \tag{12.5}$$

where C_s is the concentration at the metal/oxide interface, C_o is the initial concentration in the metal, C is the concentration at the distance z from surface, D is the diffusion coefficient, and t is time. Solution of Eq. 12.5 gives the diffusion coefficient of oxygen at a certain temperature, which can be used to determine the diffusion activation energy of oxygen in titanium or titanium alloys (Q_d) (Kofstad, 1988).

$$D = D_o \exp\left(\frac{-Q_d}{RT}\right). \tag{12.6}$$

In Eq. 12.6, D_o is the diffusion constant. Oxygen diffusion kinetics can be determined by various methods, including X-ray diffraction analysis, strain ageing, internal friction, and microhardness measurements (Chaze and Coddet, 1987; Kofstad, 1988). Since linear relation between the microhardness of the material and the concentration of the dissolved oxygen is established, Eq. 12.5 can be rewritten as (Gobel *et al.*, 2001):

$$\frac{H - H_s}{H_o - H_s} = erf\left(\frac{z}{2\sqrt{Dt}}\right), \tag{12.7}$$

where H is microhardness, and $H_o \, \alpha \, C_o$ and $H_s \, \alpha \, C_s$. Shamblen and Redden (1968) studied diffusion of oxygen in $Ti_6Al_2Sn_4Zr_2Mo$ alloy under normal atmospheric condition in the temperature range 300°C–900°C and reported Q_d as 202 kJ/mol after conducting calculations according to the microhardness method. Frangini *et al.* (1994) reported a similar Q_d value for oxygen diffusion in Ti_6Al_4V alloy (200.6 kJ/mol) between temperatures 600°C and 700°C. By using the micohardness method, Guleryuz and Cimenoglu (2009) calculated Q_d as 202 kJ/mol after studying the diffusion of oxygen in Ti_6Al_4V alloy in the temperature range 600–800°C.

3.1.3. *Structural interactions of titanium with oxygen*

The oxide film, which is generally a few nanometers thick, forms naturally at room temperature and protects the underlying titanium metal against further oxidation (Boyer *et al.*, 1994). A variety of different stochiometries of titanium oxides are known to cover a wide range of oxygen to titanium ratios, such as Ti_3O, Ti_2O, Ti_3O_2, TiO, Ti_2O_3, Ti_3O_5, and TiO_2. The most stable titanium oxide is TiO_2, which exists in three different crystallographic forms: Rutile and anatase with tetragonal and brookite with orthorhombic structures (Leyens and Peters, 2003). Oxidation at temperatures above 200°C significantly increases the thickness from a few nanometers to several tens of nanometers (Kofstad, 1988). At elevated temperatures, titanium may dissolve large amounts of oxygen up to 30 at. % (Gobel *et al.*, 2001; Kofstad, 1988). According to a Ti–O phase diagram, oxygen dissolves more in α-titanium than β-titanium (Massalski *et al.*, 1990). Dissolution of oxygen in β-titanium stabilizes α-titanium and shifts α to β transition to higher temperatures. In metallic crystal lattices, interstitially dissolved atoms may occupy two types of interstitial sites, which have octahedral and tetrahedral symmetry of the lattice atoms (Barrett, 1952). Octahedral sites are larger and may accommodate atoms like carbon, nitrogen, and oxygen (Kofstad, 1988). Weissmann and Shrier (1968) carried out a strain analysis study on high purity titanium by an X-ray diffraction technique after oxidation at 825°C. They suggested that ordering of oxygen atoms in the titanium lattice by filling the octahedral sites lead to asymmetrical strains on the 'c' and 'a' axis of the titanium lattice. They considered the fact that the c/a ratio of pure titanium was 3% smaller than the ideal HCP lattice. In order to accommodate the oxygen atom in the octahedral hole, the strain would be larger on the 'c' axis. This results in the increment of the c/a ratio and hardening of the titanium due to oxygen dissolution, which generates stress during oxidation (Weissman and Shrier, 1968). Also, Borgioli *et al.* (2001) reported the displacement of diffraction angles in the X-ray diffraction pattern of titanium after oxidation for a long time at high temperature and attributed this observation to the change of titanium lattice parameters.

The generation of stress in the oxide layer and underlying diffusion zone is an important issue during oxidation at high temperatures. Generally, the stress acting on the oxide layer is compressive and arises from the thermal expansion coefficient mismatch between the oxide layer and the substrate (Chatterjee *et al.*, 2001). However, more elaborate mechanisms have also been proposed for stress generation and cracking of the oxide layer at elevated temperatures (Garbacz and Lewandowska, 2003; Imbrie and Lagoudas, 2001; Kofstad, 1988; Krishnamurthy and Srolowitz, 2003):

i. Oxygen dissolution in metals: Large stresses may develop as a result of lattice expansion caused by the dissolution of interstitial oxygen atoms.
ii. Pilling–Bedworth ratio: This is the molar volume ratio of the formed oxide to consumed metal. If the Pilling–Bedworth ratio is higher than unity during inward growth of oxide, the growing oxide is constrained to occupy the volume of consumed metal. This situation contributes to the development of compressive stress.
iii. Oxide growth mechanisms: Due to outward migration of metal ions through the oxide layer, voids and cavities are formed at or near the metal/oxide interface. Hence, oxidation causes a buildup of stress in the metal/oxide interface. Also, counter diffusion of metal ion and oxygen leads to formation new oxide which produces large stress within the oxide layer.
iv. Metal orientation: In polycrystalline materials, stress may develop at grain boundaries due to the difference in oxidation rates between neighboring grains and a preferential diffusion and oxide formation along the grain boundaries.

v. Phase transformations: The transformation of one oxide to another changes the oxide layer density and generates stress in the oxidized layers.

Unless the stress is relieved, cracking of the oxide or detachment of the oxide layer from the substrate may occur. Cracking and rupture of the oxide layer increase oxidation rate (Imbrie and Lagoudas, 2001; Kofstad, 1988). Thin oxide scales may deform easily and remain adherent to the substrate. As the thickness of the oxide layer increases, it exhibits resistance to deformation. If the oxide/metal interface has a high adhesive strength relative to the cohesive strength of oxide, cracking of the oxide is observed. Poor interfacial adhesion leads to detachment of oxide layer before cracking (Chatterjee *et al.*, 2001; Kofstad, 1988).

During oxidation of titanium alloys, cracking and detachment of the oxide layer due to growth stresses is observed. Indeed, oxygen dissolution leads to large strain and stress in the metal (Weissman and Shrier, 1968). After the loss of the protective oxide layer, the rate of oxidation increases and thick oxide layer formation begins (Chatterjee *et al.*, 2001; Imbrie and Lagoudas, 2001; Kofstad, 1988; Weissman and Shrier, 1968). At high temperatures, enhanced diffusion of oxygen in the base metal accelerates thickening of the oxide layer. Guleryuz and Cimenoglu (2009) have reported that an oxide layer forming after oxidation of a Ti_6Al_4V alloy exhibited two different morphologies (dense and porous) depending on the oxidation temperature and time. A relatively thin and dense oxide layer formed in air after 60 hours oxidation at 600°C exhibited excellent adhesion to the substrate. On the other hand, a thick and porous oxide layer formed after 6 hours oxidation at 800°C had a multilayered structure with a limited attachment to the substrate (Guleryuz and Cimenoglu, 2009). According to Du *et al.* (1994), high stress developing due to the thermal expansion coefficient mismatch between the oxide layer and the substrate limits the adhesion of the thick oxide layer to the substrate. Coddet *et al.* (1987), who studied the oxidation of commercially pure titanium in the temperature range 500°C–700°C, claimed that the adhesion strength of the oxide layer was relatively high for temperatures below 650°C, while it tended to be zero at 700°C (Coddet *et al.*, 1987).

Guleryuz and Cimenoglu (2009) suggested that the deviation in the morphology of the oxide layer with respect to the oxidation temperature and time could be associated with the oxidation mechanisms mentioned in the previous sections. A dense oxide layer forms at oxidation temperatures (600°C–700°C) where parabolic oxidation kinetics is obeyed. At elevated temperatures (700°C–800°C) linear oxidation kinetics is dominant and promotes formation of a relatively thick and crumbly oxide layer exhibiting multilayered porous structure. Also, Guleryuz and Cimenoglu (2009) showed that oxidation at 700°C was critical for the oxide layer structure shifting from dense to porous. At 700°C and oxidation times shorter than 36 hours, parabolic kinetics dominates the oxidation process which forms a dense oxide layer. However, at oxidation times longer than 36 hours, linear kinetics becomes prominent and a porous oxide layer with a multilayered structure develops. Yu *et al.* (2007) also reported increasing oxidation rate after 20 hours oxidation at 700°C due to the failure of the oxide layer. Guleryuz and Cimenoglu (2009) demonstrated that the number of layers within the oxide layer tended to increase upon its growth at higher oxidation temperatures and/or longer oxidation times. According to Du *et al.* (1994), the formation of a multilayered oxide layer on the surface of Ti_6AlV alloy is due to alternating growth of Al_2O_3 and TiO_2 layers by outward diffusion of aluminum and inward diffusion of oxygen. At the early stages of oxidation, Al_2O_3 nucleates on the surface together with TiO_2. At extended oxidation times, Al_2O_3 grows laterally and covers TiO_2. In this case, the outermost section of the oxide layer (gas/oxide interface) is Al_2O_3, while the inner section of the oxide layer (oxide/substrate interface) is TiO_2. Until it reaches a critical thickness, the oxide layer maintains a good contact with the substrate. Once the critical thickness is exceeded, a crack develops at the interface. Guleryuz and Cimenoglu (2009) identified that oxidation of Ti_6Al_4V alloy at temperatures between 600°C and 800°C for exposure times of less than 72 hours is governed by the structure of the oxide layer. Parabolic oxidation provides a dense and adherent oxide layer on the substrate by maintaining a Q_o value of 276 kJ/mol. The oxidation rate fits linear kinetics above 700°C by forming a porous and crumbly oxide layer over the substrate and yields a Q_o value of 191 kJ/mol. However, diffusion of oxygen into the substrate beyond the oxide layer obeys parabolic kinetics between 600°C and 800°C by giving a Q_d value of 202 kJ/mol. Similarities arising between the activation energies of oxygen diffusion in the base metal and the linear oxidation stage imply that overall oxidation rate is determined by the oxygen diffusion in the base metal above 700°C (Guleryuz and Cimenoglu, 2009).

Cimenoglu and coworkers investigated the oxidation of Ti6Al7Nb alloy in an air-circulating furnace over a temperature range of 600–900°C for different time intervals ranging from 0.5 to 72 hours (Cimenoglu *et al.*, 2011; Unlu *et al.*, 2010). The rate of oxidation evaluated according to the weight gain measurements fitted parabolic kinetics and yielded a Q_o value of 226 kJ/mol (Unlu *et al.*, 2010). Cimenoglu and coworkers reported that Ti_6Al_7Nb alloy exhibited better oxidation resistance than Ti_6Al_4V alloy (Cimenoglu *et al.*, 2011; Guleryuz and Cimenoglu, 2009; Unlu *et al.*, 2010). In fact, vanadium and niobium were classified as detrimental and beneficial alloying elements, respectively, according to their effects on oxidation resistance of titanium alloys (Shida and Anada, 1996). The beneficial effect of niobium was correlated with the stabilization of the oxide layer as a consequence of the annihilation of anion vacancies in the crystal lattice of TiO_2 (Metikos-Hukovic *et al.*, 2003). In this respect, Jiang *et al.* (2002) reported that niobium in the solid solution of the oxide layer improves the oxidation resistance but high niobium levels may lead to a reduction in oxidation resistance by inducing formation of additional oxide phases such as $TiNb_2O_7$ or $AlNbO_4$.

3.1.4. *Thermal oxidation for achieving enhanced corrosion and wear performance*

In the light of the oxidation kinetics studies and microstructure examinations summarized above, the dense and adherent nature of an oxide layer forming below 700°C is supposedly very promising for protection against wear in corrosive environments. Intuitively, one can assume that long time exposure at 600°C provides an oxidation mechanism which prevents any alteration of dense and adherent oxide structure. In fact, it has been shown that the most corrosion-resistant surface is obtained after oxidation at 600°C. Corrosion tests carried out by measuring weight loss with respect to duration time in 5 M HCl solution indicated that the corrosion resistance of Ti_6Al_4V alloy was maximized after oxidation for 60 hours at 600°C (Guleryuz and Cimenoglu, 2004). Continuous dissolution of untreated alloy, which exhibited the lowest corrosion resistance among the investigated oxidation conditions, was sustained throughout the testing period. No measurable weight loss was observed on the Ti_6Al_4V alloys that were oxidized at 650°C for durations of 12 and 36 hrs. However, prolonged corrosion tests resulted in an abrupt increase in weight loss due to flaking and removal of the oxide scales. Fragments of oxide lost contact with the substrate and separated from the surface without dissolving in the acidic solution. For the samples oxidized at 600°C, weight loss gradually increased with increasing duration time. Longer oxidation times at 600°C formed a thicker protective surface layer, which did not show any weight loss in 36 hours of corrosion testing time. The surface of the alloy, which exhibited the maximum corrosion resistance, was still covered with an oxide layer. This indicated that very stable oxide formed on the surface of the examined Ti_6Al_4V alloy after oxidation at 600°C for 60 hours. Thick oxide layers (formed on the surfaces of the alloys oxidized at 650°C) resisted the attack of corrosive media for 36 hours without any weight loss. However, at longer testing times fragments of oxide layers detached from the surfaces allowing further corrosion progress at a rate similar to that for untreated alloy. Since the oxide layer is very effective in protecting the titanium and its alloys from the detrimental effects of corrosive media, the higher the stability of the oxide layer throughout the testing period, the better the corrosion resistance (Guleryuz and Cimenoglu, 2004). Increasing oxidation temperature accelerates the oxidation and allows formation of a thicker oxide layer and deeper oxygen diffusion zone (Guleryuz and Cimenoglu, 2009). However, flaking and detachment of the oxide layer occur as a consequence of increased oxidation rate (Guleryuz and Cimenoglu, 2009). Frangini *et al.* (1994) reported that oxidation of Ti_6Al_4V at 600°C yielded a thin, dense, and adherent oxide layer, and there was no evidence of cracking. The thickness of the oxide layer increases at a higher rate, when oxidation is conducted at 650°C (Guleryuz and Cimenoglu, 2004). This situation affirms the role of temperature on oxidation rate by activating diffusing species. However, accelerated oxidation due to increasing temperature may put the whole oxide layer in a more stressed condition as a result of intrinsic and thermal effects (Coddet *et al.*, 1987; Schütze, 1992). The formation of a defective oxide structure provides easy diffusion paths for oxygen and metal ions allowing oxidation progress in an uncontrollable way. Since the corrosion resistance of thermally oxidized surface layers relies on their chemical stability and defect-free structure, this observation may also be valid for explaining the corrosion behavior of oxidized samples because strong reducing acids would not dissolve a heavy oxide layer on titanium (Baboian, 1995). Small structural defects (microcracks and micropores) may be responsible for the failure of oxidized surfaces (Bloyce *et al.*, 1998). During the incubation period, aggressive ions penetrate towards the oxide/metal interface and steadily extend, undermining the oxide because of the galvanic coupling of the oxide and substrate metal. Oxide layers gradually detach from the surface as fragments. This observation points out the fact that corrosive solution enters the interface through individual defects. As soon as the oxide fragments lose their contact with the substrate, they detach. Guleryuz and Cimenoglu (2004) reported that the corrosion behavior of the alloys that were oxidized for short times at 600°C differed from alloys oxidized for a long time (Guleryuz and Cimenoglu, 2004). The relatively thin oxide layer that covered these alloys was a mixture of anatase and rutile. Anatase was readily attacked and dissolved in reducing acids whereas rutile was inert and resistant to attack (Boyer *et al.*, 1994; Bloyce *et al.*, 1998). Dissolution of anatase at the beginning of the corrosion test left some sites of oxidized samples unprotected and further corrosion continued with total removal of the oxide layer. Increasing oxidation time yielded a higher amount of rutile in the oxidized surface, which increased the protective nature of the oxide layer against the corrosive environment. Less defective structures of oxide containing more rutile formed at

600°C after longer oxidation times. This combination presented the most corrosion-resistant oxide layer that formed on Ti_6Al_4V alloy (Guleryuz and Cimenoglu, 2004).

The dry sliding reciprocating wear tests conducted by rubbing Al_2O_3 balls on the surfaces of untreated and oxidized Ti_6Al_4V alloys indicated the beneficial effect of oxidation on wear resistance (Guleryuz and Cimenoglu, 2005). On the untreated surface, formation of a wide and deep wear track was accompanied by the creation of a large amount of wear debris. Rough shear deformation features aligned to the direction of sliding, and the untreated surface was steadily worn off by shear delaminating and smearing. However, there were only minute traces of wear track on the oxidized surface even after a testing time of 300 min. On the oxidized surface, wear progressed by deformation and removal of the asperities and some local breakdown and flaking of the oxide layer. Thermal oxidation treatment conducted at 600°C for 60 hours totally suppressed the extensive wear of the Ti_6Al_4V alloy under normal atmospheric condition (Guleryuz and Cimenoglu, 2005). However, corrosion-wear tests carried out in a mild corrosive media indicated the detrimental effects of corrosion on the wear resistance of the alloy oxidized at 600°C for 60 hours (Guleryuz and Cimenoglu, 2004). Nevertheless, this oxidation condition achieved 25 times higher wear resistance than the untreated alloy during a reciprocating wear test conducted in a 0.9% NaCl solution. A typical feature of the wear tracks produced on untreated surfaces was extensive shear deformation due to the plowing action of the Al_2O_3 ball. The wear tracks on the oxidized surface were smooth and contained microcracks with traces of local material removal. Thus, on the oxidized surface wear was initiated by disruption of the oxide layer followed by the corrosion and wear of the oxygen diffusion zone, which was locally removed by cracking at extended testing times. The Al_2O_3 balls were also subjected to wear during testing (Guleryuz and Cimenoglu, 2004). Extensive wear of the ball sliding on untreated surface progressed by a grain pull-out mechanism (Dearnley *et al.*, 2004). The topography of the wear scar that developed on the ball that slid on the oxidized surface was almost similar to that of the untreated surface but smaller by a factor of 16. Thus, the size of the wear scar was proportional to the size of the wear track formed on the surface of the material being tested (Guleryuz and Cimenoglu, 2004).

Corrosion-wear test results confirm the superiority of the thermally oxidized Ti_6Al_4V alloy over untreated alloy (Guleryuz and Cimenoglu, 2004, 2005). Surface degradation of untreated alloy commences with the onset of sliding action and a large amount of wear debris is produced through the entire test duration. On the oxidized surface, the oxide layer prevents the wear of Ti_6Al_4V alloy over a certain period of testing time. The removal of the oxide layer and diffusion hardened zone occurs due to mechanical and chemical effects. Even though the oxidized (at 600°C for 60 hours) surface exhibits the best corrosion resistance in HCl solution with its less defective structure, it is subjected to mechanical stresses during corrosion-wear test. This situation causes the local breakdown of the oxide layer and allows the corrosive solution to enter the oxide/oxygen diffusion zone interface. The oxide layer is gradually removed by the combined action of corrosion and wear together. Eventually, corrosion-wear continues on the oxygen diffusion zone by producing a smaller amount of wear debris. After extended testing times, cracking of the oxygen diffusion zone causes local material removal, and thereafter the depth of the wear track reaches the substrate. When the Al_2O_3 ball comes into contact with the substrate, it is subjected to wear with the mechanism (grain pull-out), which is observed during testing of the untreated surface. Apparently, the wear mechanism of an Al_2O_3 ball on an untreated surface is maintained on oxidized surface when the depth of the wear track reaches the substrate. Grain pull-out wear mechanism is inevitable when the adhesion stresses between the sliding surfaces tend to be greater than the cohesive strength of the materials (Dearnley *et al.*, 2004).

Cimenoglu *et al.* (2011) investigated the wear resistance of untreated and thermally oxidized Ti_6Al_7Nb alloys by conducting reciprocating wear tests in SBF solutions. The worn surface of the untreated alloy exhibited characteristic features of severe wear. However, there was no evidence of plastic deformation on the worn surface of the thermally oxidized alloy with the exception of some shallow grooves. Thermally oxidized alloy exhibited a more than ten-fold increase in wear resistance compared to the untreated sample. The results of the wear tests conducted in SBF solution confirmed the superiority of the thermal oxidation process (oxidation in air at 600°C for 60 hours) providing a wear resistant surface on a Ti_6Al_7Nb alloy similar to that of a Ti_6Al_4V alloy (Cimenoglu *et al.*, 2011).

Streicher *et al.* (1991) studied the effect of oxygen diffusion hardening (ODH) treatment (conducted by means of thermal oxidation) on corrosion, wear, and fatigue performance of Ti_6Al_7Nb alloy. They reported that the wear factor and the coefficient of friction of ultra-high molecular weight polyethylene (UHMWPE) rubbing against the ODH-treated surface are reduced to half of that for the reference CoCrMo alloy. The corrosion resistance of the ODH-treated titanium alloy was equal to Cp titanium and the untreated Ti_6Al_7Nb alloy. The fatigue resistance of the ODH-treated wrought and forged titanium alloy was higher than for the same components made from a $Co_{28}Cr_6Mo$ cast alloy which had never suffered a clinical failure until then (Streicher *et al.*, 1991). ODH-treated Ti_6Al_7Nb alloy became available for clinical use in femoral knee components and clinical studies involving femoral heads for hip prostheses started in 1992 (Semlitsch *et al.*, 1995). To the authors' knowledge, the outcomes of these clinical studies were not reported.

3.1.5. *Tensile and fatigue performances of thermally oxidized titanium alloys*

As a matter of fact, surface modification by thermal oxidation treatment not only changes the tribological performance, but also alters the tensile and fatigue properties of the titanium alloys (Cingi *et al.*, 2007). Cingi *et al.* (2007) reported that thermal oxidation treatment conducted at 600°C for 60 hours considerably increased the yield strength of Ti_6Al_4V alloy. Tensile strength was also improved by a factor of 10% after oxidation treatment. They also carried out rotating bending fatigue tests in order to evaluate the effect of thermal oxidation on the fatigue strength of Ti_6Al_4V alloy. In terms of the relationship between fracture stress and number of cycles to failure, thermal oxidation treatment reduced the number of cycles to failure and affected the fatigue strength detrimentally. Particularly at a number of cycles to failure less than 10^5, fracture stress of the oxidized alloy decreased sharply. The rotating bending fatigue strength at 5×10^6 cycles of untreatedalloy was about 610 MPa, while it was about 400 MPa for the oxidized alloy. Thus, thermal oxidation caused a reduction in the fatigue strength of around 34%. Similarly, Li *et al.* (2007) reported a 24% decrease in fatigue strength of a Ti_6Al_4V alloy. Cingi *et al.* (2007) also showed that fracture surfaces of the untreated and oxidized alloys comprised distinct features. For both of the oxidized and untreated alloys, it was clearly seen that cracks initiated at the surface led to the final fracture after propagation to the inner sections. However, the number of crack initiation sites at the surface of the untreated alloy seemed to be less compared to that of the oxidized alloy. Therefore, it was suggested that a hard oxidized layer at the surface and the oxygen diffusion zone beneath it encouraged easy crack initiation, which resulted in the appearance of a relatively large final fracture region. The larger final fracture region of the oxidized alloy indicated that most of the fatigue life is spent for crack initiation. Once the crack is formed at the surface, it easily propagated to the inner sections and fracture took place rapidly by leaving a large final crack region at the center. Leinenbach and Eifler (2006) studied the fatigue behavior of Ti_6Al_7Nb alloy in an oxygen-saturated Ringer's solution and reported a loss in fatigue strength after thermal oxidation conducted at 675°C for 3 hours. Cingi (2008) showed that reduction in the fatigue strength of Ti_6Al_7Nb alloy was less than that of Ti_6Al_4V alloy after thermal oxidation treatment conducted under identical conditions. This was advocated by the better oxidation resistance of Ti_6Al_7Nb alloy (Cimenoglu *et al.*, 2011).

3.1.6. *Biocompatibility of thermally oxidized titanium alloys*

Besides corrosion-wear resistance, biological response is another issue that has to be taken into consideration because it has a crucial importance on long term bone/implant interface stability and the functional performance of the implants. There are a limited number of reports focusing on the biological response of titanium-based materials after the thermal oxidation process (Cimenoglu *et al.*, 2011; Garcia-Alonso *et al.*, 2003; Hwang *et al.*, 2002; Park *et al.*, 2007, Vanzillotta *et al.*, 2006; Wang *et al.*, 2003). Cimenoglu *et al.* (2011) evaluated the biocompatibility of the thermally oxidized Ti_6Al_7Nb alloy (at 600°C for 60 hours) by immersing it in SBF and conducting cell culture tests. Immersion tests were carried out by soaking the samples in the SBF solution for 30 days at 37°C. The SBF solution was continuously stirred with a mixer running at 80 rpm throughout the testing period. Immersion of the thermally oxidized alloys in SBF solution for 30 days produced randomly distributed, white-colored, micrometer-sized precipitates which were detected during electron microscope examination of the surface. Chemical analysis conducted on the precipitates indicated that they were composed of Ca and P. Such Ca- and P-rich precipitates were not observed on the surface of the untreated alloy soaked in the SBF. The precipitates detected on the thermally oxidized surface exhibited the characteristic flake-like morphology of hydroxyapatite with a Ca:P ratio slightly higher than 1.67. A relatively rough oxide layer favored deposition of Ca- and P-rich precipitates in the SBF solution as the primary signal of bioactivity. The results of the SBF immersion tests suggested that an oxide layer formed by the thermal oxidation process had better bioactivity compared to the surface of the untreated alloy (Cimenoglu *et al.*, 2011). Cimenoglu *et al.* (2011) also monitored cell viability/proliferation capability, alkaline phosphates, and collagen production by the cells in the presence of the untreated and thermally oxidized Ti_6Al_7Nb alloys. The results of the cell culture studies revealed that the rough oxide layer formed on the thermally oxidized alloy, which provided favorable sites for deposition of hydroxyapatite precipitates during SBF immersion tests, is a better environment for cell integration than the relatively smooth surface of the untreated alloy. Biocompatibility tests (SBF immersion and cell culture tests) indicated the promising potential of the thermal oxidation process for orthopedic implants manufactured from the Ti_6Al_7Nb alloy (Cimenoglu *et al.*, 2011).

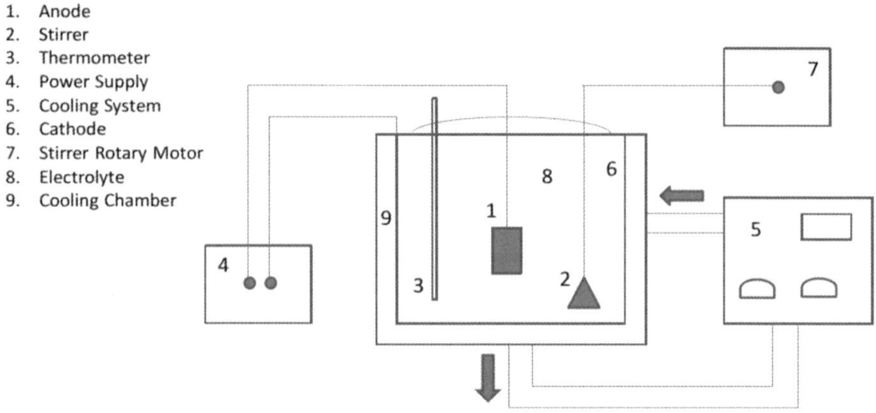

Figure 12-3. Schematic of an electrochemical cell.

3.2. *Electrolytic Oxidation Processes*

Titanium and its alloys can also be oxidized by electrochemical techniques. These techniques are based on the application of an electrical potential difference between an anode and a cathode that are immersed in an aqueous solution (electrolyte) providing cations and anions to form an oxide layer on the anode surface (Schreckenbach and Graf, 2008; Sul *et al.*, 2002). The electrolytic oxidation process is carried out in an electrochemical cell presented schematically in Figure 12-3. An electrochemical cell mainly consists of an anode, a cathode, a power supply, and an electrolyte (Li and Zhao, 2009). A titanium oxide layer with a thickness ranging from a few nanometers to hundreds of micrometers can be grown on titanium and its alloys by electrolytic oxidation processes. The nature of the oxide layer strongly depends on the level of the applied voltage, current density, and electrolyte composition (Liu *et al.*, 2004; Sul *et al.*, 2002). For a successful oxidation process, the temperature of the electrolyte should be kept relatively low. For this purpose, a thermometer and a cooling system with a cooling chamber is attached to the electrochemical cell shown in Figure 12-3. During the oxidation process, the electrolyte is continuously stirred in order to achieve a homogeneous oxide layer.

3.2.1. *Anodic oxidation*

Conventionally, an electrolytic oxidation process carried out at voltages lower than 100 V in an acidic electrolyte (H_2SO_4, H_3PO_4, acetic acid, and others) is referred to as 'anodic oxidation'. The most important advantages offered by anodic oxidation for titanium based implants are (Liu *et al.*, 2004):

i. Strong adhesion at the oxide/substrate interface, which is free of discontinuities.
ii. Better wear and corrosion performance.
iii. Minimized release of alloying elements into the body fluid.
iv. Permanent color coding of implants.

Although anodic oxidation of titanium has been investigated extensively, studies reporting the tribological performance of the oxidized surfaces have remained scarce. Games *et al.* (2012) carried out anodic oxidation of Cp-titanium in ammonium phosphate and ammonium fluoride solutions at 20–30 V for 60 min and conducted nanoscratch tests after treatment. Nanoscratch tests showed a very ductile behavior and good adhesion of the oxide layers, without any apparent signs of cracks or delamination. Besides, hardness of the bare substrate was improved with the formation of oxide layers, which also increased the corrosion resistance (Games *et al.*, 2012). Kumar *et al.* (2010) reported that surface modification by anodic oxidation at 20 V for 60 min in an electrolyte solution of 1 M H3PO4 containing 0.3 wt% HF provided improvement in the fretting wear performance of Cp-titanium in a corrosive medium. Chen *et al.* (2013) carried out anodic oxidation of Ti_6Al_4V alloy at 20 V for 20 min in a mixture of sodium hydroxide and sodium silicate electrolyte containing aminopropyl trimethoxysilane. The wear resistance was improved with the addition of aminopropyl trimethoxysilane due to its toughening effects and serving as lubricants in the oxide layers as measured by a ball-on-disk friction test (Chen *et al.*, 2013).

When the crucial role of the surface on the biological performance of an implant is a matter of concern, anodic oxidation appears to be an attractive surface modification technique compared to other mechanical and chemical methods (such as sandblasting and acid etching, respectively) and thermal oxidation processes. The superior biological performance provided by anodic oxidation is generally attributed to mechanical interlocking and biochemical fixation maintained by a titanium oxide layer with desired roughness, porosity, and composition (Geetha *et al.*, 2009). The porous nature of the oxide layer provides mechanical interlocking and better osseointegration when the bone cells grow into the pores of the oxide layer (Yao *et al.*, 2010). Incorporation of biologically important constituents (such as calcium- and phosphorous-containing chemicals added to the electrolyte) in the composition of the oxide layer induce much better bonding with the surrounding tissues. In fact, calcium and phosphorous tend to form biocompatible compounds (such as hydroxyapatite, calcium phosphate, and calcium titanate) which precipitate within the titanium oxide layer to provide rapid biochemical fixation (Gao *et al.*, 2009).

Since the growth rate of the oxide layer is determined by the formation and dissolution of the oxide during the anodic oxidation process, it is possible to alter the thickness, phase structure (amorphous to crystalline), and the morphology of the oxide layer (nano- to microporous) by precisely controlling the process parameters including applied voltage, current density, and electrolyte composition (Bayati *et al.*, 2010). Utilization of strong acids (chromic acid, hydrofluoric acid, etc.) in the electrolyte promotes formation of a nanoporous (nanotubular) titanium oxide layer which may be very beneficial for biomedical applications. A nanoporous titanium oxide layer may provide antibacterial activity by reducing the adhesion of bacteria and better integration with the surrounding cells and proteins (Liu *et al.*, 2004). In Figure 12-4, a scanning electron microscope (SEM) image of a thin (in nanometer range), nanoporous and amorphous titanium oxide layer generated on Cp-titanium at 10 V is presented. The diameter of the pores observed in Figure 12-4 is around 50 nm. It should be noted that an annealing treatment is required to crystallize this nanoporous titanium oxide layer. At low annealing temperatures, anatase and rutile structures of titanium oxide forms in the oxide layer. However, at annealing temperatures higher than 600°C the anatase structure becomes prominent (Ozturk and Baydogan, 2012).

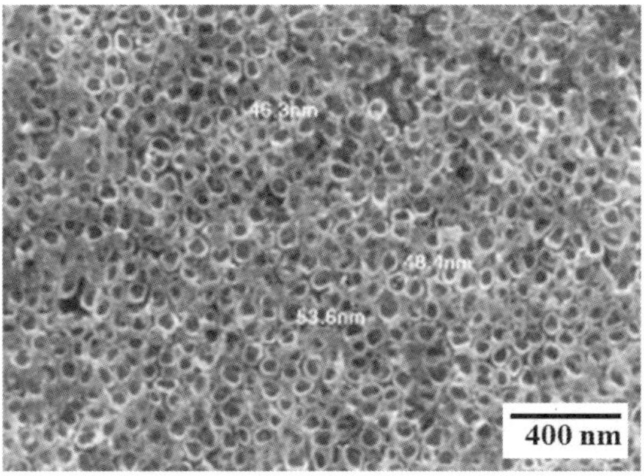

Figure 12-4. SEM micrograph of a nanoporous titanium oxide layer formed on Cp-titanium at 10 V (Ozturk and Baydogan, 2012).

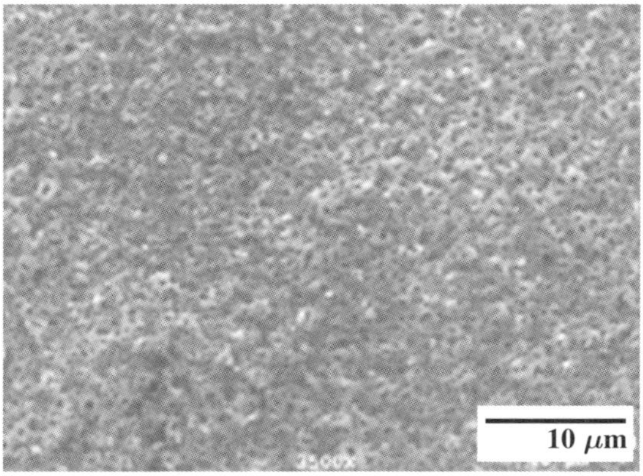

Figure 12-5. SEM micrograph of titanium oxide layer formed on Cp-titanium at 150 V (Cimenoglu, 2008).

3.2.2. *Micro-arc oxidation*

Electrolytic oxidation at higher voltages (>100 V) and current densities (>200 A/m^2) produces microporous and thicker (in micrometer range) titanium oxide layers. Such an oxide layer produced on Cp-titanium at 150 V is presented in Figure 12-5. Further increase of voltage combines anodic oxidation with a high-voltage anodic spark deposition treatment, which is named 'plasma electrolytic oxidation' or 'micro-arc oxidation' (MAO) in the literature. These plasma evolutions increase surface temperature and pressure up to 10,000 K and 1,000 MPa, respectively. It should be noted that the electrolytes of the MAO process are non-toxic and environmentally benign, in contrast to the anodic oxidation process (Shen *et al.*, 2009). When the applied voltage exceeds a critical value (i.e. 200 V) during the MAO process, microplasma discharge occurs on the surface of the substrate, resulting in a microporous, rough, strictly adherent, thick (up to 200 μm), crystalline (anatase and/or rutile) titanium oxide layer (Yerokhin *et al.*, 1999).

Tribological studies showed that oxide layers formed on Ti_6Al_4V alloy by MAO can change the wear mechanisms from adhesive/abrasive to an asperity deformation one. Oxide layers produced in a phosphate solution can drastically reduce the unlubricated friction coefficient against steel from 0.6 to 0.2. Hard and thick oxide layers formed in an aluminate/phosphate electrolyte provided the minimum wear rate; however, the friction coefficient remained in the range 0.6–0.7 due to material transfer from the steel counterface to the oxidized surface (Yerokhin *et al.*, 2000). Lin *et al.* (2010) reported that MAO treatment alleviated fretting wear of Ti_6Al_4V alloy and the friction coefficient of the oxidized alloy was lower than that of the untreated alloy due to the hard oxidized surface preventing the plastic deformation of the alloy. Khorasanian *et al.* (2011) carried out MAO treatment of Ti_6Al_4V alloy in an electrolyte containing starch. The presence of starch in the electrolyte formed a thick gel layer beyond the gaseous film around the anode, which helped the gas film to be stable. Therefore, the plasma envelope around the anode was more stable and uniform. The surface and cross-sectional morphology of the coatings had a very dense structure with no significant crack or porosity. The friction coefficient and the weight loss of the MAO-treated material were very low compared with the untreated alloy (Khorasanian *et al.*, 2011). Cheng *et al.* (2013) reported that the oxide layer surface morphology and thickness could be manipulated by controlling the MAO process parameters such as starting current density. They showed that the oxidized surfaces with large pores and high roughness would lead to a higher friction coefficient. On the other hand, a smooth and uniform oxide surface reduced the friction coefficient and led to a better performance during the wear tests. It was emphasized that the SBF solution used during the wear tests reduced the friction coefficient for the relatively smooth and porous surface but an obvious lubricating effect was not shown for highly porous and rough surfaces at the tested boundary-lubricating conditions under a high load (Cheng *et al.*, 2013). Durdu and Usta (2014) showed that MAO treatment time could affect the tribological performance of the oxidized Ti_6Al_4V alloy. The wear resistance of alloy treated for 60 min was higher than alloy treated for 90 min. They pointed to the fact that the oxide layer produced at 90 min was much more porous and looser than the one produced at 60 min (Durdu and Usta, 2014). Chen *et al.* (2013) indicated that the roughness of the oxide layers had a very significant effect on the sliding wear behavior of the MAO-treated Ti_6Al_4V alloy. They stated that the high surface roughness of the oxide would result in no advantage other than increasing the coating thickness. In fact, the rough surface caused early failure and a large mass loss on the counterface material (Chen *et al.*, 2013). More recently, Muhaffel *et al.* (2014) reported that incorporation of zirconia particles into the microporous titania layer increases its wear resistance by 20%. Zirconia particles were introduced into the titania layer by conducting MAO in an electrolyte containing zirconia particles. In Figure 12-6, micrographs of contact surfaces of the titania layers and counterface (alumina ball) after sliding wear testing in SBF at 37°C are presented. Although wear developed by local delamination on the titania layers, material transfer to the contact surface of the alumina ball was not evident in contrast to the unoxidized surface (Figure 12-1). Zirconia particles present in the titania layer provided extra resistance against delamination and therefore enhanced the wear resistance of the titania layer.

Rough and porous surfaces produced after MAO treatment may have a beneficial contribution to the biocompatibility of titanium and its alloys. In Figure 12-7, the topography and composition of the titanium oxide layer formed on Cp-titanium by MAO at 400 V are shown (Cimenoglu, 2013). Micropores are around 2 μm in diameter and evenly distributed in the oxide layer. Energy dispersive

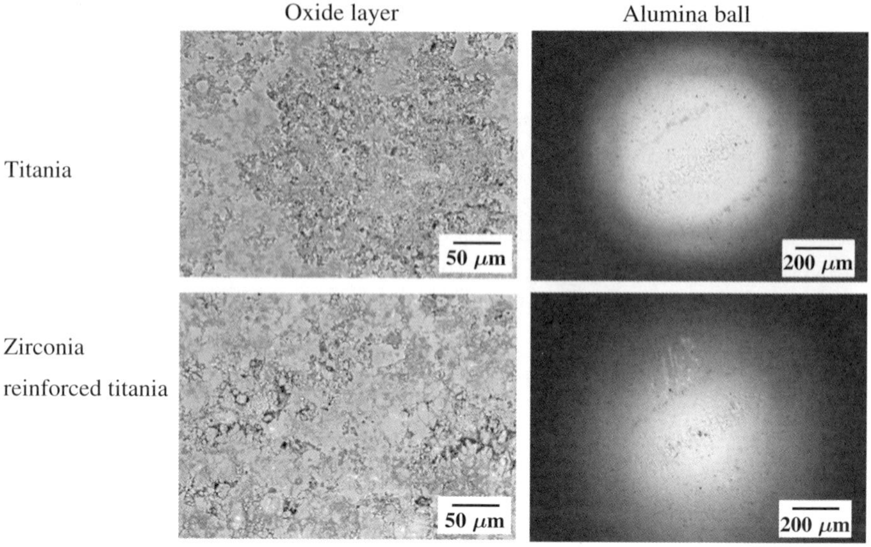

Figure 12-6. Micrographs of contact surfaces of oxide layers produced by MAO on Cp-Ti and the counterface (alumina ball) after sliding wear tests conducted in SBF at 37°C (Muhaffel *et al.*, 2014).

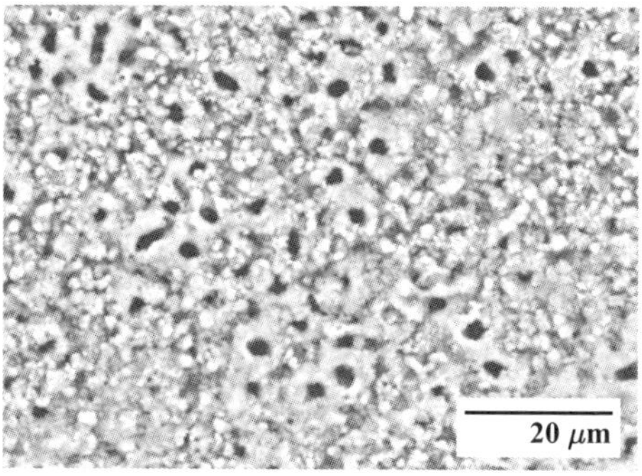

(a)

Elements	(wt%)
P	16.9
Ca	62.9
Ti	20
Ag	2.2

(b)

Figure 12-7. (a) SEM micrograph, and (b) chemical composition of the titanium oxide layer produced on Cp-titanium at 380 V (Cimenoglu, 2013).

spectroscopy (EDS) analyses revealed incorporation of biologically important (calcium and phosphorous) and antibacterial (silver) constituents of the electrolyte into the titanium oxide layer. As a result of calcium and phosphorous incorporation, biocompatible compounds

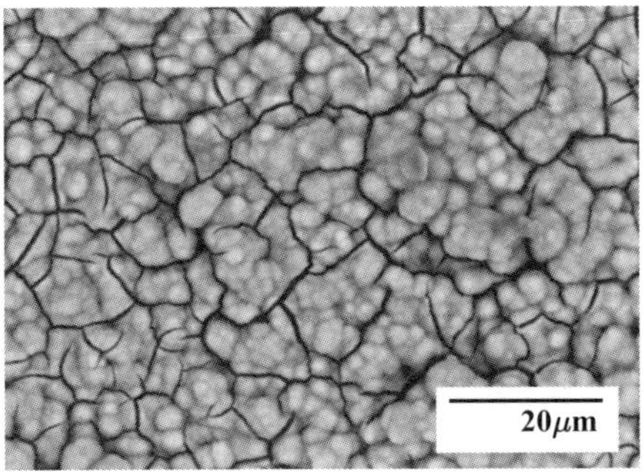

(a)

Elements	(wt%)
P	16
Ca	75.1
Ti	0.8
Ag	0.7

(b)

Figure 12-8. (a) SEM micrograph, and (b) chemical composition of the titanium oxide layer shown in Figure 12-5 after immersion in SBF for 24 hours (Cimenoglu, 2013).

(hydroxyapatite and calcium titanate) formed within the titanium oxide layer. As can be seen in Figure 12-8, this oxide layer was fully covered with hydroxyapatite after immersion in SBF for 24 hours. This is a good indicator of enhanced bioactivity.

The presence of 2% silver along with these biocompatible compounds provided superior antimicrobial effect by preserving the bioactivity of the oxide layer. The interaction of silver ions with thiol groups plays a crucial role in blocking the bacteria proliferation. It should be noted that the microporous nature of the titanium oxide layer can provide further improvement in antimicrobial activity when the pores are filled with wide spectrum antibiotics. Antimicrobial tests revealed that release of antibiotics reduced bacterial activity remarkably against Escherichia coli (Aral *et al.*, 2012).

In vivo tests conducted on New Zealand rabbits confirmed the outstanding contribution of the MAO process on the biocompatibility of titanium-based implants (Cimenoglu, 2008). Histology studies conducted on the surfaces of the screws implanted in the jaw bones of New Zealand rabbits are depicted in Figure 12-9. Histological characteristics were quite different for MAO-treated (Figure 12-9b) and original implant (Figure 12-9a) after eight weeks of implantation. Histological findings showed that mature lamellar bone (blue stained area) grew extensively on the MAO treated screw. Hence,

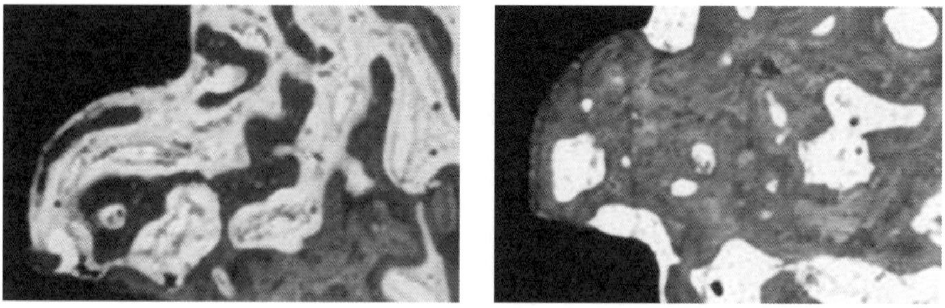

(a) (b)

Figure 12-9. Histological images of (a) untreated and (b) MAO treated Ti_6Al_4V screw surfaces after eight weeks of implantation in a rabbit jaw bone (Cimenoglu, 2008).

after the MAO process, better bone formation and bone ingrowth was achieved. In contrast to the original surface, the titanium oxide layer produced by the MAO process induced rapid healing after surgery.

Cimenoglu *et al.* (2011) compared *in vitro* biological responses of two competitive titanium alloys (Ti_6Al_4V and Ti_6Al_7Nb) after MAO in $(CH_3COO)_2Ca{\cdot}H_2O$ and Na_3PO_4 containing electrolyte at 500 V for 5 min and reported generation of biocompatible titanium oxide layers with different characteristics. The oxide layer of the Ti_6Al_4V alloy was microporous and contained hydroxyapatite precipitates whereas the oxide layer of the Ti_6Al_7Nb alloy showed a more grainy appearance and contained calcium titanate precipitates. Although the oxidized alloys exhibited similar bioactivity during SBF tests, SAOS-2 cells displayed a higher rate of attachment on the oxide layer of the Ti_6Al_4V alloy than that of the Ti_6Al_7Nb alloy. However, it should be noted that there is a possibility of Ti_6Al_7Nb alloy obtaining a titanium oxide layer exhibiting similar characteristics with that of Ti_6Al_4V alloy by adjusting the MAO process parameters.

4. Conclusion

In this chapter, various oxidation treatments used for modifying surfaces of biomedical grade titanium and its alloys have been discussed. These are thermal oxidation, anodic oxidation, and MAO treatments, which have been developed enough to be applied in biomedical practices. However, more research focusing on the *in vivo* performance of the oxidized titanium surfaces must be carried out.

Electrolytic oxidation processes (anodic oxidation and MAO) can produce a porous oxide structure for promoting biomineralization, cell attachment, and cell growth. As compared to anodic oxidation, MAO offers excellent biocompatibility and induces better bioactivity for titanium implant surfaces. Antibacterial and antimicrobial properties can be achieved by using novel electrolyte formulations during the MAO process and/or by post-processing treatments. Corrosion-wear resistance can also be improved by applying MAO but thermal oxidation seems to be more promising due to the formation of a dense and adherent oxide layer which is supported by an oxygen diffusion zone. Such an oxide layer and diffusion zone elevate surface hardness of the titanium implants and provide gradual hardness transition between the surface and the bulk of the implant. Therefore, after the failure of the oxide layer, a relatively hard diffusion zone protects titanium from the catastrophic corrosion-wear stage which necessitates immediate revision of the implant. The thermally oxidized titanium surface exhibits better biocompatibility and bioactivity than an untreated titanium surface but thermal oxidation treatment diminishes the fatigue strength of titanium. Nevertheless, thermal oxidation parameters can be optimized for relevant titanium alloys to achieve better fatigue strength and corrosion-wear resistance after oxidation.

The performance of oxidized titanium alloys which will be used for orthopedic bearing surfaces can be enhanced profoundly by developing an appropriate oxidation procedure that will increase wear resistance and lower the coefficient of friction between the mating surfaces. Hence, it is suggested that in future greater focus should be placed on the areas of development of hard oxidized surface with low roughness in order to mitigate the abrasive wear of the counterface material. In addition, tailoring the surface chemistry of the oxide layer may improve the lubrication characteristics and be beneficial for decreasing the coefficient of friction between sliding surfaces.

Acknowledgments

As the contributing author of this chapter, Hüseyin Çimenoğlu expresses his gratitude for the financial support of The Turkish Scientific and Technological Research Council (TUBITAK) through the projects 105M062 and 111M517.

References

Aral, A., Gunyuz, M., Baydogan, M., Karaguler, N.G., Olcay, E. and Cimenoglu, H. (2012). Anti-bacterial microporous ceramic coating for Ti6Al4V alloys, *Key Eng Mat*, **493–494**, 916–919.

Atar, E. (2013). A study on wear testing of orthopedic implant materials in simulated body fluid, *Mater Test*, **55**, 103–108.

Baboian, R. (1995). *Corrosion Tests and Standards: Application and Interpretation*, ASTM, Philadelphia.

Barrett, C.S. (1952). *Structure of Metals. Crystallographic Methods, Principles, and Data*, McGraw Hill, New York.

Bayati, M.R., Zargar, H., Molaei, R., Golestani-Fard, F., Kajbafvala, E. and Zanganeh, S. (2010). One step growth of WO_3-loaded Al_2O_3 micro/nano-porous films by micro arc oxidation,*Colloid Surface A*, **355**, 187–192.

Bertrand, G., Jarraya, K. and Chaix, J.M. (1983). Morphology of oxide scales formed on titanium, *Oxid Met*, **21**, 1–19.

Bhushan, B. (2013). *Principles and applications of tribology*, John Wiley and Sons, New York.

Bloyce, A., Qi, P.-Y., Dong, H. and Bell, T. (1998). Surface modification of titanium alloys for combined improvements in corrosion and wear resistance, *Surf Coat Tech*, **107**, 125–132.

Boettcher, C., Bell, T. and Dong, H. (2002). Surface engineering of Timet 550 with oxygen to form a rutile-based, wear resistant coating, *Metall Mater Trans A*, **33**, 1201–1211.

Borgioli, F., Galvanetto, E., Galliano, F.P. and Bacci, T. (2001). Air treatment of pure titanium by furnace and glow-discharge processes, *Surf Coat Tech*, **141**, 103–107.

Boyer, R., Welsch, G. and Collings, E.W. (1994). *Materials properties handbook: Titanium alloys*, ASM International, Ohio.

Brunette, D.M., Tengwall, B., Textor, M. and Thomsen, P. (2001). *Titanium in medicine*, Springer, Heidelberg.

Buckley, D.H. (1981) *Surface effects in adhesion, friction, wear, and lubrication*, Elsevier, Amsterdam.

Buckley, D.H. and Miyoshi, K. (1984). Friction and wear of ceramics, *Wear*, **100**, 333–353

Chatterjee, U.K., Bose, S.K. and Roy, S.K. (2001). *Environmental degradation of metals*, Marcel Dekker, New York.

Chaze, A.M. and Coddet, C. (1987). Influence of alloying elements on the dissolution of oxygen in the metallic phase during the oxidation of titanium alloys, *J Mater Sci*, **22**, 1206–1214.

Chen, J., Wang, J. and Yuan, H. (2013). Morphology and performances of the anodic oxide films on Ti6Al4V alloy formed in alkaline-silicate electrolyte with aminopropyl silane addition under low potential, *Appl Surf Sci*, **284**, 900–906.

Chen, Y., Cheng, T. and Nie, X. (2013). Wear failure behaviour of titanium-based oxide coatings on a titanium alloy under impact and sliding forces, *J Alloy Comp*, **578**, 336–344.

Cheng, T., Chen, Y. and Nie, X. (2013). Surface morphology manipulation and wear property of bioceramic oxide coatings on titanium alloy, *Surf Coat Tech*, **215**, 253–259.

Cimenoglu, H. (2008). *Advanced surface modification of titanium and its alloys used as implant materials: Investigation of cost effective production of high quality implants*, Turkish Scientific and Technological Research Council (TUBITAK), Project Nr: 105M062.

Cimenoglu, H. (2013). *Deposition of bioactive, antibacterial and micrro-porous oxide layer on titanium and its alloys for biomedical applications*, Turkish Scientific and Technological Research Council (TUBITAK), Project Nr: 111M517.

Cimenoglu, H., Gunyuz, M., Kose, G.T., Baydogan, M., Ugurlu, F. and Sener, C. (2011). Micro-arc oxidation of Ti6Al4V and Ti6Al7Nb alloys for biomedical applications, *Mater Char*, **62**, 304–311.

Cimenoglu, H., Meydanoglu, O., Baydogan, M., Bermek, H., Huner, P. and Kayali, E.S. (2011). Characterization of thermally oxidized Ti6Al7Nb alloy for biological applications, *Met Mater Int*, **17**, 765–770.

Cingi, M. (2008). *Investigation of the effect of oxidation on the fatigue strength of titanium and its alloys*, PhD thesis, Istanbul Technical University, Istanbul.

Cingi, M., Meydanoglu, O., Güleryüz, H., Baydogan, M., Çimenoğlu, H. and Kayali, E.S. (2007). High cycle fatigue behavior of thermally oxidized Ti6Al4V alloy, *Mater Sci Forum*, **561–565**, 2179–2182.

Coddet, C., Chaze, A.M. and Beranger, G. (1987). Measurement of the adhesion of thermal oxide films: Application to the oxidation of titanium, *J Mater Sci*, **22**, 2969–2974.

Dearnley, P.A. (1999). A review of metallic, ceramic and surface-treated metals used for bearing surfaces in human joint replacements, *Proc Inst Mech Eng H*, **213**, 107–135.

Dearnley, P.A. (2005). A brief review of test methodologies for surface-engineered biomedical implant alloys, *Surf Coat Tech*, **198**, 483–490.

Dearnley, P.A., Dahm, K.L. and Cimenoglu, H. (2004). The corrosion-wear behaviour of thermally oxidised Cp-Ti and Ti-6Al-4V, *Wear*, **256**, 469–479.

Donachie, M.J. (1989). *Titanium: A Technical Guide*, ASM International, Ohio.

Dong, H. and Bell, T. (1999). Tribological behavior of alumina sliding against Ti6Al4V in unlubricated contact, *Wear*, **225–229**, 874–884.

Dong, H. and Bell, T. (2000). Enhanced wear resistance of titanium surfaces by a new thermal oxidation treatment, *Wear*, **238**, 131–137.

Dong, H. and Li, X.Y. (2000). Oxygen boost diffusion for the deep-case hardening of titanium alloys, *Mater Sci Eng*, **280**, 303–310.

Dong, H., Bloyce, A. and Bell, T. (1999). Slurry abrasion response of surface engineered Ti6Al4V ELI, *Tribol Int*, **32**, 517–526.

Du, H.L., Datta, P.K., Lewis, D.B. and Burnell-Gray, J.S. (1994). Air oxidation behaviour of Ti-6Al-4V alloy between 650 and 850°C, *Corrosion Sci*, **36**, 631–642.

Durdu, S. and Usta, M. (2014). The tribological properties of bioceramic coatings produced on Ti6Al4V alloy by plasma electrolytic oxidation, *Ceram Int*, **40**, 3627–3635.

Frangini, S., Mignone, A. and De Riccardis, F. (1994). Various aspects of the air oxidation behaviour of a Ti6Al4V alloy at temperatures in the range 600-700°C, *J Mater Sci*, **29**, 714–720.

Games, L.A., Sanchez, A.G., Jimenez-Pique, E., Schreiner, W.H, Ceré, S.M. and Ballarre, J. (2012). Chemical and mechanical properties of anodized cp-titanium in NH_4 H_2PO_4/NH_4F media for biomedical applications, *Surf Coat Tech*, **206**, 4791–4798.

Galliano, F., Galvanetto, E., Mischler, S. and Landolt, D. (2001). Tribocorrosion behavior of plasma nitrided Ti-6Al-4V alloy in neutral NaCl solution, *Surf Coat Tech*, **145**, 121–131.

Garbacz, H. and Lewandowska, M. (2003). Microstructural changes during oxidation of titanium alloys, *Mater Chem Phys*, **81**, 542–547.

Gao, Y., Zou, S., Liu, X., Bao, C. and Hu, J. (2009). The effect of surface immobilized bisphosphonates on the fixation of hydroxyapatite-coated titanium implants in ovariectomized rats, *Biomaterials*, **30**, 1790–1796.

Garcia-Alonso, M.C., Saldana, L., Valles, G., Gonzalez-Garrasco, J.L., Gonzalez-Cabrero, J., Martinez, M.E. *et al.* (2003). *In vitro* corrosion behavior and osteoblast response of thermally oxidised Ti6Al4V alloy, *Biomaterials*, **24**, 19–26.

Geetha, M., Singh, A.K., Asokamani, R. and Gogia, A.K. (2009). Ti based biomaterials, the ultimate choice for orthopaedic implants — a review. *Prog Mater Sci*, **54**, 397–425.

Gobel, M., Haannappel, V.A.C. and Stroosnijder, M.F. (2001). On the determination of diffusion coefficients of oxygen in one-phase Ti (α-Ti) and two-phase (α-and β-Ti) by micro-hardness measurement, *Oxid Met*, **55**, 137–151.

Guclu, F.M., Cimenoglu, H. and Kayali, E.S. (2006). The recrystallization and thermal oxidation. behavior of cp-titanium, *Mat Sci Eng C*, **56**, 1367–1372.

Guleryuz, H. and Cimenoglu, H. (2004). Effect of thermal oxidation on corrosion and corrosion-wear behaviour of a Ti-6Al-4V alloy, *Biomaterials*, **25**, 3325–3333.

Guleryuz, H. and Cimenoglu, H. (2005). Surface modification of a Ti-6Al-4V alloy by thermal oxidation, *Surf Coat Tech*, **192**, 164–170.

Guleryuz, H. and Cimenoglu, H. (2009). Oxidation of Ti-6Al-4V alloy, *J Alloy Comp*, **472**, 241–246.

Hwang, K.S., Yun, Y.H., Min, S.S., Lee, Y.R. and Par, Y.J. (2002). Calcium phosphate forming ability of thermally oxidized titanium implant, *Met Mater Int*, **8**, 411–415.

Imam, M.A. and Fraker, A.C. (1996). Titanium alloys as implant materials, in Brown, S.A. and Lemons, J.E. (eds), *Medical applications of titanium and its alloys*, ASTM, Philadelphia, 3–15.

Imbrie, P.K. and Lagoudas, D.C. (2001). Morphological evolution of TiO_2 scale formed on various 1D and 2D geometries of titanium, *Oxid Met*, **55**, 359–399.

Jiang, H., Hirohasi, M., Lu, Y. and Imanari, H. (2002). Effect of Nb on the high temperature oxidation of Ti-(0–50 at.%)Al, *Scripta Mater*, **46**, 639–643.

Khorasanian, M., Dehghan, A., Shariat, M.H., Bahrololoom, M.E. and Javadpour, S. (2011). Microstructure and wear resistance of oxide coatings on Ti-$_6$Al-$_4$V produced by plasma electrolytic oxidation in an inexpensive electrolyte, *Surf Coat Tech*, **206**, 1495–1502.

Kofstad, P. (1988). *High Temperature Corrosion*, Elsevier Applied Science, London.

Komotori, J., Lee, B.J., Dong, H. and Dearnley, P.A. (2001). Corrosion response of surface engineered titanium alloys damaged by prior abrasion, *Wear*, **251**, 1–11.

Krishnamurthy, R. and Srolovitz, D.J. (2003). Stress distributions in growing oxide films, *Acta Mater*, **51**, 2171–2190.

Kumar, S., Narayanan, T.S.N.S., Raman, S.G.S. and Seshadri, S.K. (2010). Surface modification of CP-Ti to improve the fretting-corrosion resistance: Thermal oxidation vs. anodizing, *Mat Sci Eng C*, **30**, 921–927.

Leinenbach, C. and Eifler, D. (2006). Fatigue and cyclic deformation behaviour of surface-modified titanium alloys in simulated physiological media, *Biomaterials*, **27**, 1200–1208.

Leyens, C. and Peters, M., (2003). *Titanium and Titanium Alloys: Fundamentals and applications*, Wiley-VCH, Weinheim.

Li, J. and Zhao, Y. (2009). Biocompatibility and antibacterial performance of titanium by surface treatment, *J Coating Tech Res*, **9**, 223–228.

Li, C.X., Horspool, D. and Dong, H. (2007). Effect of ceramic conversion surface treatment on fatigue properties of Ti_6Al_4V alloy, *Int J Fatigue*, **29**, 2273–2280.

Lin, X., Zhu, M., Zheng, J., Luo, J. and Mo, J. (2010). Fretting wear of micro-arc oxidation coating prepared on Ti_6Al_4V alloy, *Trans Nonferrous Met Soc China*, **20**, 537–546.

Liu, X., Chu, P. and Ding, C. (2004). Surface modification of titanium, titanium alloys, and related materials for biomedical applications, *Mat Sci Eng R Rep*, **47**, 49–121.

Long, M. and Rack, H.J. (1998). Titanium alloys in total joint replacement-a materials science perspective, *Biomaterials*, **19**, 1621–1639.

Long, M. and Rack, H.J. (2001). Friction and surface behavior of selected titanium alloys during reciprocating-sliding motion, *Wear*, **249**, 158–168.

Lopez, M.F., Jimenez, J.A. and Gutierrez, A. (2003). Corrosion study of surface-modified vanadium-free titanium alloys, *Electrochim Acta*, **48**, 1395–1401.

Massalski, T.B., Okamoto, H., Subramarian, P.R. and Kaczprzak, L. (1990). *Binary Alloy Phase Diagrams*, ASM International, Ohio.

Metikos-Hukovic, M., Kwokal, A. and Piljac, J. (2003). The influence of niobium and vanadium on passivity of titanium-based implants in physiological solution, *Biomaterials*, **24**, 3765–3775.

Molinari, A., Straffelini, G., Tesi, B. and Bacci, T. (1997). Dry sliding wear mechanism of the Ti6Al4V alloy, *Wear*, **208**, 105–112.

Muddugangadhar, B.C., Amarnath, G.S., Tripathi, S., Dikshit, S. and Diva, M.S. (2011). Biomaterials for Dental Implants: An Overview, *Int J Oral Impl Clin Res*, **2**(12.1), 13–24.

Muhaffel, F., Teker, D., Cimenoglu, H. (2014). Tribological behaviour of micro arc oxidation coatings on Cp-Ti for biomedical applications, *Proc Int Conf BioTribology 2014*, Toronto.

Ozturk, T. and Baydogan, M. (2012). Fabrication and characterization of TiO_2 nanotubes on Cp titanium surface, *Int Mater Symp 2012*, Denizli, 103–107.

Park, Y.J., Song, H.J., Kim, I. and Yang, H.S. (2007). Surface characteristics and bioactivity of oxide film on titanium metal formed by thermal oxidation, *J Mater Sci Mater Med*, **18**, 565–575.

Qi, P.-Y., Li, X.Y., Dong, H. and Bell, T. (2002). Characterization of the palladium-modified thermal oxidation-treated titanium, *Mat Sci Eng*, **326**, 330–342.

Rabinowicz, E. (1955). Lubricants for titanium, *Met Prog*, **67**, 112–114.

Schreckenbach, J.P. and Graf, H.-L. (2008). Preparation and characterization of selenium incorporated anodic conversion coatings on titanium surfaces for biomedical applications. *J Mater Sci Mater Med*, **19**, 233–238.

Schütze, M. (1992). Failure of oxide scales on advanced materials due to presence of stresses, in Saito, Y., Onay, B. and Maruyama, T. (eds), *High Temperature Corrosion of Advanced Materials and Protective Coatings*, Elsevier, Amsterdam, 39–49.

Semlitsch, M.F., Weber, H. and Steger, R. (1995). Fifteen years of experience with a Ti6Al7Nb alloy for joint replacements, *Biomed Tech (Berl)*, **40**, 347–355.

Semlitsch, M.F., Weber, H., Streicher, R.M. and Schön, R. (1992). Joint replacement components made of hot-forged and surface-treated Ti-6Al-7Nb alloy, *Biomaterials*, **13**, 781–788.

Shamblen, J.E. and Redden, T.K. (1968). Air contamination and embrittlement of titanium alloys, in Jaffee, R.I., Promisel, N.E. (eds), *The science, technology and application of titanium*, Pergamon Press, London, 199–208.

Shapiro, A. and Gisser, H. (1963). Lubrication of titanium surfaces modified by metallic diffusion, *ASLE Trans*, **6**, 40–48.

Shen, L., Kong, L.Y., Xiong, T.Y., Du, H. and Li, T.F. (2009). Preparation of $TiAl_3$-Al composite coating by cold spraying, *T Nonferr Metal Soc*, **19**, 879–882.

Shida, Y. and Anada, H. (1996). The effect of various ternary additives on the oxidation behavior of TiAl in high-temperature air, *Oxid Met*, **45**, 197–219.

Stachowiak, G.W. and Bachelor, A.W. (2001). *Engineering Tribology*, Butterworth Heinemann, Boston.

Streicher R.M., Weber H., Schlin R. and Semlitsch M. (1991). New surface modification for Ti6Al7Nb alloy: Oxygen diffusion hardening (ODH), *Biomaterials*, **12**, 125–129.

Sul, Y.T., Johansson, C. B., Petronis, S., Krozer, A., Jeong, Y., Wennerberg, A. *et al.* (2002). Characteristics of the surface oxides on turned and electrochemically oxidized pure titanium implants up to dielectric breakdown: The oxide thickness, micropore configurations, surface roughness, crystal structure and chemical composition, *Biomaterials*, **23**, 491–501.

Unlu, M.D., Meydanoglu, O. and Cimenoglu, H. (2010). Air oxidation behaviour of a Ti-6Al-7Nb alloy, *Defect Diffus Forum*, **297–301**, 1389–1394.

Unnam, J., Shenoy, R.N. and Clark, R.K. (1986). Oxidation of commercial purity titanium, *Oxid Met*, **26**, 231–252.

Vanzillotta, P.S., Sader, M.S., Bastos, I.N. and Soares, G.D.A. (2006). Improvement of in vitro titanium bioactivity by three different surface treatments, *Dent Mater*, **22**, 275–282.

Wang, X.X., Yan, W., Hayakawa, S., Tsuru, K. and Osaka, A. (2003). Apatite deposition on thermally and anodically oxidized titanium surfaces in a simulated body fluid, *Biomaterials*, **24**, 4631–4637.

Weissman, S. and Shrier, A. (1968). Strain distribution in oxidized alpha titanium crystals, in Jaffee, R.I. and Promisel, N.E (eds), *The Science, Technology and Application of Titanium*, Pergamon Press, London, 441–458.

Wiklund, U. and Hutchings, I.M. (2001). Investigation of surface treatments for galling protection of titanium alloys, *Wear*, **251**, 1034–1041.

Yao, Z.Q., Ivanisenko, Y., Diemant, T., Caron, A., Chuvilin, A., Jiang, J.Z. *et al.* (2010). Synthesis and properties of hydroxyapatite-containing porous titania coating on ultrafine-grained titanium by micro-arc oxidation, *Acta Biomater*, **6**, 2816–2825.

Yerokhin, A.L., Nie, X., Leyland, A. and Matthews, A. (2000). Characterisation of oxide films produced by plasma electrolytic oxidation of a Ti6Al4V alloy, *Surf Coat Tech*, **130**, 197–206.

Yerokhin, A.L., Nie, X., Leyland, A., Matthews, A. and Dowey, S.J. (1999). Plasma electrolysis for titanium surface engineering, *Surf Coat Tech*, **122**, 73–93.

Yu, C., Zhu, S., Wei, D. and Wang, F. (2007). Oxidation and H_2O/NaCl-induced corrosion behavior of sputtered Ni-Si coatings on Ti6Al4V at 600–650°C, *Surf Coat Tech*, **201**, 7530–7537.

Chapter 13

Diamond-Like Carbon Coatings for Joint Arthroplasty

So Nagashima, Myoung-Woon Moon and Kwang-Ryeol Lee
Materials and Life Science Research Division, Korea Institute of Science and Technology

1. Introduction

With the increase in the average human lifespan, there is an increased demand for high quality health-related products. Biomedical implants such as hip joints, vascular grafts, and dental roots have proven to be effective for the treatment of major injuries to improve the overall quality of life. Joint replacement is a common orthopedic procedure wherein dysfunctional joints, including hips and knees, are replaced with implants. These implants are primarily composed of metals (e.g. titanium, stainless steel), metal alloys (e.g. titanium–aluminum–vanadium alloys, cobalt–chromium–molybdenum alloys), ceramics (alumina-based), or polymeric materials (e.g. ultra-high molecular weight polyethylene (UHMWPE)). Such implants demonstrate adequate short-term biocompatibility and mechanical properties; however, they are far from being completely biostable or inert. Accordingly, these implants suffer from several drawbacks with respect to long-term use, such as cytotoxicity to surrounding tissues, the release of metal ions or wear debris that causes allergic reactions, corrosion, and frictional wear. To reduce such risks, the biological compatibility and long-term stability of joint replacement implants need to be improved.

Surface properties significantly affect the overall performance of implants, and surface modification with biologically, mechanically, and chemically stable materials is an effective method for overcoming the aforementioned drawbacks. Diamond-like carbon (DLC) is an amorphous carbon that possesses outstanding properties, including high hardness, a low friction coefficient, chemical inertness, high wear, and corrosion resistance, and biological compatibility. Since Aisenberg and Chabot (1971) first reported the synthesis of DLC, it has gained considerable attention as a functional coating material, and its biomedical applications have been actively explored, including coatings for hip and knee implants to prevent or minimize wear, inhibit corrosion, and maintain biological compatibility. Wear debris from joint implants can induce adverse biological reactions and cause bone loss and implant loosening. Therefore, the wear behavior of implants should be carefully examined. This chapter includes a brief, fundamental introduction to DLC, a review of recent studies on the evaluation of wear performance of various DLC joint implant coatings, and a discussion on issues to be solved for the effective development of DLC-coated implants with satisfactory performance.

2. DLC

DLC is an amorphous carbon comprising a mixture of sp^3 and sp^2 carbon bonds with various levels of hydrogen. Owing to its attractive properties, DLC has attracted a great deal of attention as a promising material for use in a range of applications. DLC can be synthesized by a variety of methods, and its properties can be controlled by altering the synthesis method and parameters. This allows one to synthesize DLC with the properties required for a particular application by selecting the appropriate synthesis method and optimizing the parameters. In this section, the fundamental properties of DLC will be described, with an explanation of approaches to tuning them.

2.1. *Deposition Methods and Fundamental Properties*

A number of techniques based on physical vapor deposition (PVD) or chemical vapor deposition (CVD) have been developed for the synthesis of DLC, including filtered cathodic vacuum arc (FCVA), ion plating, plasma immersion ion implantation and deposition (PIIID), magnetron sputtering, ion beam sputtering, pulsed laser deposition, and radio frequency plasma enhanced CVD (r.f.-PECVD) (Cuong *et al.*, 2003; He *et al.*, 1994; Leu *et al.*, 2004; Sánchez *et al.*, 2000; Shim *et al.*, 2000; Sui *et al.*, 2006; Zou *et al.*, 2004). Figure 13-1 shows schematics of representative systems for the synthesis of DLC (Robertson, 2002), and detailed explanations of the systems can be found in the corresponding reference. The properties of DLC vary based on the synthesis method and parameters. The precise control of the synthesis parameters directly affects the chemical structure of DLC, such as the sp^3:sp^2 ratio and hydrogen content, to produce DLC with properties that range from polymer like to diamond like.

As shown in Figure 13-2, there are various forms of amorphous carbon. DLC is the general term used to describe a broad range of amorphous carbon that can be categorized into several types according to its properties (Robertson, 2002). Amorphous carbon (a-C) has a high sp^3 bond content (40–80%), and hydrogenated amorphous carbon (a-C:H) contains up to approximately 40% sp^3 bonds (Donnet *et al.*, 1999). Tetrahedral amorphous carbon (ta-C) is a type of a-C with a significant quantity of sp^3 bonds (>70%) (McKenzie, 1996). The fraction of sp^3 bonds in amorphous carbon is closely related to the mechanical properties, including hardness, elastic modulus, and residual stress. The hardness of ta-C measures as high as 80 GPa, and that of a-C:H is in the range 10–30 GPa (Robertson, 1992). Although the friction coefficient of a-C:H is reportedly lower than that of ta-C in dry conditions, the wear rate for a-C:H is higher than that for ta-C in various testing conditions (Erdemir and Donnet, 2006). The residual stress in DLC is an intrinsic nature and is strongly correlated with the kinetic energy of the deposited carbon atoms, which is dependent on the bias voltage, pressure, and precursor gas molecules (Lee *et al.*, 1994). When the stress in a DLC film deposited on a substrate exceeds the interfacial adhesion strength, the film can delaminate from the substrate, which eventually degrades the overall performance. Thus, residual stress should be lowered, which can be accomplished by incorporating an appropriate third element, such as

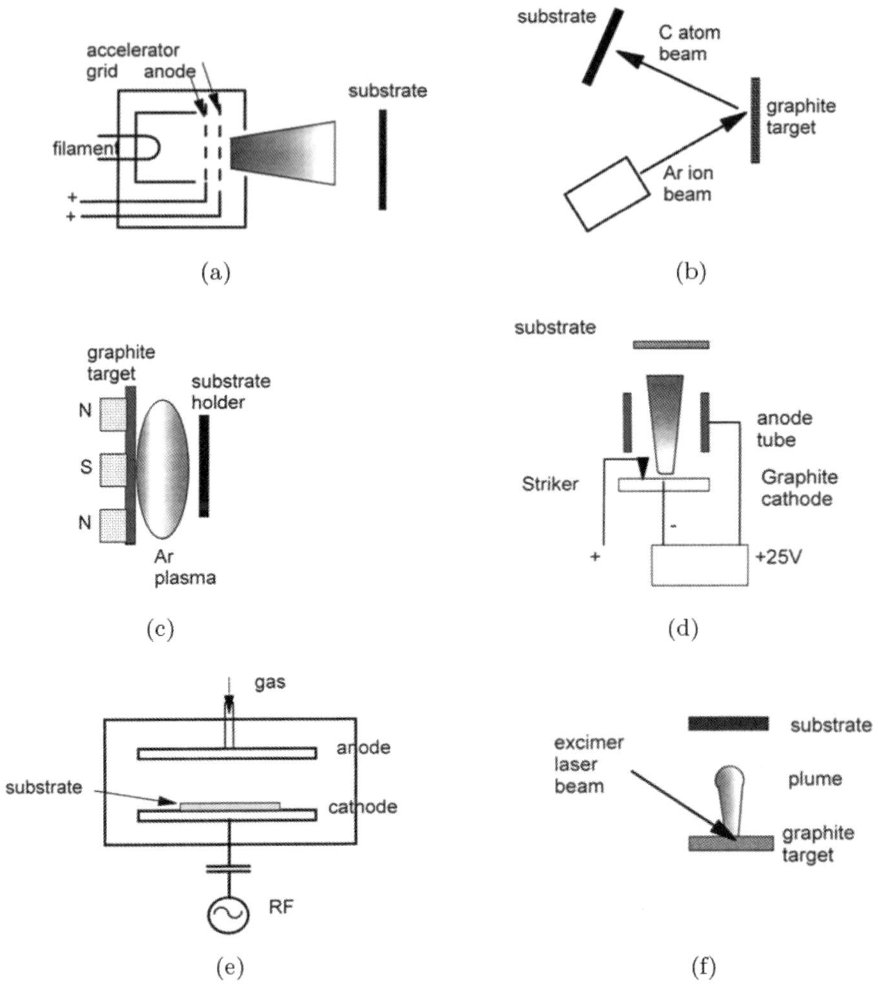

Figure 13-1. Schematics of representative systems for the synthesis of DLC (Robertson, 2002). Reprinted with permission from Elsevier. (a) Ion deposition, (b) Ion assisted sputtering, (c) Sputtering, (d) Cathodic Vacuum Arc, (e) Plasma deposition, (f) Pulsed laser deposition.

Si or Ti, into the film or depositing an interlayer onto the substrate prior to film deposition.

The biological properties, including hemocompatibility and cell compatibility, of DLC have been actively studied in *in vitro* and *in vivo* systems for biomedical applications, and numerous researchers

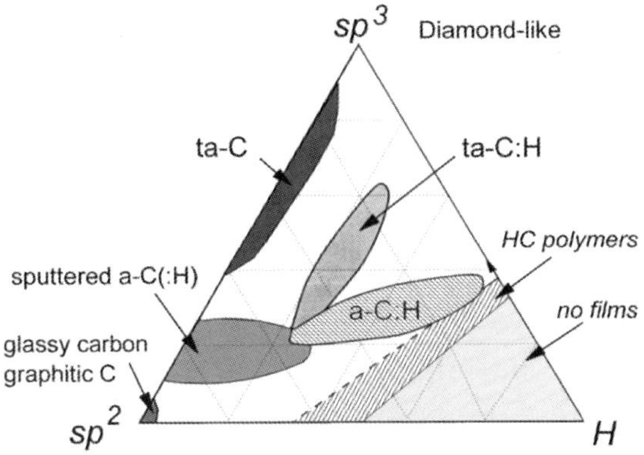

Figure 13-2. Ternary phase diagram of amorphous carbon materials (Robertson, 2002). Reprinted with permission from Elsevier.

have reported its excellent biocompatibility. For example, Mohanty *et al.* (2002) implanted bare Ti substrates, commercially used biomaterials, and DLC-coated Ti substrates in the skeletal muscle of rabbits and investigated the surrounding tissue response. DLC was synthesized by r.f.-PECVD, and the specimens were explanted after 1, 3, 6, and 12 months. The results from this study demonstrated that the DLC-coated substrates were as biocompatible as the uncoated substrates, even after long-term implantation, indicating the good biocompatibility of DLC.

2.2. *Incorporation of a Third Element*

Several attempts have been made to further improve the properties of DLC. The amorphous nature of DLC allows for incorporation of a third element, such as Si (Jones *et al.*, 2010; Kim *et al.*, 2005; Lee *et al.*, 1997, 2002; Maguire *et al.*, 2005; Ogwu *et al.*, 2008; Okpalugo *et al.*, 2004; Papakonstantinou *et al.*, 2002), F (Hasebe *et al.*, 2006, 2007; Saito *et al.*, 2005), P (Kwok *et al.*, 2005), Ag (Ahmed *et al.*, 2009; Choi *et al.*, 2007, 2008; Kwok *et al.*, 2007), N (Okpalugo *et al.*, 2008; Yokota *et al.*, 2007), or Ti (Bui *et al.*, 2008; Gilmore and Hauert, 2001; Ouyang and Sasaki, 2005; Pandiyaraj *et al.*, 2012), the concentration of which significantly affects the resulting DLC properties. For example, Choi *et al.* (2007) prepared Ag-incorporated DLC films using ion beam deposition and investigated the effect of the Ag content on the residual stress. Their results demonstrated that increasing the Ag content up to 9.7 at. % resulted in a decrease in stress from >3.0 to 1.3 GPa, indicating that the residual stress was strongly dependent on the Ag content. Lee *et al.* (2002) synthesized ta-C films using a filtered vacuum arc of graphite with simultaneous sputtering of Si and measured the residual stress as a function of the varied Si content. They reported that the residual stress decreased from 6.0 to 3.3 GPa by incorporating 1 at. % of Si, and further increases in the Si content to 50 at. % resulted in stress decreases to 0.8 GPa. The incorporation of a third element also changes the biological compatibility of DLC. Saito *et al.* (2005) synthesized F-incorporated DLC (F-DLC) using an r.f.-PECVD apparatus and demonstrated that F-DLC dramatically suppressed platelet adhesion and activation compared with DLC alone. Ogwu *et al.* (2008) prepared Si-incorporated DLC (Si-DLC) using an r.f.-PECVD system and showed the improved adhesion of human microvascular endothelial cells compared with unmodified DLC.

3. Wear Behavior

The wear debris released from joint implants can induce adverse biological reactions and cause both bone loss and implant loosening. Therefore, the wear behavior of the implants should be carefully examined, and the wear properties of DLC-coated joint implants have been studied *in vitro* using several different methods, including pin-on-disk, hip joint simulators, and self-made simulators (Affatato *et al.*, 2000; Dong *et al.*, 1999; Dowling *et al.*, 1997; Fisher *et al.*, 2004; Lappalainen *et al.*, 1998, 2003; Oñate *et al.*, 2001; Platon *et al.*, 2001; Saikko *et al.*, 2001; Sheeja *et al.*, 2001; Shi *et al.*, 2003; Thorwarth *et al.*, 2010; Tiainen, 2001; Xu and Pruitt, 1999).

3.1. *Pin-On-Disk*

Pin-on-disk is the most commonly used method for evaluating wear behavior, wherein a flat or sphere-shaped indenter is located on a test plate with a precisely known force and the wear coefficients for the pin and the plate are calculated from the volume of material lost during a given friction run. Several parameters can be controlled in this process, including contact pressure, temperature, humidity, and lubrication. This method provides basic information on the properties and tribological performance of materials. Hip prostheses are ball-in-socket joints that consist of an acetabular cup (socket) that is usually made of UHMWPE and a femoral head that is made of metallic alloys (e.g. CoCr) or ceramics (e.g. Al_2O_3). DLC coatings have been applied to the materials used for the femoral head of hip prostheses. Comparative tribological tests using ball-on-disk and pin-on-disk methods have been developed to investigate the wear of different materials used for hip joint prostheses. Platon *et al.* (2001) compared the wear rate of stainless steel, titanium alloy, alumina, zirconium dioxide, DLC-coated stainless steel, and DLC-coated titanium and demonstrated the superior wear resistance of the DLC-coated materials. The DLC coating was prepared using a PECVD method in that study, but no detailed description of the process was provided. Lappalainen *et al.* (1998) prepared DLC-coated substrates, including CoCrMo and Ti_6Al_4V, using a filtered pulsed arc discharge method and investigated the wear resistance of UHWMPE with a NaCl solution as a lubricant. The resistance was found to be improved by a factor of up to 600 (Lappalainen *et al.*, 1998). Conversely, Sheeja *et al.* (2001) evaluated the wear properties of DLC-coated CoCrMo against UHMWPE, where the DLC coating was synthesized using a FCVA, and found no favorable improvement in the wear behavior of the DLC-coated specimen (Table 13-1). Sheeja *et al.* (2005) conducted a study on the tribological properties of DLC-coated CoCrMo using a pin-on-disk method in simulated body fluid, where the DLC coating was fabricated using the filtered cathodic vacuum arc method, and found that coating the surface of both UHMWPE and CoCrMo with DLC enhanced the lifetime of the implants to a considerable extent.

3.2. *Joint Simulators*

Simulators have also been widely utilized to investigate the performance of DLC-coated specimens. Lappalainen *et al.* (2003) performed a study on DLC-coated hip joints using a commercially available hip joint simulator, where the DLC coating was prepared

Table 13-1. The short- and long-term tribological behavior of DLC-coated and uncoated CoCrMo alloys sliding against UHMWPE in simulated body fluid evaluated using a pin-on-disk tribometer (Sheeja *et al.*, 2001). Reprinted with permission from Elsevier.

Sample	Test condition	No. of cycles	Friction coefficient	Wear of UHMWPE pin (mm^3/Nm)
Uncoated Co–Cr–Mo alloy	Load = 10 N Speed = 6 cm/s Environment = SBF Track radius = 8 mm	30 000 120 000	0.08 ± 0.01 0.05 ± 0.00	4.97×10^{-7} 1.65×10^{-7}
DLC coated Co–Cr–Mo alloy	Load = 10 N Speed = 6 cm/s Environment = SBF Track radius = 8 mm	30 000 120 000	0.17 ± 0.02 0.14 ± 0.01	5.31×10^{-7} 2.02×10^{-7}

by filtered pulsed plasma arc discharge. This study revealed that the wear rates measured for 15 million walking cycles, corresponding to approximately 15 years of clinical use, in serum lubrication were 10^6 times lower than the clinical values for conventional metal-on-metal or UHMWPE-on-metal pairs (Lappalainen *et al.*, 2003). Tiainen (2001) used a hip simulator to study the mechanical properties of ta-C coatings prepared with filtered pulsed arc discharge for biomechanical applications. The wear of ta-C coated metal-on-polyethylene joints was found to be 10^5–10^6 times smaller than metal-on-polyethylene or metal-on-metal joints. Dowling *et al.* (1997) evaluated the wear performance of DLC-coated orthopedic implants, where DLC films with 40–50% sp^3 content were synthesized using a saddle beam deposition system. The stainless steel femoral head coated with the DLC film showed a significantly lower level of UHMWPE wear after 6 million cycles compared with the uncoated femoral head. Saikko *et al.* (2001) conducted a study on the wear of polyethylene acetabular cups against CoCr, alumina, and DLC-coated CoCr using a hybrid vapor deposition process with a biaxial hip wear simulator and diluted calf serum as the lubricant. Figure 13-3 shows scanning electron microscopic (SEM) images of

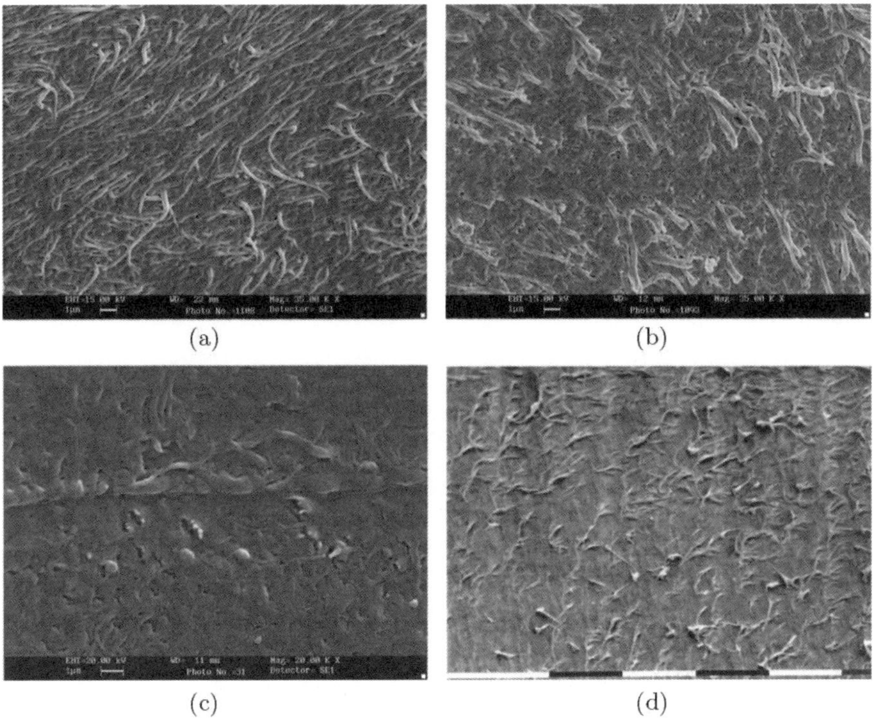

Figure 13-3. SEM images of the bearing surface of polyethylene acetabular cups used in a hip wear simulator for 3 million cycles against (a) alumina, (b) CoCr, and (c) DLC-coated heads, and (d) used *in vivo* for 97 months against a CoCr head (Saikko *et al.*, 2001). Each scale bar section in (d) corresponds to 10 μm. Reprinted with permission from Elsevier.

the bearing surface of a polyethylene acetabular cup tested in the hip wear simulator for 3 million cycles against (a) alumina, (b) CoCr, and (c) DLC-coated heads and a polyethylene acetabular cup after (d) 97 months *in vivo* against a CoCr head. Figure 13-4 presents SEM images of polyethylene wear particles produced against (a) alumina, (b) CoCr, and (c) DLC-coated heads. Although the authors noted that the wear resistance of the DLC coating did not markedly differ from those of CoCr and alumina against polyethylene, detailed information on the DLC coating was not provided in the study, which prevents a careful interpretation of their results.

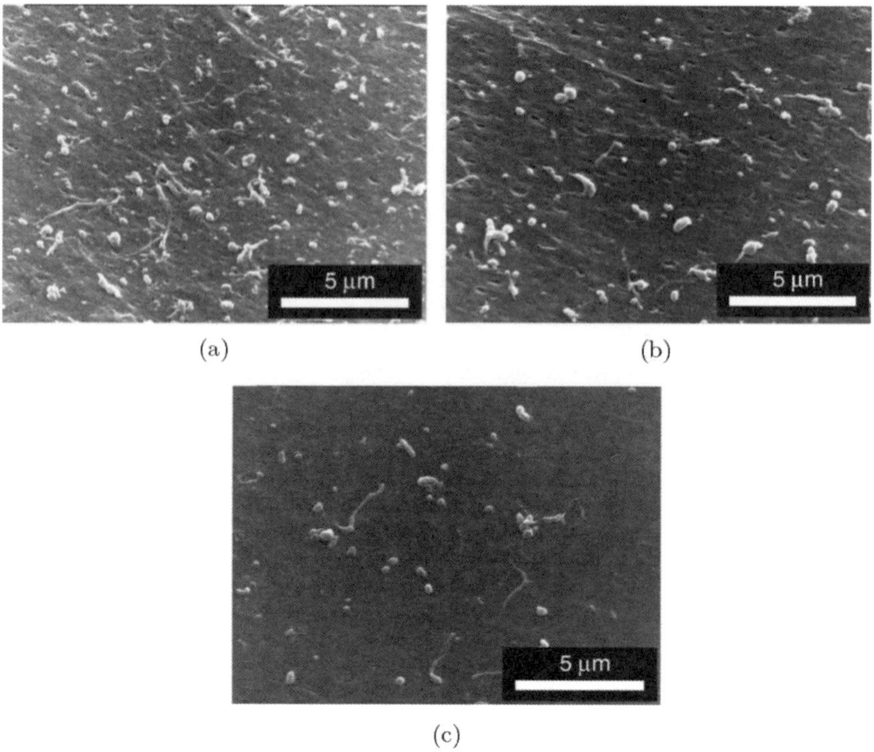

Figure 13-4. SEM images of polyethylene wear particles produced in a hip wear simulator against (a) alumina, (b) CoCr, and (c) DLC-coated heads (Saikko *et al.*, 2001). Reprinted with permission from Elsevier.

3.3. *Self-Made Simulators*

Wear behavior should be evaluated under conditions that resemble *in vivo* situations; to this end, self-made simulators have been employed to evaluate DLC-coated specimen performance (Oñate *et al.*, 2001; Thorwarth *et al.*, 2010). Oñate *et al.* (2001) used a special knee wear simulator to investigate the wear performance of UHMWPE plates against DLC-coated CoCr and Al_2O_3 balls. The simulator was used with a combined rolling-sliding movement that corresponded to the most unfavorable wear situation in the knee. The DLC film in this study was synthesized by r.f. glow discharge of C_2H_2 gas, and the coated and uncoated samples were tested against UHMWPE

Table 13-2. Weight loss of UHMWPE tested in a knee wear simulator at 5 million wear cycles (Oñate *et al.*, 2001). Asterisks indicate contacting materials with statistically significant differences. Reprinted with permission from Elsevier.

Test No.	Ball material (femoral head)	Plate material	Average UHMWPE wear (mg)	Standard deviation
1	Co–Cr–Mo	UHMWPE	−0.690*	0.078
2	Co–Cr–Mo coated with TiN	UHMWPE	−3.531**	0.330
3	Co–Cr–Mo treated with N^+ implantation	UHMWPE	−0.130	0.049
4	Co–Cr–Mo coated with DLC	UHMWPE	−0.150	0.090
5	Co–Cr–Mo	UHMWPE treated with N^+ implantation	−0.244	0.183
6	Ceramic Al_2O_3	UHMWPE	−0.253	0.002

plates. This study revealed that the DLC coating led to a reduction in UHMWPE wear at up to 5 million wear cycles, representing approximately 3 years of implant life (Table 13-2). Thorwarth *et al.* (2010) employed a simulator that induced a simplified spinal motion for the evaluation of wear performance of DLC-coated ball-on-socket implant pairs made from $Co_{28}Cr_6Mo$. The DLC coating was prepared with an r.f.-PECVD system using C_2H_2 gas, and the DLC-coated pairs and uncoated reference samples were subjected to wear tests in a simplified linear spinal simulator setup. The authors found that uncoated samples began to generate metal wear after 7 million loading cycles, with the wear volume eventually exceeding 20 times that of the DLC-coated samples (Figure 13-5). This volume corresponds to approximately two to three years *in vivo*, which demonstrates a significant improvement in wear resistance.

4. Delamination

Delamination is the instability of the coating layer that is commonly observed in DLC-coated specimens, which impairs their overall

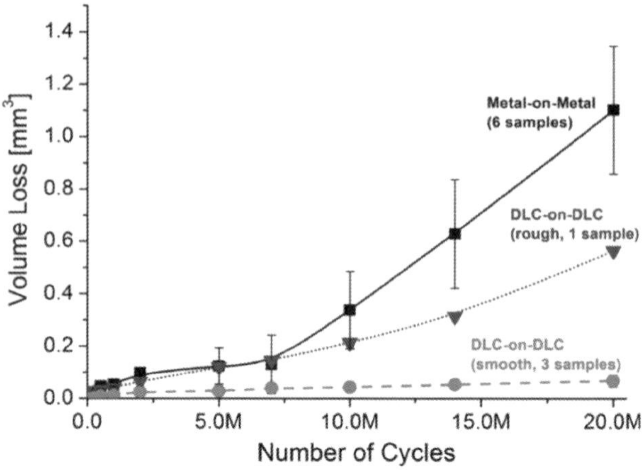

Figure 13-5. Wear volumes for metal-on-metal and smooth and rough DLC-on-DLC pairs tested in protein-containing simulated body fluid (Thorwarth *et al.*, 2010). The load and motion frequency were 1200 N and 3 Hz, respectively. Reprinted with permission from Elsevier.

performance and long-term stability. The high residual stress of DLC and poor substrate adhesion are implicated in early delamination. Thus, lowering the residual stress by incorporating a third element, such as Si or Ti, or depositing an interlayer has attracted much attention as a method for reducing delamination. Specifically, a thin layer of amorphous hydrogenated silicon or amorphous silicon has been used as an interlayer between Ti_6Al_4V substrates and DLC or Si-DLC to promote improved adhesion (Chandra *et al.*, 1995a, 1995b; Kim *et al.*, 2005, 2008). Although these interlayers appear to work effectively *in vitro*, they do not necessarily ensure long-term performance *in vivo*. Recently, delamination that occurs many years after implantation has been the focus of in-depth discussion (Hauert *et al.*, 2012a, 2012b, 2013). This delayed delamination can be ascribed to slow corrosion processes related to the crevice corrosion (CC) of a Si-based interlayer and the stress corrosion cracking (SCC) of a reactively formed interface. The *in vitro* testing methods that are commonly used prior to implantation only evaluate the wear properties and cannot approximate the corrosion properties of the interlayer or the reactively formed interface, which hinders an accurate understanding of the *in vivo* behavior. Delayed delamination is considered a serious issue in developing DLC-coated joint implants. Therefore, detailed investigations on the properties of the interlayer and interface should be carefully performed to better guarantee the long-term *in vivo* stability of these implants.

5. Concluding Remarks

DLC possesses outstanding physical and biological properties and has thus been a focus of active research for the development of highly functionalized joint implants. Here, the wear properties of DLC-coated specimens have been discussed. Many research groups have performed *in vitro* and *in vivo* studies and reported that DLC coatings can significantly reduce implant wear, suggesting that DLC coatings can be effectively applied to conventional joint implants. However, it should be noted that several important issues hinder the practical application of DLC coatings. First, there is no well-established, standardized procedure for evaluating the coating properties. Thus, researchers must determine the experimental methods and conditions independently. Their results can be affected by the properties of the coating and by the chosen experimental setup, and it is therefore difficult to directly compare data among different groups and to properly judge the efficiency of their respective DLC coatings. Second, the properties of DLC coatings are widely varied. Although these properties are largely dependent on the synthesis method and parameters, detailed information on DLC coating properties is not typically provided in studies. This inconvenience also significantly hinders the direct comparison of data presented by different groups. Finally, DLC coatings can spontaneously delaminate from their substrates. Such delamination not only negates the beneficial effects of the coatings but also further degrades the implants. This issue becomes especially significant after long-term use. The aforementioned drawbacks should be addressed in future research to promote the effective use of DLC coatings in joint implants.

The current situation provides information on the importance of careful interpretation of the reported results and the necessity of developing a universal experimental procedure for accurately predicting *in vivo* performance. In addition, although the focus of this chapter has been on the wear behavior of DLC-coated specimens, corrosive and biological properties should also be carefully examined. Comprehensive assessment and precise understanding of the *in vivo* properties are vital to the successful development of DLC-coated implants.

References

Affatato, S., Frigo, M. and Toni, A. (2000). An *in vitro* investigation of diamond-like carbon as a femoral head coating, *J Biomed Mater Res*, **53**, 221–226.

Ahmed, S.F., Moon, M.W. and Lee, K.R. (2009). Effect of silver doping on optical property of diamond like carbon films, *Thin Solid Films*, **517**, 4035–4038.

Aisenberg, S. and Chabot, R. (1971). Ion-beam deposition of thin films of diamondlike carbon, *J Appl Phys*, **42**, 2953–2958.

Bui, X.L., Pei, Y.T. and De Hosson, J.T.M. (2008). Magnetron reactively sputtered Ti-DLC coatings on HNBR rubber: The influence of substrate bias, *Surf Coat Tech*, **202**, 4939–4944.

Chandra, L., Allen, M., Butter, R., Rushton, N., Lettington, A.H. and Clyne, T.W. (1995a). The effect of biological-fluids on the adhesion of diamond-like carbon-films to metallic substrates, *Diam Relat Mater*, **4**, 852–856.

Chandra, L., Allen, M., Butter, R., Rushton, N., Lettington, A.H. and Clyne, T.W. (1995b). The effect of exposure to biological-fluids on the spallation resistance of diamond-like carbon coatings on metallic substrates, *J Mater Sci Mater M*, **6**, 581–589.

Choi, H.W., Choi, J.H., Lee, K.R., Ahn, J.P. and Oh, K.H. (2007). Structure and mechanical properties of Ag-incorporated DLC films prepared by a hybrid ion beam deposition system, *Thin Solid Films*, **516**, 248–251.

Choi, H.W., Dauskardt, R.H., Lee, S.C., Lee, K.R. and Oh, K.H. (2008). Characteristic of silver doped DLC films on surface properties and protein adsorption, *Diam Relat Mater*, **17**, 252–257.

Cuong, N.K., Tahara, M., Yamauchi, N. and Sone, T. (2003). Diamond-like carbon films deposited on polymers by plasma-enhanced chemical vapor deposition, *Surf Coat Tech*, **174**, 1024–1028.

Dong, H., Shi, W. and Bell, T. (1999). Potential of improving tribological performance of UHMWPE by engineering the Ti_6Al_4V counterfaces, *Wear*, **225**, 146–153.

Donnet, C., Fontaine, J., Lefèbvre, F., Grill, A., Patel, V. and Jahnes, C. (1999). Solid state 13C and 1H nuclear magnetic resonance investigations of hydrogenated amorphous carbon, *J Appl Phys*, **85**, 3264–3270.

Dowling, D.P., Kola, P.V., Donnelly, K., Kelly, T.C., Brumitt, K., Lloyd, L. *et al.* (1997). Evaluation of diamond-like carbon-coated orthopaedic implants, *Diam Relat Mater*, **6**, 390–393.

Erdemir, A. and Donnet, C. (2006). Tribology of diamond-like carbon films: Recent progress and future prospects, *J Phys Appl Phys*, **39**, R311–R327.

Fisher, J., Hu, X.Q., Stewart, T.D., Williams, S., Tipper, J.L., Ingham, E. *et al.* (2004). Wear of surface engineered metal-on-metal hip prostheses, *J Mater Sci Mater M*, **15**, 225–235.

Gilmore, R. and Hauert, R. (2001). Control of the tribological moisture sensitivity of diamond-like carbon films by alloying with F, Ti or Si, *Thin Solid Films*, **398**, 199–204.

Hasebe, T., Shimada, A., Suzuki, T., Matsuoka, Y., Saito, T., Yohena, S. *et al.* (2006). Fluorinated diamond-like carbon as antithrombogenic coating for blood-contacting devices, *J Biomed Mater Res*, **76A**, 86–94.

Hasebe, T., Yohena, S., Kamijo, A., Okazaki, Y., Hotta, A., Takahashi, K. *et al.* (2007). Fluorine doping into diamond-like carbon coatings inhibits protein adsorption and platelet activation, *J Biomed Mater Res*, **83A**, 1192–1199.

Hauert, R., Thorwarth, K. and Thorwarth, G. (2013). An overview on diamond-like carbon coatings in medical applications, *Surf Coat Tech*, **233**, 119–130.

Hauert, R., Falub, C.V., Thorwarth, G., Thorwarth, K., Affolter, C., Stiefel, M. *et al.* (2012a). Retrospective lifetime estimation of failed and explanted diamond-like carbon coated hip joint balls, *Acta Biomater*, **8**, 3170–3176.

Hauert, R., Thorwarth, G., Muller, U., Stiefel, M., Falub, C.V., Thorwarth, K. *et al.* (2012b). Analysis of the *in-vivo* failure of the adhesive interlayer for a DLC coated articulating metatarsophalangeal joint, *Diam Relat Mater*, **25**, 34–39.

He, X., Li, W. and Li, H. (1994). Bonding structure and tribological properties of DLC films synthesized by dual ion beam sputtering, *Vacuum*, **45**, 977–980.

Jones, B.J., Mahendran, A., Anson, A.W., Reynolds, A.J., Bulpett, R. and Franks, J. (2010). Diamond-like carbon coating of alternative metal alloys for medical and surgical applications, *Diam Relat Mater*, **19**, 685–689.

Kim, H.G., Ahn, S.H., Kim, J.G., Park, S.J. and Lee, K.R. (2005). Effect of Si-incorporation on wear-corrosion properties of diamond-like carbon films, *Thin Solid Films*, **482**, 299–304.

Kim, H.G., Ahn, S.H., Kim, J.G., Park, S.J. and Lee, K.R. (2005). Corrosion performance of diamond-like carbon (DLC)-coated Ti alloy in the simulated body fluid environment, *Diam Relat Mater*, **14**, 35–41.

Kim, J.G., Lee, K.R. and Yang, S.J. (2008). Wear-corrosion performance of Si-DLC coatings on Ti-$_6$Al-$_4$V substrate, *J Biomed Mater Res*, **86A**, 41–47.

Kwok, S.C.H., Wang, J. and Chu, P.K. (2005). Surface energy, wettability, and blood compatibility phosphorus doped diamond-like carbon films, *Diam Relat Mater*, **14**, 78–85.

Kwok, S.C.H., Zhang, W., Wan, G.J., McKenzie, D.R., Bilek, M.M.M. and Chu, P.K. (2007). Hemocompatibility and anti-bacterial properties of silver doped diamond-like carbon prepared by pulsed filtered cathodic vacuum arc deposition, *Diam Relat Mater*, **16**, 1353–1360.

Lappalainen, R., Heinonen, H., Anttila, A. and Santavirta, S. (1998). Some relevant issues related to the use of amorphous diamond coatings for medical applications, *Diam Relat Mater*, **7**, 482–485.

Lappalainen, R., Selenius, M., Anttila, A., Konttinen, Y.T. and Santavirta, S.S. (2003). Reduction of wear in total hip replacement prostheses by amorphous diamond coatings, *J Biomed Mater Res B Appl Biomater*, **66**, 410–413.

Lee, C.S., Lee, K.R., Eun, K.Y., Yoon, K.H. and Han, J.H. (2002). Structure and properties of Si incorporated tetrahedral amorphous carbon films prepared by hybrid filtered vacuum arc process, *Diam Relat Mater*, **11**, 198–203.

Lee, K.R., Baik, Y.J., Eun, K.Y. and Han, S. (1994). Precursor gas effect on the structure and properties of diamond-like carbon-films, *Diam Relat Mater*, **3**, 1230–1234.

Lee, K.R., Kim, M.G., Cho, S.J., Eun, K.Y. and Seong, T.Y. (1997). Structural dependence of mechanical properties of Si incorporated diamond-like carbon films deposited by RF plasma-assisted chemical vapour deposition, *Thin Solid Films*, **308**, 263–267.

Leu, M.S., Chen, S.Y., Chang, J.J., Chao, L.G. and Lin, W. (2004). Diamond-like coatings prepared by the filtered cathodic arc technique for minting application, *Surf Coat Tech*, **177**, 566–572.

Maguire, P.D., McLaughlin, J.A., Okpalugo, T.I.T., Lemoine, P., Papakonstantinou, P., McAdams, E.T. *et al.* (2005). Mechanical stability, corrosion performance and bioresponse of amorphous diamond-like carbon for medical stents and guidewires, *Diam Relat Mater*, **14**, 1277–1288.

McKenzie, D.R. (1996). Tetrahedral bonding in amorphous carbon, *Rep Progr Phys*, **59**, 1611–1664.

Mohanty, M., Anilkumar, T.V., Mohanan, P.V., Muraleedharan, C.V., Bhuvaneshwar, G.S., Derangere, F. *et al.* (2002). Long term tissue response to titanium coated with diamond like carbon, *Biomol Eng*, **19**, 125–128.

Ogwu, A.A., Okpalugo, T.I.T., Ali, N., Maguire, R.D. and McLaughlin, J.A.D. (2008). Endothelial cell growth on silicon modified hydrogenated amorphous carbon thin films, *J Biomed Mater Res B Appl Biomater*, **85**, 105–113.

Okpalugo, T.I.T., Ogwu, A.A., Maguire, P.D. and McLaughlin, J.A.D. (2004). Platelet adhesion on silicon modified hydrogenated amorphous carbon films, *Biomaterials*, **25**, 239–245.

Okpalugo, T.I.T., Ogwu, A.A., Okpalugo, A.C., McCullough, R.W. and Ahmed, W. (2008). The human micro-vascular enclothelial cells in vitro interaction with atomic-nitrogen-doped diamond-like carbon thin films, *J Biomed Mater Res B Appl Biomater*, **85**, 188–195.

Oñate, J.I., Comin, M., Braceras, I., Garcia, A., Viviente, J.L., Brizuela, M. *et al.* (2001). Wear reduction effect on ultra-high-molecular-weight polyethylene by application of hard coatings and ion implantation on cobalt chromium alloy, as measured in a knee wear simulation machine, *Surf Coat Tech*, **142**, 1056–1062.

Ouyang, J.H. and Sasaki, S. (2005). Friction and wear characteristics of a Ti-containing diamond-like carbon coating with an SRV tester at high contact load and elevated temperature, *Surf Coat Tech*, **195**, 234–244.

Pandiyaraj, K.N., Heeg, J., Lampka, A., Junge, F., Barfels, T., Wienecke, M. *et al.* (2012). *In vitro* cyto and blood compatibility of titanium containing diamond-like carbon prepared by hybrid sputtering method, *Plasma Sci Tech*, **14**, 829.

Papakonstantinou, P., Zhao, J.F., Lemoine, P., McAdams, E.T. and McLaughlin, J.A. (2002). The effects of Si incorporation on the electrochemical and nanomechanical properties of DLC thin films, *Diam Relat Mater*, **11**, 1074–1080.

Platon, F., Fournier, P. and Rouxel, S. (2001). Tribological behaviour of DLC coatings compared to different materials used in hip joint prostheses, *Wear*, **250**, 227–236.

Robertson, J. (1992). Properties of diamond-like carbon, *Surf Coat Tech*, **50**, 185–203.

Robertson, J. (2002). Diamond-like amorphous carbon, *Mater Sci Eng R Rep*, **37**, 129–281.

Saikko, V., Ahlroos, T., Calonius, O. and Keränen, J. (2001). Wear simulation of total hip prostheses with polyethylene against CoCr, alumina and diamond-like carbon, *Biomaterials*, **22**, 1507–1514.

Saito, T., Hasebe, T., Yohena, S., Matsuoka, Y., Kamijo, A., Takahashi, K. *et al.* (2005). Antithrombogenicity of fluorinated diamond-like carbon films, *Diam Relat Mater*, **14**, 1116–1119.

Sánchez, N.A., Rincón, C., Zambrano, G., Galindo, H. and Prieto, P. (2000). Characterization of diamond-like carbon (DLC) thin films prepared by r.f. magnetron sputtering, *Thin Solid Films*, **373**, 247–250.

Sheeja, D., Tay, B.K. and Nung, L.N. (2005). Tribological characterization of surface modified UHMWPE against DLC-coated Co–Cr–Mo, *Surf Coat Tech*, **190**, 231–237.

Sheeja, D., Tay, B.K., Lau, S.P. and Nung, L.N. (2001). Tribological characterisation of diamond-like carbon coatings on Co–Cr–Mo alloy for orthopaedic applications, *Surf Coat Tech*, **146**, 410–416.

Shi, B., Ajayi, O.O., Fenske, G., Erdemir, A. and Liang, H. (2003). Tribological performance of some alternative bearing materials for artificial joints, *Wear*, **255**, 1015–1021.

Shim, K.S., Kim, S.M., Bac, S.H., Lee, S.Y., Jung, H.S. and Park, H.H. (2000). Fabrication and characterization of diamond-like carbon thin films by pulsed laser deposition, *Appl Surf Sci*, **154**, 482–484.

Sui, J.H., Cai, W. and Zhao, L.C. (2006). Surface modification of NiTi alloys using diamond-like carbon (DLC) fabricated by plasma immersion ion implantation and deposition (PIIID), *Nucl Instrum Meth B*, **248**, 67–70.

Thorwarth, G., Falub, C.V., Muller, U., Weisse, B., Voisard, C., Tobler, M. *et al.* (2010). Tribological behavior of DLC-coated articulating joint implants, *Acta Biomater*, **6**, 2335–2341.

Tiainen, V.M. (2001). Amorphous carbon as a bio-mechanical coating — mechanical properties and biological applications, *Diam Relat Mater*, **10**, 153–160.

Xu, T. and Pruitt, L. (1999). Diamond-like carbon coatings for orthopaedic applications: An evaluation of tribological performance, *J Mater Sci Mater Med*, **10**, 83–90.

Yokota, T., Terai, T., Kobayashi, T., Meguro, T. and Iwaki, M. (2007). Cell adhesion to nitrogen-doped DLCs fabricated by plasma-based ion implantation and deposition method using toluene gas, *Surf Coat Tech*, **201**, 8048–8051.

Zou, Y.S., Wang, W., Song, G.H., Du, H., Gong, J., Huang, R.F. *et al.* (2004). Influence of the gas atmosphere on the microstructure and mechanical properties of diamond-like carbon films by arc ion plating, *Mater Lett*, **58**, 3271–3275.

Chapter 14

Nanocrystalline Diamond Coatings on Silicon Nitride Bioceramic Bearings

M. Amaral, S.P. Rodrigues, F.J. Oliveira and R.F. Silva
CICECO, Department of Materials and Ceramic Engineering, University of Aveiro, Aveiro, Portugal

1. The Idea of Applying Nanocrystalline Diamond (NCD) Coatings to Articular Prosthesis

The present chapter describes a new proposal of a tribopair material for articular joint prosthesis, namely to be used in total hip replacement (THR): all-nanocrystalline diamond coated silicon nitride ceramic hip joints.

The materials solution here proposed comprises a NCD-coated silicon nitride (Si_3N_4) ceramic femoral head working against an NCD/Si_3N_4 acetabular cup. As the probability of fracture is correlated with the mechanical strength it is expected that the *in vivo* reliability will be improved by using silicon nitride-based ceramics for femoral heads and acetabular components. On the other hand, the NCD/NCD tribopair will improve the wear resistance.

The improved mechanical properties of Si_3N_4 ceramics, namely fracture toughness (5–10 MPa $m^{1/2}$ (Petzow and Herrmann, 2002)) and bending strength values (500–1200 MPa (Petzow and Herrmann, 2002)) higher than those presented by alumina (4–5 MPa $m^{1/2}$ and 300–400 MPa, respectively (Bal *et al.*, 2008)), configure Si_3N_4

ceramics as a superior structural ceramic. Furthermore, from the biological point of view, they provide excellent biocompatibility (Amaral *et al.*, 2002; Guedes e Silva *et al.*, 2004; Howlett *et al.*, 1989). Moreover, due to the low thermal expansion coefficient mismatch and grain-to-grain epitaxial relationships between Si_3N_4 and diamond crystals, which assist the interface strength (Almeida *et al.*, 2011), this ceramic ensures the best adhesion properties to CVD diamond coatings (Almeida *et al.*, 2007). NCD is a unique material maintaining the exceptional properties of diamond combined with very smooth surfaces. By providing a very low surface roughness, coating with NCD is an alternative to polishing microcrystalline diamond (MCD), a time-consuming, expensive task and impractical in the case of complex geometries. Previous studies have also demonstrated the excellent biological behaviour of NCD films with no cytotoxic effects (Amaral *et al.*, 2008a, 2009).

In the following sections, the characteristics of NCD coatings and their relationship with the tribo and biotribological behaviour are explored in more detail.

2. The Advantage of NCD Coatings in Tribological Applications

2.1. *Synthesis of NCD Coatings by Hot-Filament Chemical Vapour Deposition (HFCVD)*

NCD can be grown by chemical vapour (CVD) technique, using hot filament (HFCVD) or microwave plasma (MWCVD) reactors. Prior to deposition, the Si_3N_4 ceramic substrates are typically scratched for 30–60 min in an ultrasonic suspension of nanometric to micrometric diamond powder in alcohol media, for diamond seeding purposes. The HFCVD technique is the most suitable to achieve conformal coatings in convex and concave surfaces, as those of the hip joint components. As such, the tribological characterization below reported is solely that of the coatings produced using HFCVD technique. Typical NCD deposition parameters are as follows (Almeida *et al.*, 2007; Amaral *et al.*, 2006, 2009): CH_4/H_2 flow ratio $= 0.04$;

Ar/H_2 flow ratio = 0.10; total pressure, P = 5.0 kPa; substrate temperature, T_s = 750°C; filament temperature, T_f = 2300°C; total flow, Q = 50 mL·min^{-1}. These conditions allow NCD growth rates near 1.5 μm·h^{-1}. Partial substitution of hydrogen by argon and relatively high methane concentration in hydrogen promote the continuous renucleation of diamond, resulting in tiny diamond grains with an intrinsic ultra-smooth film surface (Figure 14-1(a)). A final average crystallite size of about 28 nm was estimated from X-ray low incident beam angle diffraction (LIBAD) measurements (Amaral *et al.*, 2006). Raman spectroscopy (λ = 325 nm) permits the identification of diamond, graphitic, and other phases (Figure 14-1(b)). Deconvolution of the Raman spectrum depicts a very small diamond peak (1336 cm^{-1}), and the graphitic D (~1370 cm^{-1}) and G (1580 cm^{-1}) bands (Ferrari and Robertson, 2001). The noticeable graphite bands reflect the incorporation of the sp^2 carbon phase at the grain boundaries, in an extensive amount due to the very small diamond crystallite size of NCD. The dispersive D band is shifted to higher wavenumbers from its common position (~1350cm^{-1}) in visible Raman, as a result of the 325 nm UV excitation wavelength (Zhang *et al.*, 2002). Bands centred at 1,183, 1,249, and 1,512 cm^{-1} are assigned to C–H polymeric structures that appear at the diamond crystallite boundaries (Fernandes *et al.*, 2007; Ferrari and Robertson, 2001; Pfeiffer *et al.*, 2003).

2.2. *The Tribological Behaviour of Homologous NCD/NCD Sliding Contacts*

The first step towards the envisaged biotribological application of NCD coatings consisted of their extensive characterization as self-mated (homologous) NCD/NCD sliding contacts in dry conditions (Abreu *et al.*, 2006a, 2006b; Salgueiredo *et al.*, 2013) and in water-lubricated contacts (Abreu *et al.*, 2009; Mubarok *et al.*, 2008), in order to appraise the mechanical integrity of the proposed tribopair. The tribological characterization was carried out by reciprocating ball-on-flat experiments using, typically, Si_3N_4 balls with 5 mm diameter and squared Si_3N_4 substrates (10 × 10 × 3 mm^3).

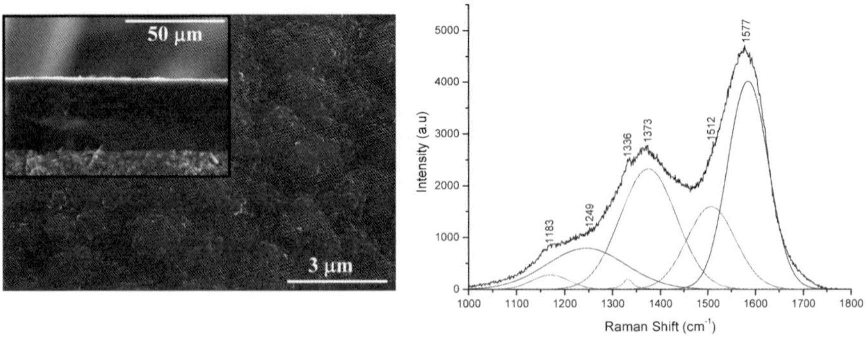

(a) (b)

Figure 14-1. (a) SEM micrographs of top and cross-section (inset) views (Reprinted from Almeida *et al.* (2007), with permission from Elsevier) and (b) micro-Raman spectrum of the as-grown NCD films.

A study was conducted in order to select the best surface finishing state for the Si_3N_4 substrates (Abreu *et al.*, 2006a). Three different conditions were compared: (i) flat lapping with 15 μm diamond slurry (FL samples); (ii) hard cloth polishing with 15 μm diamond slurry (PP); and, (iii) polishing to a mirror-like finish with colloidal silica (P). The tribological tests were conducted with a constant stroke of 6 mm and frequency of 1 Hz (average velocity of 9 mm$\cdot$s^{-1}), and sliding distances of 86 m (regular tests) and 690 m (endurance tests), which correspond to 2 and 16 hours of uninterrupted sliding, respectively. Normal loads varied in the range 10–40 N. AFM scans, and the respective surface roughness value, Rq (rms), of the NCD films corresponding to the distinct surface finishing conditions, are depicted in Figure 14-2a–14-2c. Differences are clearly evidenced: In the FL sample, grooves from the lapping operation are still present; for the PP sample, grooves disappear; finally, for the P sample, the highest smoothness was achieved. The higher value of the surface roughness of the NCD films comparing to the crystallite size ($\sim$28 nm) is the outcome from the overlapping effect of the substrate surface finishing with the intrinsic surface roughness of the NCD agglomerates.

The corresponding friction coefficient evolution during the very beginning of the tests can be seen in the plots of Figure 14-2d–14-2f.

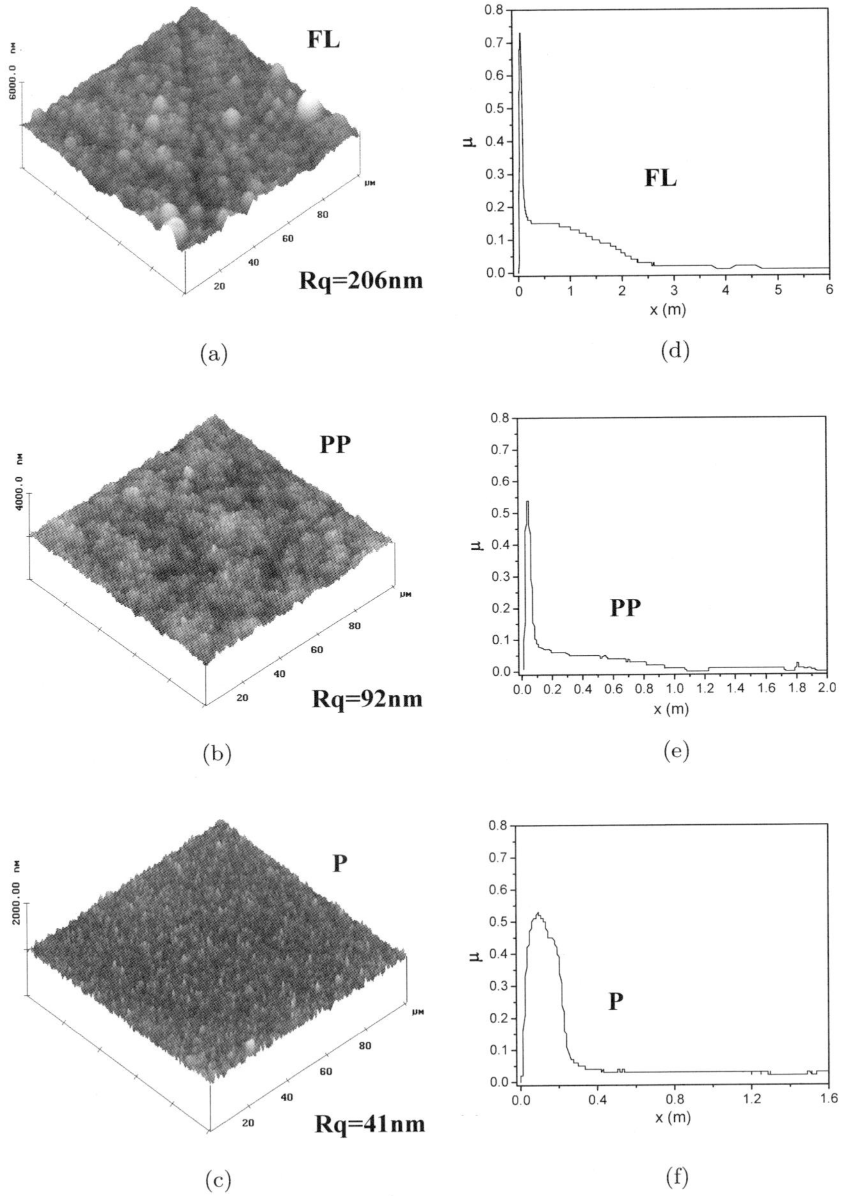

Figure 14-2. 3D AFM images of pristine NCD coated substrates (left column) and the corresponding friction curves (right column) in testing of self-mated pairs under 10–20 N of applied load, obtained for the various surface conditions. FL: flat lapped substrate; PP: pre-polished; P: polished. (Reprinted from Abreu *et al.* (2006a), with permission from Elsevier).

Curves for FL and PP samples start by an intense ephemeral friction coefficient above 0.5, originated from the mechanical interlocking of the film asperities, followed by a relatively short transition stage associated with the flattening of asperities, until the accommodation of the antagonist surfaces, reaching low friction values of ~0.03. In contrast, the very smooth P sample reveals an enlarged friction peak resulting from premature film detachment. Wear coefficient values of about 5×10^{-8} $mm^3 \cdot N^{-1} \cdot m^{-1}$ were calculated taking data for the endurance tests, denoting a mild wear regime. Further optimization of the adhesion levels of the diamond coatings led to the implementation of hydrogen plasma (Abreu *et al.*, 2006b) or CF_4 pretreatments (Salgueiredo *et al.*, 2013) of the ceramic surfaces prior to deposition. By doing this treatment, the threshold loads prior to film delamination for mirror polished substrates, as observed by optical and scanning electron microscopy, almost triple to 30 N for the same film thickness (~25 μm) (Abreu *et al.*, 2006b).

A distinct strategy to improve adhesion and to further enhance the tribological behaviour was recently reported (Salgueiredo *et al.*, 2013): The multilayer multigrade coatings, starting with the deposition of a MCD layer onto the Si_3N_4 ceramic surface in order to assure a high adhesion strength (Almeida *et al.*, 2007), then intercalating NCD with MCD layers to prevent excessive MCD grain growth, and ending with a smooth NCD layer on the top. Multigrade diamond films have been explored by others in coating of tungsten carbide-cobalt (WC-Co) substrates, namely for application in cutting tool inserts and wear resistant components (Kadlečíková *et al.*, 2007; Schäfer *et al.*, 2006; Sun *et al.*, 2009; Vojs *et al.*, 2005), resulting in significant improvements in the mechanical resistance and in the working lifetime of the tools. Figure 14-3a displays a cross-section SEM image of an as-deposited four-fold multilayer on the flat component of a ball-on-plate tribological pair, a similar morphology being obtained on the spherical counterbody (Salgueiredo *et al.*, 2013). Endurance tests (690 m of total sliding, as above referred) carried out under a constant applied load of 60 N, just below the delamination load, resulted in the typical worn track appearance of Figure 14-3b: Very smooth polished surfaces characteristic of a fine-scale

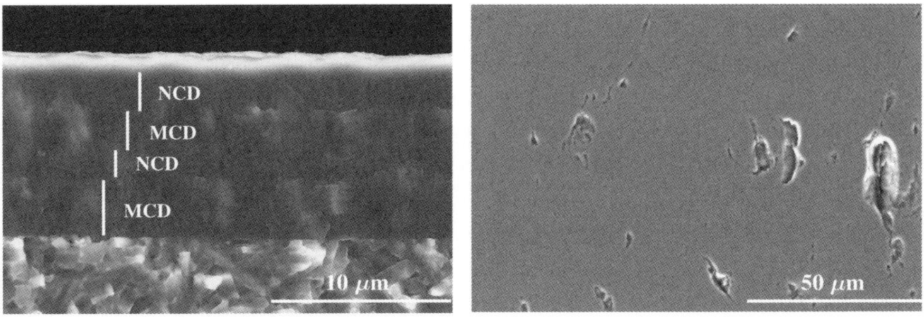

(a) (b)

Figure 14-3. SEM micrographs of (a) cross-section of the pristine multilayered MCD/NCD/MCD/NCD diamond coating; (b) aspect of the worn morphology, after ball-on-plate self-mated endurance tests (~690 m) at a constant load of 60 N. (Reprinted from Salgueiredo *et al.* (2013), with permission from Elsevier).

abrasive wear mechanism. Due to the high initial Hertzian stresses (~3.5 GPa), some interspersed grain pull-out took place. Wear coefficient values within the 10^{-8}–10^{-7} $mm^3{\cdot}N^{-1}{\cdot}m^{-1}$ order of magnitude were calculated for this tribopair, with no net difference between the monolayer and bilayer coatings. But, a distinct feature of the multilayer four-fold configuration is the outstanding threshold load of 200 N prior to gross film detachment from a FL substrate subjected to CF_4 plasma for 10 mins (Salgueiredo *et al.*, 2013).

In an approach closer to biotribological applications of NCD-on-NCD bearing contacts, water-lubricated systems were also characterized (Abreu *et al.*, 2009). Silicon nitride spheres and plates were coated with NCD monolayers using the same deposition parameters as for the dry experiments. Similarly, reciprocating ball-on-flat endurance tests were accomplished. Water lubrication allowed the threshold load to be increased before delamination to 85 N (30 N for the same coating in dry conditions). The water film contributed in reducing local contact stresses, therefore improving the load-supporting capability of the coating. Two different classes of wear debris are the outcome of the tribological interaction: (i) long blunted agglomerates (Figure 14-4a) originated from the initial truncation of NCD clusters and smeared due to repeated traversals inside the contact interface; (ii) nano-sized near spherical debris

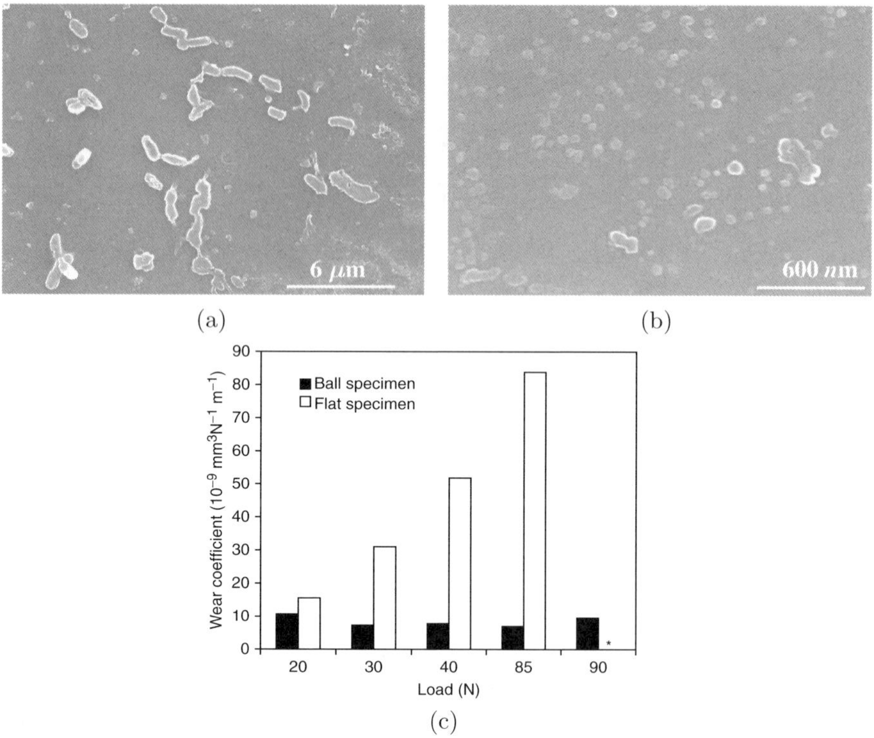

Figure 14-4. SEM images of the (a) morphology of the wear debris and (b) of the smallest wear particles after ball-on-plate self-mated endurance tests (~690 m) at a constant load of 60 N; (c) wear coefficient values as a function of applied load for ball and flat specimens. *omitted value due to film delamination. (Reprinted from Abreu *et al.* (2009), with permission from Elsevier).

(Figure 14-4b) resulting from removal of NCD nanocrystallites. In fact, water was not renewed during the test, therefore acting as a reservoir for the abrasive debris particles, contrarily to the dry experiments where the debris are expelled away from the contact region (Abreu *et al.*, 2009). Under water lubrication, the wear coefficient values fall in the range 10^{-9}–10^{-8} mm^3·N^{-1}·m^{-1} (Figure 14-4(c)), which correspond to very mild (at low loads) to mild (at high loads) wear regimes. The flat specimens exhibit wear coefficient values one order of magnitude higher than the ball counterparts at high loading, due to fatigue effects in the former. For all loading conditions below the threshold load of 85 N, a steady state very low friction regime ($\mu \sim 0.02-0.05$) followed a running-in regime with initial sharp peak ($\mu \sim 0.33$) related to the mechanical interlocking among salient NCD clusters. It is worth mentioning that a similar tribopair tested with water lubrication but in conformal plan-on-plan configuration, simulating mechanical seals, attained stable friction coefficient values of 0.01 without any measurable wear (Mubarok *et al.*, 2008).

3. The Biotribological Behaviour of NCD

The biotribological characterization was conducted with a reciprocating pin-on-plate test configuration like that reported in the previous sub-section, but with the pins flat-ended (cylinders of 4 mm diameter and 3 mm thickness) (Amaral *et al.*, 2008b) to permit contact stress levels similar to those of working human joints. Again, self-mated tribopairs were tested, anticipating the articulating surfaces of the hip prosthesis, acetabular cup and femoral head, both to be coated with NCD films. Two sets of samples were used regarding the Si_3N_4 surface preparation: Polished samples until colloidal silica finishing (P); and polished followed by CF_4 plasma etching (PE). Simulated physiological conditions of lubrication were compared: (i) Hank's balanced salt solution (HBSS, Cambrex, Belgium) containing 8 $g{\cdot}L^{-1}$ NaCl, 1 $g{\cdot}L^{-1}$ glucose, 0.4 $g{\cdot}L^{-1}$ KCl, 0.35 $g{\cdot}L^{-1}$ $NaHCO_3$, 0.09 $g{\cdot}L^{-1}$ $Na_2HPO_4.7H_2O$ and 0.06 $g{\cdot}L^{-1}$ KH_2PO_4 as the main components; (ii) fetal bovine serum (FBS, Cambrex, Belgium) diluted to 50% to contain 18.5 $mg{\cdot}ml^{-1}$ of protein, which is the concentration present in the synovial fluid (Tercic and Bozic, 2001), plus 0.2 wt% of a biocide (NaN_3, Merck, Germany). The applied normal load was 45 N, corresponding to the nominal contact stress of 3.5 MPa, a value compatible with *in vivo* hip and knee joint stress conditions (Dumbleton, 1981). By measuring the true contact area after testing, the real contact stresses were recalculated yielding values of about 25 MPa, still below the upper limit suffered by hip joints loaded at different axes (Szivek *et al.*, 1996). The experiments lasted for 500,000 cycles corresponding to a total sliding distance of 6 km.

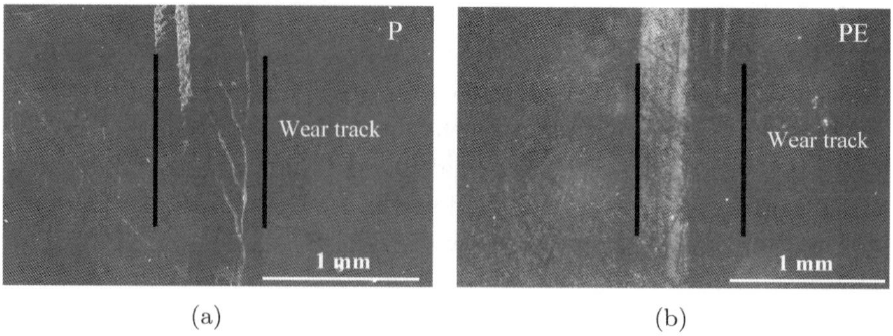

Figure 14-5. SEM micrographs of the wear tracks of (a) the P sample showing delamination cracks (Reprinted from Amaral *et al.* (2008), with permission from Elsevier) and (b) the PE sample with improved adhesion.

As for the dry experiments, the P samples revealed a poor mechanical resistance for tribological applications as depicted by the cracking pattern inside the wear track (Figure 14-5a), in contrast to the PE samples where the NCD coating appears unbroken (Figure 14-5b). The fracture of the films on P substrates at nominal loads as low as 25 MPa is due to low adhesion that induces interfacial failure and finally breakage. One way of increasing adhesion is to chemically attack the Si_3N_4 grains by CF_4 plasma, as said in the previous section. The increase of the surface roughness at the micrometre level due to Si_3N_4 grain attack by F radicals enables the mechanical interlocking between coating and substrate (Amaral *et al.*, 2010).

In the PE NCD-coated pairs, and only with FBS fluid, SEM microscopy operating at 1 mbar of total pressure allowed an extensive deposition of organic compounds to be observed on the NCD surface (Figure 14-6(a)). Figure 14-6(b) is an image of the same coating but after cleaning in acetone and ethanol, where only the flat plateaus of the NCD clusters and unfilled valleys are observed. In Figure 14-6(c), a higher magnification of those deposits is depicted and the corresponding EDS analysis is shown in Figure 14-6(d), evidencing the presence of carbon (C), nitrogen (N), oxygen (O), and sodium (Na) as major components. C is mostly from the NCD film, whereas N and O are possibly from the aminoacids that constitute the proteins

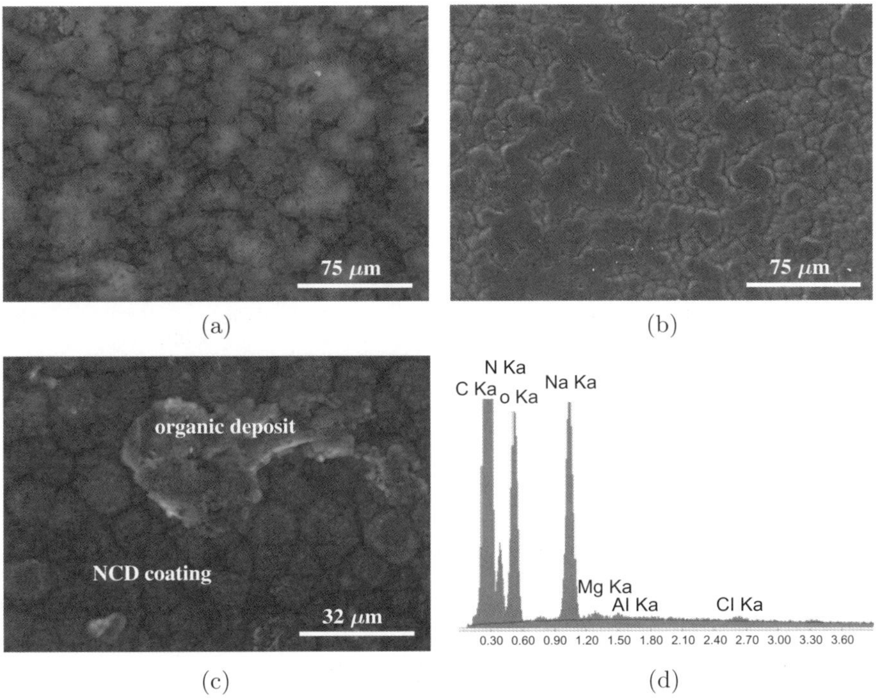

Figure 14-6. SEM micrographs of NCD-coated PE substrates after tribological testing under FBS showing the presence of a surface smeared film (a) and (c) rich in N, O, and Na as detected by EDS (d) and after cleaning in acetone and ethanol (b). (Reprinted from Amaral *et al.* (2008), with permission from Elsevier).

structure. Sources of Na are the biocide (0.2 wt% NaN_3) but, most likely, the aqueous saline solution that constitutes the serum base.

The distinct tribological behaviour under HBSS and FBS is reflected by the plots of the friction coefficient evolution during the tests (Figure 14-7a, 14-7b). In both media, initial friction peaks, due to the truncation of surface asperities in the first moments of sliding, are very clear in the insets of these figures. The steady state friction value is larger when the tribological tests are carried out with the FBS liquid (0.10) than with HBSS (0.06). This result is in line with the above SEM observations (Figure 14-6) and it has already been observed with other materials combinations, namely alumina-on-alumina and alumina-on-UHMWPE (Gispert *et al.*, 2006; Hall

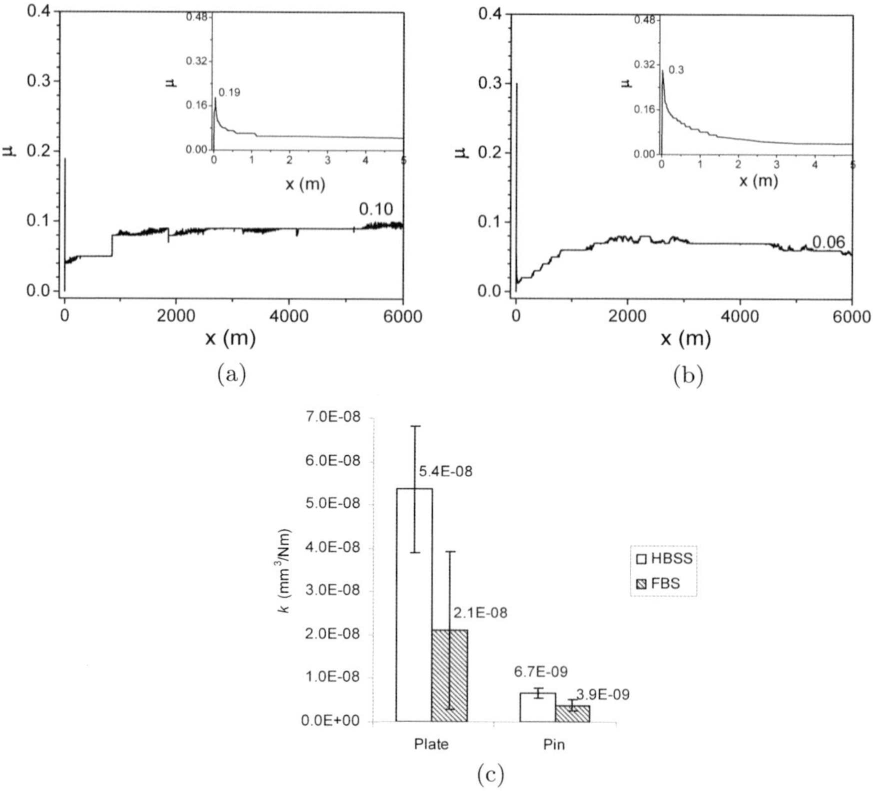

Figure 14-7. Evolution of the friction coefficient of NCD self-mated contacts tested under HBSS (a) and FBS lubrication (b). Inset charts evidence the running-in stage. (c) Wear coefficient values of NCD tribopair tested under HBSS and FBS fluids. (Reprinted from Amaral *et al.* (2008), with permission from Elsevier.)

et al., 2001; Scholes *et al.*, 2000). The reasons for the higher friction coefficient value with FBS are not fully understood because for metal-on-metal bearings, the friction coefficient is smaller when using protein-containing fluids than when using protein-free ones. Some explanations are based on wetting differences, as proteins tend to adsorb more strongly on hydrophobic surfaces producing more stable adsorbed layers (Gispert *et al.*, 2006). Alumina is less hydrophobic than metals and thus proteins are less stable and may contribute to the increase of friction. Another possible explanation is the fact that adsorbed proteins act to increase the surface roughness of the originally smooth ceramic surface, leading to a predominantly mixed lubrication regime and therefore to an increase of the friction coefficient (Scholes *et al.*, 2000).

The steady state friction coefficient values are slightly higher than the values found for bearings for artificial hip joints in the presence of bovine serum, namely ceramic-on-ceramic and ceramic-on-metal (0.002–0.07), but are considerably lower than the values for metal-on-metal combinations (0.22–0.27) (Jin *et al.*, 2006). The main reason for the observed differences between the present NCD/NCD tribosystem and those involving ceramics is the high starting surface roughness values compared to 5–10 nm for the ceramics (Jin *et al.*, 2006). However, the wear coefficient values measured for NCD self-mated pairs under physiological liquid lubrication are of the order of $\sim 10^{-9}$–10^{-8} $mm^3 \cdot N^{-1} m^{-1}$ (mild to very mild wear regime), values that equal or are even better than the wear factors assessed in similar test conditions for metal-on-metal ($\sim 10^{-7}$ $mm^3 \cdot N^{-1} m^{-1}$), UHMWPE-on-metal ($\sim 10^{-7}$ $mm^3 \cdot N^{-1} m^{-1}$), and ceramic-on-ceramic ($\sim 10^{-8} mm^3 \cdot N^{-1} m^{-1}$) contacts (Jin *et al.*, 2006).

The reported biotribological performance of NCD-on-NCD bearings may reduce the amount of wear debris generated by all-NCD coated hip implants. In order to investigate the cytotoxicity and biocompatibility of NCD, *in vitro* cell cultures were accomplished (Amaral *et al.*, 2008a, 2009). Two fibroblast cell culture systems were used to address the cytotoxicity of NCD-coated samples: L929 cells, a mouse permanent cell line, and human gingival fibroblasts. The seeded NCD film allowed reproduction of the typical features of the two tested cell culture systems, further suggesting the lack of cytotoxicity of these coatings (Amaral *et al.*, 2009). The biocompatibility test was performed concerning the human cell system characteristic of the tissue that NCD will encounter *in vivo*. Considering the coating of hip prostheses, NCD films were exposed to MG63 osteoblast-like cells for screening toxicity and in a second stage seeded with human bone marrow cells. This work revealed that NCD films induced human osteoblast proliferation and stimulated specific metabolic activities such as ALP activity and matrix mineralization (Amaral *et al.*, 2008a).

4. Next Step: Wear Simulation Tests of NCD-Coated Silicon Nitride Hip Joints

Impelled by the evidence of NCD-coated Si_3N_4 ceramic as a superior tribopair, this novel combination of materials for hip joint prosthesis is here proposed. The system is composed of an acetabular cup with a Si_3N_4 inlay and a Si_3N_4 ceramic femoral head, i.e. concave and convex surfaces, respectively, coated with NCD (Figure 14-8). The HFCVD coating of the hip joint implant components was performed using a special approach of filament arrangement.

The novel hip prosthesis is designed to have an improved lifetime in highly demanding conditions when compared to common joint implants that are used in THR. The production of dense high-strength Si_3N_4 ceramics and the coating with well-adhered NCD films are part of the strategy to achieve that goal.

Papo *et al.* (2004) tested NCD-coated Ti_6Al_4V substrates imitating the condyle and fossa components of the temporomandibular joint in a mandibular movement simulator. The damage in both

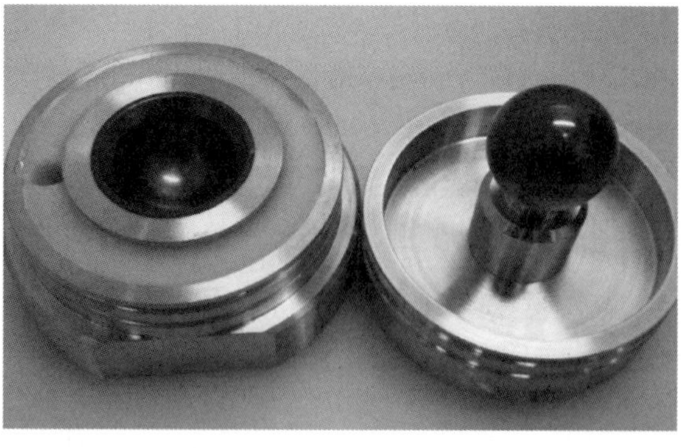

Figure 14-8. Acetabular cup (left) and femoral head (right) components made of NCD coatings on the Si_3N_4 ceramic mounted in their respective holders for wear simulating hip joint testing.

the films was minimal and, when compared with an uncoated condyle/fossa pair, the wear performance was improved. In a more recent study, finite element analysis (FEM) was used to calculate the wear at the bearing surfaces of a diamond-on-diamond hip joint prosthesis (Uddin and Zhang, 2013). Even though the model was applied to bulk PCD (sintered diamond grains with a metallic binder), a material less hard than NCD coatings, lower wear was still predicted in comparison to other hard-on-hard combinations of metals or ceramics. In addition, higher resistance to bacterial colonization of NCD is reported compared to medical steel and titanium, a very important property since infection due to microbial occupation of the implant surface is a significant clinical problem (Jakubowski *et al.*, 2004).

A hip joint wear simulator will be used to test NCD coated acetabular cups and femoral heads. The joint simulator reproduces the three-dimensional loading and motion pattern experienced by hip joints and provides a lubricant environment similar to synovial fluid. The machine for the wear tests is an AMTI-Boston 6 station (at Inmetro, Brazil). The same axial force and motions are applied to all work stations by a unique servo-hydraulic system monitored and controlled by load and position sensors. Experiments will be carried out following ISO 14242-1 standard. The surface morphology will be investigated by a set of methods (optical and SEM microscopy, Raman spectroscopy, surface roughness) to evaluate wear and the wear debris will be characterized with respect to size, number, and biological reactivity. The absence of toxicity and excellent biocompatibility of NCD films has already been proved, but some uncertainty remains about NCD particles. Cell cultures assays will be carried out to assess the biocompatibility and the macrophages behaviour.

Ackowledgements

This work was conducted under the framework of FCT projects MULTIDIACOAT PTDC/EME-TME/100689/2008 and HipCer-Diam PTDC/EME-PME/112910/2009. M. Amaral acknowledges

FCT for the Grant SFRH/BPD/26787/2006. The authors also acknowledge the financing programme PEst-C/CTM/LA0011/2013.

References

Abreu, C.S., Amaral, M., Oliveira, F.J., Gomes, J.R. and Silva, R.F. (2009). HFCVD nanocrystalline diamond coatings for tribo-applications in the presence of water, *Diam Relat Mater*, **18**, 271–275.

Abreu, C.S., Amaral, M., Fernandes, A.J.S., Oliveira, F.J., Silva, R.F. and Gomes, J.R. (2006a). Friction and wear performance of HFCVD nanocrystalline diamond coated silicon nitride ceramics, *Diam Relat Mater*, **15**, 739–744.

Abreu, C.S., Amaral, M., Oliveira, F.J., Fernandes, A.J.S., Gomes, J.R. and Silva, R.F. (2006b). Enhanced performance of HFCVD nanocrystalline diamond self-mated tribosystems by plasma pretreatments on silicon nitride substrates, *Diam Relat Mater*, **15**, 2024–2028.

Almeida, F.A., Amaral, M., Oliveira, F.J., Fernandes, A.J.S. and Silva, R.F. (2007). Nano to micrometric HFCVD diamond — adhesion strength to Si_3N_4, *Vacuum*, **81**, 1443–1447.

Almeida, F.A., Oliveira, F.J., Silva, R.F., Baptista, D.L., Peripolli, S.B. and Achete, C.A. (2011). High resolution study of the strong diamond/silicon nitride interface, *Appl Phys Lett*, **98**, 171913.

Amaral, M., Fernandes, A.J.S., Vila, M., Oliveira, F.J. and Silva, R.F. (2006). Growth rate improvements in the hot-filament CVD deposition of nanocrystalline diamond, *Diam Relat Mater*, **15**, 1822–1827.

Amaral, M., Abreu, C.S., Oliveira, F.J., Gomes, J.R. and Silva, R.F. (2007). Biotribological performance of NCD coated Si_3N_4 — bioglass composites by HFCVD, *Diam Relat Mater*, **16**, 790–795.

Amaral, M., Abreu, C.S., Oliveira, F.J., Gomes, J.R. and Silva, R.F. (2008b). Tribological characterization of NCD in physiological fluids, *Diam Relat Mater*, **17**, 848–852.

Amaral, M., Costa, M.A., Lopes, M.A., Silva, R.F., Santos, J.D. and Fernandes, M.H. (2002). Si_3N_4 — bioglass composites stimulate the proliferation of MG63 osteoblast-like cells and osteogenic differentiation of human bone marrow cells, *Biomaterials*, **23**, 4897–4906.

Amaral, M., Gomes, P.S., Lopes, M.A., Santos, J.D., Silva, R.F. and Fernandes, M.H. (2009). Cytotoxicity evaluation of nanocrystalline diamond (NCD) coatings by fibroblast cell cultures, *Acta Biomater*, **5**, 755–763.

Amaral, M., Almeida, F., Fernandes, A.J.S., Costa, F.M., Oliveira, F.J. and Silva, R.F. (2010). The role of surface activation prior to seeding on CVD diamond adhesion, *Surf Coat Techn*, **204**, 3585–3591.

Amaral, M., Gomes, P.S., Dias, A.G., Lopes, M.A., Silva, R.F., Santos, J.D. *et al.* (2008a). Nanocrystalline diamond: *In vitro* biocompatibility assessment by MG63 and human bone marrow cells cultures, *J Biomed Mater Res*, **87A**, 91–99.

Amedica Corporation. Available at: http://www.amedicacorp.com/ [Accessed 10 July 2013].

Bal, B.S., Khandkar, A., Lakshminarayanan, R., Clarke, I., Hoffman, A.A. and Rahaman, M.N. (2008). Testing of Silicon nitride ceramic bearings for total hip arthroplasty, *J Biomed Mater Res B Appl Biomater*, **87**, 447–454.

Dumbleton, J.H. (1981). *Tribology of natural and artificial joints*, Tribology Series, Elsevier, Amsterdam.

Fernandes, A.J.S., Neto, M.C., Almeida, F.A., Silva, R.F. and Costa, F.M. (2007). Nano- and micro-crystalline diamond growth by MPCVD in extremely poor hydrogen uniform plasmas, *Diam Relat Mater*, **16**, 757–761.

Ferrari, A.C. and Robertson, J. (2001). Origin of the 1150 cm^{-1} Raman mode in nanocrystalline diamond, *Phys Rev B Condens Matter*, **63**, 121405-1–121405-4.

Gispert, M.P., Serro, A.P., Colaço, R., Saramago, B. (2006). Friction and wear mechanisms in hip prosthesis: Comparison of joint materials behaviour in several lubricants, *Wear*, **260**, 149–158.

Guedes e Silva, C.C., Higa, O.Z. and Bressiani, J.C. (2004). Cytotoxic evaluation of silicon nitride-based ceramics, *Mater Sci Eng C*, **24**, 643–646.

Hall, R.M., Bankes, M.J.K. and Blunn, G. (2001). Biotribology for joint replacement, *Curr Orthop*, **15**, 281–290.

Howlett, C.R., McCartney, E. and Ching, W. (1989). The effect of silicon-nitride ceramic on rabbit Skeletal cells and tissue — an *in vitro* and *in vivo* investigation, *Clin Orthop Relat R*, **244**, 293–304.

International Standard ISO 14242-1, *Implants for surgery — Wear of total hip-joint prostheses — Part 1: Loading and displacement parameters for wear-testing machines and corresponding environmental conditions for test.*

Jakubowski, W., Bartosz, G., Niedzielski, P., Szymanski, W. and Walkowiak, B. (2004). Nanocrystalline diamond surface is resistant to bacterial colonization, *Diam Relat Mater*, **13**, 1761–1763.

Jin, Z.M., Stone, M., Ingham, E. and Fisher, J. (2006). Biotribology, *Curr Orthop*, **20**, 32–40.

Kadlečíková, M., Vojs, M., Breza, J., Veselý, M., Frgala, Z., Michalka, M. *et al.* (2007). Microwave and hot filament chemical vapour deposition of diamond multilayers on Si and WC-Co substrates, *Microelectron J*, **38**, 20–23.

Mubarok, F., Almeida, F.A., Fernandes, A.J.S., Carrapichano, J.M and Silva, R.F. (2008). Enhanced sealing performance of CVD nanocrystalline diamond coated mechanical seals, *Diam Relat Mater*, **17**, 1132–1136.

Papo, M.J., Catledge, S.A., Vohra, Y.K. and Machado, C. (2004). Mechanical wear behaviour of nanocrystalline and multilayer diamond coatings on temporomandibular joint implants, *J Mater Sci Mater Med.*, **15**, 773–777.

Petzow, G. and Herrmann, M. (2002). Silicon nitride ceramics, in Jansen, M. (ed), *High Performance Non-Oxide Ceramics II, Structure and Bonding*, Springer, Berlin, 47–167.

Pfeiffer, R., Kuzmany, H., Knoll, P., Bokova, S., Salk, N. and Günther, B. (2003). Evidence for trans-polyacetylene in nano-crystalline diamond films, *Diam Relat Mater*, **12**, 268–271.

Salgueiredo, E., Abreu, C.S., Amaral, M., Oliveira, F.J., Gomes, J.R. and Silva, R.F. (2013). Self-mated tribological systems based on multilayer micro/nanocrystalline CVD diamond coatings, *Wear*, **303**, 225–234.

Schäfer, L., Höfer, M. and Kröger, R. (2006). The versatility of hot-filament activated chemical vapor deposition, *Thin Solid Films*, **515**, 1017–1024.

Scholes, S.C., Unsworth, A., Hall, R.M. and Scott, R. (2000). The effects of material combination and lubricant on the friction of total hip prostheses, *Wear*, **241**, 209–213.

Sun, F., Ma, Y., Shen, B., Zhang, Z. and Chen, M. (2009). Fabrication and application of nano–microcrystalline composite diamond films on the interior hole surfaces of Co cemented tungsten carbide substrates. *Diam Relat Mater*, **18**, 276–282.

Szivek, J.A., Anderson, P.L. and Benjamin, J.B. (1996). Average and peak contact stress distribution evaluation of total knee arthroplasties, *J Arthroplasty*, **11**, 952–963.

Tercic, D and Bozic, B. (2001). The basis of the synovial fluid analysis. *Clin Chem Lab Med*, **39**, 1221–1226.

Uddin, M.S. and Zhang, L.C. (2013). Predicting the wear of hard-on-hard hip joint prostheses, *Wear*, **301**, 192–200.

Vojs, M., Veselý, M., Redhammer, R., Janík, J., Kadlečíková, M., Daniš, T. *et al.* (2005). Double bias HF CVD multilayer diamond films on WC–Co cutting tools. *Diam Relat Mater*, **14**, 613–616.

Chapter 15

Coatings of Transition Metal Nitrides and Carbides

C. Fabry, C. Zietz, R. Dammer and R. Bader

Biomechanics and Implant Technology Research Laboratory, Department of Orthopaedics, University Medical Center Rostock, Rostock, Germany

1. History

The historical origin of thin film technology is in the glass industry. At the beginning of the last century, surfaces were coated primarily for optical purposes. However, in the 1930s thin coatings were also used for the production of carbon resistors in electronics (Bobzin *et al.*, 2008). The main field of application remained optical products until the 1960s when microelectronics became popular. Further developments of coating technology led to the first wear-resistant ceramic coatings on different cutting tools in the early 1980s (Buhl *et al.*, 1981). In particular, drills, milling cutters, and turning tools were refined with different functional coatings (Odrey *et al.*, 1981). The most commonly adopted coating was the gold-coloured titanium nitride coating (TiN). Drills and indexable inserts with thin TiN layers showed an up to ten-fold improvement in durability compared to uncoated ones (Zhang and Zhu, 1993). In addition to the extended durability, coated drills yield holes with a higher surface quality (Thornley and Upton, 1997). The wear resistance of TiN coatings was also used for tailoring the surface of watch cases, trinkets, and tools in the fields of extrusion moulding and deep drawing (Buhl *et al.*, 1981). Due to the excellent biocompatibility and the aesthetic aspect of the golden colour, titanium nitride layers found their way into dentistry in the mid-1980s (Jabbari *et al.*, 2012). Crowns, partially fixed and removable prostheses, as well as dental instruments were coated with TiN (Mezger and Creugers, 1992).

The first carbide coatings were developed in the late 1950s (Kim and Chun, 1985) and found various applications in the tooling industry in subsequent years. The high hardness of the deposits as well as resistance to wear and corrosion at high temperatures improved the performance of different cutting tools and also enhanced the durability of fusion reactors (Benarioua *et al.*, 2006).

The success of ceramic coatings for wear reduction attracted interest in the orthopaedic sector. For many years, metals, as basic materials for endoprosthetic joint replacement, have been applied in combination with polyethylene in both total knee and hip joint replacement. Due to the different structures of the involved materials, wear is dominated by abrasion and adhesion mechanisms of the softer polyethylene component. This effect is significantly enhanced by roughening of the gliding surfaces and insufficient wettability of the tribological pairing (Gispert *et al.*, 2008). The clinical interest of ceramic coatings used for joint replacements is inspired by improved long-term wear resistance and reduced metal ion release. With the help of functional coatings, surface properties can be achieved which are superior compared to the uncoated surface. Thereby, the mechanical and functional properties of the bulk material remain unchanged.

The higher demands of younger and more active patients led to increased polyethylene wear debris and early implant failure due to aseptic loosening (Revell *et al.*, 1978). Therefore, improved surface properties, which lead to lower wear rates are necessary. For total hip replacements, hard-on-hard bearings like ceramic-on-ceramic (CoC) and metal-on-metal (MoM) were developed to further improve the wear resistance. CoC bearings showed excellent wear resistance and biocompatibility (Zywiel *et al.*, 2011); however, ceramics are sensitive to brittle fracture and chipping (Clarke and Willmann, 1994). MoM bearings are resistant to breakage, produce a lower volume of wear debris compared to metal-on-polyethylene (MoP) bearings, and are considered to be cost effective in manufacturing. A cause for concern is the small particle size generated in MoM bearings, which is typically in the range 10–60 nm (Isaac *et al.*, 2006). Thus, the surface area for metal ion release from debris is increased (Fisher *et al.*, 2004). Another drawback is that small particles may enter many different cell types, as well as being phagocytosed by macrophages (Williams *et al.*, 2003).

In order to reduce the total volume of wear debris thin ceramic coatings on the surface of metallic components are applied, which enhance the wear resistance of total joint replacements. Furthermore, the coatings act as a diffusion barrier for potentially allergenic metal ions and also act as protection for fretting-assisted crevice corrosion at the sliding interfaces of various substrates (Hendry and Pilliar, 2001). Different ceramic coatings were used for this purpose. By the end of the 1980s, TiN coatings were already being utilised on titanium femoral knee components and femoral heads (Coll and Jaquot, 1988). At the turn of the millennium, implants were coated with TiNbN (Neumann *et al.*, 1998). CrCN and CrN layers were deposited to total hip implants starting in 2002 and 2004 (Fisher *et al.*, 2002, 2004). TiC and TiCN coatings were tested for biomedical applications a few years later (Gispert *et al.*, 2007).

2. Technical Background

Joint endoprostheses are exposed to load bearing and component articulation. Therefore, the surface coatings of joint endoprostheses have to meet various quality standards. The coating process should not adversely change the mechanical properties and the dimensions of the bulk material. In addition to an excellent adhesive strength, the coating itself has to be homogeneous and free of pores. Popular coating methods available are physical vapour deposition (PVD) and chemical vapour deposition (CVD). Both methods create a coating on the surface of the metallic substrate but differ in the mechanism of layer deposition and in process temperatures. PVD utilises preferred ion-based processes and CVD uses chemical reactions in order to deposit the layer. CVD requires substrate temperatures in the range 800–1100°C (Rieu, 1993) and is therefore restricted to temperature-stable substrates. For instance, the annealing temperature of a common titanium alloy (Ti_6Al_4V) is 700°C (Brunette *et al.*, 2001); any higher temperature will reduce the fatigue strength and must be avoided. As a consequence, titanium alloys cannot be coated by standard CVD. Due to lower process temperatures (typically $<500°C$), PVD is the most common coating process for articulating implant components. The PVD process is quite flexible in terms of layer and substrate materials, whereas conducting materials are preferred in practice. Many different PVD variants exist, but most of them follow a similar working principle. In a vacuum chamber, the coating material (target) is evaporated or sputtered and subsequently partly ionised. The ions are accelerated in an electric field to the substrate surface to be coated. By adding a reactive gas such as nitrogen or a hydrocarbon to the chamber volume at the same time, different surface reactions can be triggered. The ionised metallic vapours can condensate on the substrate surface and react with the gas forming the coating.

Regardless of the type of coating, before starting the coating process, the substrate has to be prepared accordingly. Because PVD coatings are usually thin coatings (layer thickness about $5\,\mu m$) the resultant coating roughness is closely related to substrate roughness. Therefore, the desired surface finish must be achieved mainly prior to the coating process, for example by polishing. Another important preparation step is the pre-cleaning of the substrate in an ultrasonic bath in order to remove contaminations due to lipids or polish residues. Suitable mountings (e.g. rotating spindles) are necessary to provide an effective substrate position relative to the target and to achieve a homogeneous coating on the substrate surface.

2.1. *Pure Vacuum Evaporation*

The main difference between various PVD variants is the way in which the target material is vaporised. In this regard, the three main PVD processes are pure vacuum evaporation, magnetron sputtering,

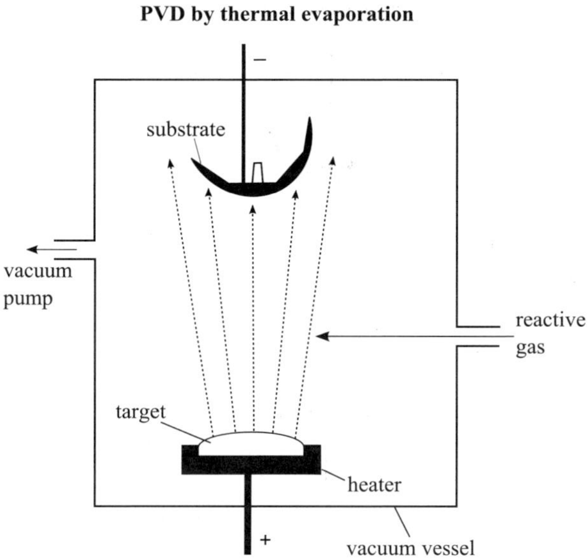

Figure 15-1. Basic principle of thermal evaporation PVD process.

and ion plating with thermal arcs. At pure vacuum evaporation (Figure 15-1), the target material is placed in a crucible and therein heated, melted, and vaporised by a thermal evaporator or any other vacuum compatible energy source (e.g. an electron beam evaporator). The evaporated atoms reach the substrate directly and condensate at the surface of the substrate and partly on the vacuum chamber walls. The benefits of this method are the easy handling and the possible high deposition rates (Kienel and Röll, 1995).

2.2. *Sputtering*

In PVD by magnetron sputtering (Figure 15-2), a glow discharge is created in an argon reactive-gas atmosphere at the negatively charged target and confined by a magnetic field. As a result, the target material is bombarded by high-energy, positively charged gas ions and atoms from the target surface suffer energetic collisions which push them out of the target surface. Emitted electrons are forced by the magnetic field into a helical orbit directly in front of the target. The effect of the electron trapping by the magnetic field is a fairly

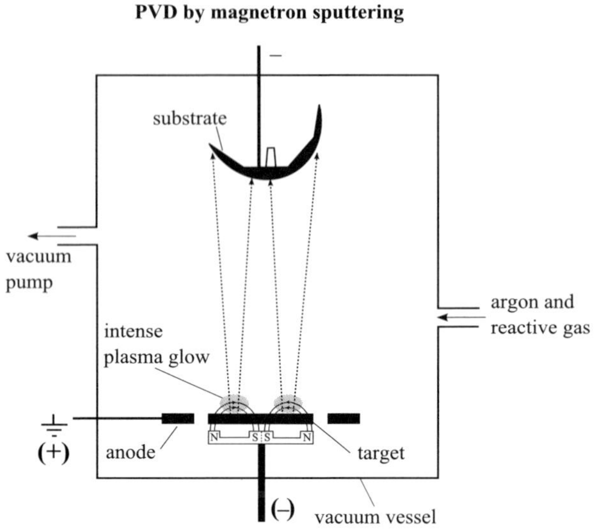

Figure 15-2. Basic principle of magnetron sputtering PVD process.

high electron density and, consequently, an enhanced ion density (Collins and Shaw, 2000). In comparison to thermally evaporated metal atoms, sputtered atoms have a higher kinetic energy. Substrates bombarded with these particles have more areas of increased binding energy because of a disordered crystal structure and thus, a higher nucleation density compared to a non-bombarded surface (Kienel and Röll, 1995). The inert gas argon in the atmosphere not only serves the glow discharge, it also helps by sputtering the target to avoid the premature and unintentional contamination of the target surface with a nitride or carbide coating. Furthermore, argon ions are accelerated to the biased substrate and densified via collisions the substrate coating. Therefore, sputtered films are typically denser and have a better adhesion on the substrate than simply evaporated films (Gotman *et al.*, 2011).

2.3. *Ion Plating*

For the coating of bearing surfaces with ceramics, ion plating with thermal arcs (Figure 15-3) is a widely used PVD process. In this

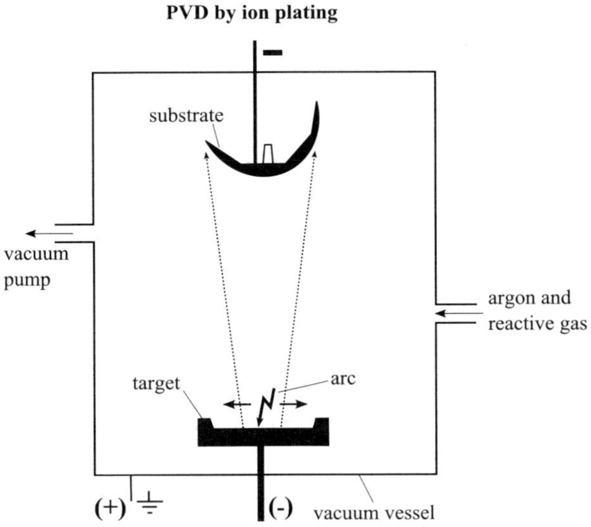

Figure 15-3. Basic principle of the ion plating PVD process with thermal arcs.

procedure, cathodic arcs evaporate and partly ionise the target material. In the first steps of the coating process, the substrate surface is cleaned by ion bombardment (sputtering) in order to remove possible contamination layers; a voltage of several kilovolts between the substrate and the vessel is applied and a glow discharge in argon gas is initiated, which cleans the substrate surface by argon ion bombardment. Subsequent to ion cleaning, the target material is evaporated by confined thermal arcs. The evaporated conducting material becomes partially ionised, crosses the vacuum chamber towards the substrate and will be accelerated before condensation by a bias between the target and the substrate. During the first condensation steps, the sputter cleaning process persists in order to obtain optimal adherence of the atomic layers. Adding the reactive gas into the chamber, the desired chemical compound arises at the surface of the substrate. The main advantages of the arc PVD process are the very high degree of ionisation of the evaporated material, which is close to 100% (Xin *et al.*, 2009), right next to the target surface, and the much higher kinetic energy of the particles (Kienel and

Röll, 1995). Therefore, the coatings gain a high adhesive strength and hardness compared to other deposition methods.

2.4. *Multilayer Coatings*

In recent years, multilayer coatings have become commercially available for femoral knee components (Reich *et al.*, 2010), which have already been used experimentally for some time (Neumann *et al.*, 1998). The idea of multilayer coating is to realise a combination of different single layer properties within one coating stack in order to optimise and adapt the hardness to toughness ratio between the substrate and the coating. The amount of interfaces limits the ion diffusion and grain growth and acts as a number of energy absorbers and crack deflections (Reich *et al.*, 2010). This should lead to an extended lifetime of joint endoprostheses. A load-resistant multilayer is made of several single layers which are deposited successively onto the substrate in a non-stop technological process. One method of creating different coating compositions is to alternate the reactive gas atmosphere without interrupting the process (Knotek *et al.*, 1993). A widely used technology to produce multilayer coatings is to process with different targets. At any given time, only the vaporisation of a selected target is active. Optionally, the reactive gas composition can be varied during deposition. These possibilities enable a wide range of individual and/or alternated layers in the stack.

3. Characterisation of Different Coatings

Different demands require different coatings. The current most important coatings for joint endoprostheses and their specific properties are listed in Table 15-1. The properties of the coatings are influenced by several process parameters such as bias and temperature of the substrate surface, coating time, degree of ionisation as well as the type of the reactive gas (Kienel and Röll, 1995). Due to the variety of process parameters in PVD, every manufacturer has specific process conditions to generate coatings. Therefore, a direct comparison between coatings with the same stoichiometric properties from

Table 15-1. Summary of general properties of different ceramic coatings.

	Hardness (HV)	Elastic modulus (GPa)	Corrosion resistance measured in simulated body fluid (SBF) or Hank's solution (HS)	Biocompatibility	Key features	Colour
TiN	2100 (Wei *et al.*, 2001) 2200 (Nevelos, 2004) 2300 (Gispert *et al.*, 2007) 2382 (Vancoille *et al.*, 1993) 2550 (Fisher *et al.*, 2002)	600 (Gispert *et al.*, 2007) 370 (Vancoille *et al.*, 1993)	SBF (Bolton and Hu, 2002)	Cytotoxicity tests with human fibroblasts (Vanraay *et al.*, 1995) Cytotoxicity according to ISO10993 (Paschoal *et al.*, 2003)	General-purpose coating with good all-round properties	Golden yellow
TiNbN	2818 (Vancoille *et al.*, 1993)	452 (Gispert *et al.*, 2007) 375 (Vancoille *et al.*, 1993)	SBF (Baumann, 2006)	Cytotoxicity according to ISO10993 (Serro *et al.*, 2009)	Improved hardness, denser than TiN, improved ion release behaviour, expensive	Light golden yellow
TiC	2800 (Wei *et al.*, 2001) 3100 (VDI Guideline 3824, 2001) 3456 (Zhang and Zhu, 1993)	420 (Gispert *et al.*, 2007) 234 (Zhang and Zhu, 1993)	HS (Cheng and Zheng, 2007)	Cytotoxicity tests at human fibroblasts (Vanraay *et al.*, 1995) Genotoxicity tests with human osteoblasts (Brama *et al.*, 2007)	Very good resistance to abrasion, harder than TiN	Anthracite to black

(*Continued*)

Table 15-1. (*Continued*)

	Hardness (HV)	Elastic modulus (GPa)	Corrosion resistance measured in simulated body fluid (SBF) or Hank's solution (HS)	Biocompatibility	Key features	Colour
TiCN	3000 (Gispert *et al.*, 2007) 4000 (Nevelos, 2004)	300–356 (Vancoille *et al.*, 1993)	HS (Cheng and Zheng, 2007)	Cytotoxicity according to ISO10993 (Serro *et al.*, 2009) Genotoxicity tests with human osteoblasts (Balazsi *et al.*, 2013) Genotoxicity according to ISO10993 (Antunes *et al.*, 2010)	Harder than TiC, excellent wear resistance and enhanced toughness compared to TiN, strong adhesion	Copper to violet, bluish grey to finally grey (depends on C/N ratio)
CrN	1800 (Warcholinski and Gilewicz, 2003) 1900 (VDI Guideline 3824, 2001) 2500 (Nevelos, 2004)	221–276 (Shah *et al.*, 2011) 201 (Jagielski *et al.*, 2006) 202 (Fuentes *et al.*, 2009)	SBF (Bolton and Hu, 2002)	Cytotoxicity tests with U936 macrophages and L929 fibroblasts (Williams *et al.*, 2004)	Low residual stresses, ductile, improved corrosion and oxidation resistance compared to TiN	Metallic silver

(*Continued*)

Table 15-1. (*Continued*)

	Hardness (HV)	Elastic modulus (GPa)	Corrosion resistance measured in simulated body fluid (SBF) or Hank's solution (HS)	Biocompatibility	Key features	Colour
CrCN	2050 (Fisher *et al.*, 2002)	137.9–185.4 (Tillmann *et al.*, 2012)		Cytotoxicity tests with U936 macrophages and L929 fibroblasts (Williams *et al.*, 2003)	Low residual stresses, good adhesion, high toughness and corrosion resistance	Silver to dark grey
ZrN	2800 (Hendry and Pilliar, 2001) 2300 (Kertzman *et al.*, 2008)	375 (Kertzman *et al.*, 2008)	pH 5.6 acetic acid and sodium acetate buffer solution (Hubler *et al.*, 2001) 0.5 M H_2SO_4 (Chou *et al.*, 2003)	Cytotoxicity tests at HEPAlClC7 cells and CCD cells (Chang *et al.*, 1999)	Excellent abrasion resistance, improved corrosion resistance compared to TiN, less ductile	Pale yellow

different manufacturers can show different layer properties. Coatings for medical purposes are characterised by the following: Adhesion strength, hardness, elastic modulus, corrosion resistance, and biocompatibility. All of these parameters are measured with the help of defined test specimens which are placed side by side with the implants in the vacuum chamber and undergo the same coating process.

The most crucial parameter for the suitability of a coating is its adhesion to the substrate. The precondition for good adhesion is a small atomic mismatch between the layer and the substrate. Therefore, coatings are primarily selected according to the basic elements of the substrate. If a specific coating property is desired regardless of the substrate material and the atomic mismatch, an adapted interface has to be created, which provides a transition between the substrate and the coating properties on an atomic level. This interface can be influenced by the PVD method, the energy input, or the type of layer (monolayer or multilayer). Thus, the adhesion of a specific PVD coating depends mainly on the substrate material and can be improved with different process parameters interface design.

The adhesive strength of coatings used for articulating implant surfaces can be assessed qualitatively by using a Mandrel bending test according to EN ISO 1519 (2003) or a Rockwell C test according to VDI guideline 3198 (1992). The induced layer damage is examined with regard to crack formation and delamination by means of a light microscope or a scanning electron microscope (up to 250-fold magnification (Reich *et al.*, 2010)). Pull-off tests are only meaningful to a limited extent in this area, caused by the low layer thickness (< 2–$10\,\mu$m) and surface roughness ($R_a \leq 0.05\,\mu$m), resulting in glue bonding failures.

Another important coating parameter for tribological applications is hardness. If the substrate hardness is insufficient, the thin coating will fail at low contact stresses even if the coating has very high hardness. Furthermore, increased hardness is associated with reduced ductility of the coating, which is not always desired. The hardness of the layer can be influenced by atomic or process-related modifications. TiC shows a higher hardness in comparison to TiN (Table 15-1). This difference may be caused by the different binding capabilities of the elements used. Carbon has a higher stoichiometric valence in contrast to nitrogen and thereby causes a more branched crystal lattice, which results in a higher hardness. Another way in which to increase the hardness of a coating is based on the distortion of the crystal lattice by substitution. With TiCN, for example, small nitrogen atoms will be replaced by bigger carbon atoms, leading to a more distorted lattice. As a result, the hardness of TiCN increases in contrast to TiC. A further option to achieve high hardness is to introduce compressive stresses into the coating with ion bombardment in order to increase the density of the microstructure and to distract cracks. The power of ion bombardment can be controlled, for example, with the bias between target and substrate. Excessive compression stresses may lead to poor coating adhesion and should be avoided. Therefore, it is essential to find the best compromise between hardness and ductility. Another possibility for increasing the hardness is to decrease the grain size of the crystal structure according to the Hall–Petch relation (Davis, 1995). In multilayer coatings, the large number of layers prevents grain growth and therefore causes an increase in hardness and ductility.

Instrumented indention according to ISO 14577 (2012) is a widely used method for measuring hardness and elastic modulus of PVD coatings. Its attractiveness can be mainly attributed to the fact that mechanical properties can be determined directly from indentation load and displacement measurements without the need to image the hardness impression (Oliver and Pharr, 2004). During the indention process, with a depth of 1/10 of the total layer thickness ($h_{\max}$) in order to determine exclusively the layer hardness, the coating is deformed elastically and plastically. At the same time, the load-displacement data are recorded for both loaded and unloaded cases. Hardness can be calculated using the maximum load $P_{\max}$ and the projected area of the indenter (Jelinek, 1997). Parallel to the determination of hardness, the modulus of elasticity can also be analysed with the help of the load-displacement data, recorded with instrumented indention. The young's modulus is defined as the slope of the upper portion of the unloading curve during the initial stages of unloading (Figure 15-4) (Oliver and Pharr, 2004). Its variation

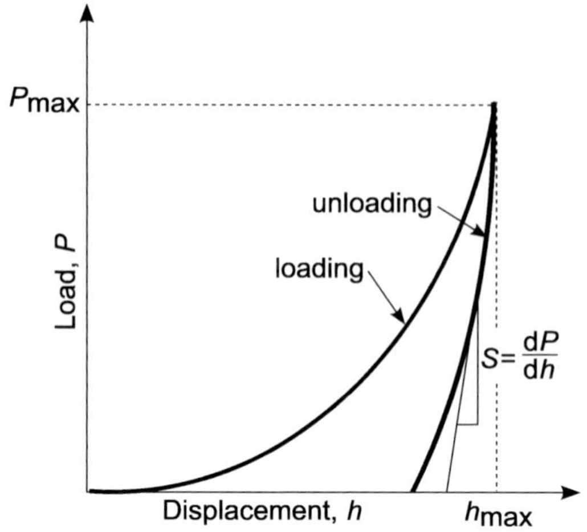

Figure 15-4. Load-displacement curve with important measurement parameters according to Oliver and Pharr (2004).

is similar to the variation of hardness owing to changing process parameters.

In addition to mechanical stresses, coated implants are also subjected to corrosion. Coatings of transition metal nitrides and carbides are mostly more noble than the substrate material, which means that their electrochemical potential is more positive. Therefore, the coating exerts an anodic protection for the substrate (Friedrich *et al.*, 1999). However, coating defects such as included microparticles (droplets from arc PVD), microcracks, or wear-through areas enable the penetration of body fluids like blood or synovial fluid. There is also a risk of ion penetration along the crystal boundaries of the columnar layer structure of selected coatings (Dobrzanski *et al.*, 2009). As a result, an ion exchange starts between the base substrate and the precious coating. A high potential difference causes an increase in the susceptibility to corrosion. Due to their low electrochemical potential, coatings of CrN and CrCN show an improved resistance to corrosion. In multilayer coatings, the ion exchange is more prevented caused by the number of interfaces and different arranged layer defects. The corrosion stability of biomedical coatings is mostly evaluated *in vitro* in simulated body fluid (SBF) or Hank's solution (HS) at 37°C using electrochemical impedance spectroscopy. All of the coatings included in this paper, with the exception of CrCN due to the lack of literature, evidence their character as ion diffusion barriers (Table 15-1).

A basic requirement of the coating for successful application onto the implant is to provide the evidence of biocompatibility. In particular, this property can be proven by two *in vitro* test methods: Cytotoxicity tests according to ISO 10993-5 (2009) and genotoxicity tests according to ISO 10993-3 (2003). In cytotoxicity tests, coated test specimens directly contact definite cultured cells. After a defined incubation time, the test specimens were picked up and inked. Cell cultures were analysed in terms of vitality. In genotoxicity tests, the coated specimens were also colonised with cells, primarily from humans. Subsequently, the cells were examined with regard to genetic alteration. Several publications describe biocompatibility for the coatings TiN, TiNbN, CrN, CrCN, TiC, TiCN, and ZrN in the cytotoxicity test (Table 15-1). However, the genotoxicity test was proven in the literature only for the coatings TiC (Brama *et al.*, 2007) and TiCN (Balazsi *et al.*, 2013) (Table 15-1).

4. Tribology

4.1. *Tribometer Tests*

Coatings of transition metal nitrides and carbides were tested in different *in vitro* studies. Before testing the coatings on implant systems, different tribometers were used to analyse the wear behaviour and other surface characteristics concerning friction properties. In order to simulate (MoP) or MoM bearings, uncoated samples of CoCrMo alloys, stainless steel (SS), and Ti_6Al_4V were used, articulating against UHMWPE and CoCrMo alloys as well as coated components.

TiN-coated Ti_6Al_4V pins and disks were tested without lubricant (Kim *et al.*, 2010). The coated surfaces showed better wear properties with lower wear rates than the uncoated Ti_6Al_4V samples. The initial higher surface roughness of the coated samples did not lead to higher wear rates. Gispert *et al.*, (2007) analysed TiN-, TiCN-, and

TiNbN-coated AISI 316L SS substrates with a ball-on-disk tribometer with balanced salt solution as a lubricant. In general, the surface roughness of the coated samples was increased before testing compared with uncoated reference SS. After completion of the tribometer tests, the resulting lower surface roughness and better material properties of the TiN- and TiCN-coated samples showed a better tribological performance than the TiNbN samples against themselves. A further ball-on-disk test with TiN- and TiCN-coated steel disks against alumina balls from Hsieh *et al.* (2006) showed higher wear rates at the TiN-coated disks. TiN, CrN, and CrCN coatings on CoCr substrates articulating against themselves in a pin-on-plate tribometer were tested by Williams *et al.* (2003). Bovine serum was used as a lubricant. The CrN- and CrCN-coated pins and plates showed lower wear rates than the uncoated CoCr reference. However, the wear of the TiN-coated samples was increased and the coating failed, while other coatings remained undamaged. The TiN-coated samples showed a higher initial surface roughness, which is associated with the above-mentioned results.

Galetz *et al.* (2010) tested TiN-coated CoCr wheels against UHMWPE in a wheel-on-flat tribometer and simulated loads and movements similar to a knee endoprosthesis. The uncoated CoCr samples showed scratches while the TiN-coated surfaces showed no scratches. Wear of UHMWPE was not analysed.

Kamali *et al.* (2005) tested TiN-coated CoCr plates against UHMWPE pins on a pin-on-plate tribometer with bovine serum as a lubricant, as well as the contact angle of the coated plates. Wear of UHMWPE was similar to the uncoated CoCr plates, but significantly lower than intentionally scratched TiN-coated plates. The TiN-coated plates were more hydrophilic than the CoCr control. TiN, TiC, and TiNbN seemed to have the same wear behaviour as UHMWPE tested from Serro *et al.* (2009) in a pin-on-disk tribometer. Onate *et al.* (2001) analysed an increase of wear of UHMWPE in a ball-on-plate tribometer with TiN-coated CoCr samples in distilled water compared to uncoated samples while DLC-coated and alumina balls led to lower wear of UHMWPE. A multilayer coating of Ti-TiN was tested against UHMWPE by Cho *et al.* (2013) in a pin-on-disk tribometer. Test data showed lower wear rates compared to uncoated CoCr samples.

4.2. *Simulator Tests*

As well as the tribometer tests, coatings for orthopaedic bearing surfaces have to be investigated according to their wear resistance under more physiological conditions. For this purpose, wear joint simulators have been used for wear testing. Here, the geometries of the components, loads, movements, and test conditions (lubricant, temperature) were in line with the physiology but differed from those of simple tribometer tests. Unfortunately, the test parameters of the below-mentioned studies were different, for example in terms of head size, lubricant, and type of joint simulator. Therefore, a direct comparison of the amount of wear was not possible. Simulator studies with different coatings of transition metal nitrides and carbides in combination with MoM and MoP bearings are available, whereas hip simulator studies dominate (Table 15-2).

In a hip simulator study by Fisher *et al.* (2004), TiN-, CrN-, and CrCN-coated femoral heads (28 mm) and inserts showed lower wear rates than the uncoated CoCrMo prostheses. After 2 million load cycles, the coated femoral heads and the coated inserts showed 23-fold and 6-fold lower wear than the uncoated CoCrMo components, respectively. The initial surface roughness of the coated components was higher than the uncoated components. During testing the surface roughness of the smooth coated bearing surfaces decreased due to a polishing mechanism. This effect can be confirmed with the authors' own measurements (Figure 15-5).

The decreased wear results for CrN-coated heads against CrN inserts compared to uncoated CoCrMo–CoCrMo were also found by Williams *et al.* (2004) (femoral head size 28 mm) and Leslie *et al.* (2009) (femoral head size 39 mm and 55 mm). Ortega-Saenz *et al.* (2013) tested 31.5 mm CrN- and multi-layered (TiN/CrN)-coated femoral heads against CoCr inserts. Wear of the coated heads was lower than the CoCr heads, but the CoCr inserts showed higher wear when articulating against the coated heads. Surface analyses of the coated heads showed rounded pits and droplets and exhibited a

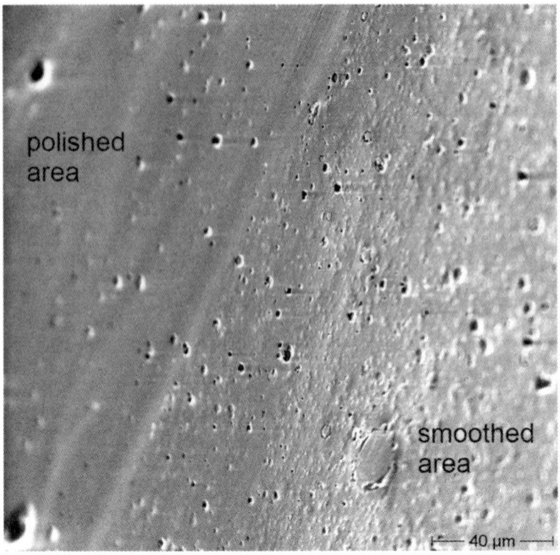

Figure 15-5. SEM image of the border area at a worn TiN-coated acetabular insert. The central bearing area is more polished in contrast to the opening area of the insert.

higher surface roughness. The harder coatings produced higher wear at the smoother CoCrMo inserts. In contrast, Weisenberger *et al.* (2011) have shown increased wear rates for large TiN-coated MoM hip bearings (femoral head size 44 mm) in comparison to the same uncoated specimens. Over 5 million cycles, the uncoated heads displayed a wear rate of 1.84 ± 0.18 mg/Mc while the coated femoral heads wore at 4.37 ± 2.01 mg/Mc. The wear rates were similar for the uncoated and coated metal acetabular liners (1.35 ± 0.11 mg/Mc and 4.16 ± 2.06 mg/Mc, respectively).

Simulator studies with coated heads against UHMWPE are also available. An investigation by Galvin *et al.* (2008) compared alumina ceramic and CoCr heads as well as TiN- and CrN-coated femoral heads against UHMWPE in a hip simulator. The coated heads produced higher wear of the UHMWPE inserts as articulating with alumina as well as CoCr heads and however, these heads showed a higher surface roughness at the beginning of the test. Gutmanas and Gotman (2004) as well as Pappas *et al.* (1990) found a reduction of UHMWPE wear combined with TiN-coated Ti_6Al_4V heads than with 316L SS and CoCr heads. Under tougher test conditions with Ringer's solution and distilled water, the TiN-coated heads remain undamaged; the same was found by Pappas *et al.* (1995). A TiC coating on Ti_6Al_4V heads was investigated in a hip simulator by Luo *et al.* (2009). Thereby, the coated heads led to a reduction of UHMWPE wear.

Peterson *et al.* (1988) found no visible damage of the TiN coating on Ti_6Al_4V femoral components after a knee simulator test with combined level walking and ascending/descending stairs activities. Wear measurement of the used UHMWPE was not possible, but the wear mechanisms on the UHMWPE were not dependent on the used material of the femoral component (CoCrMo, Ti_6Al_4V, Ti_6Al_4V+TiN). In a knee simulator study by Reich *et al.* (2010), a multilayer coating of five alternate CrN and CrCN layers with a cover of a ZrN coating was investigated on a bicondylar knee endoprosthesis system under standard conditions (ISO 14243-1, 2002) and third-body wear conditions. The coated components caused less wear at the UHMWPE tibial insert compared to the uncoated CoCrMo components. Even under third-body wear conditions with bone and bone cement particles, the multilayer coating remained undamaged. Furthermore, the Co, Cr, Mo, and Ni ion concentration in the lubricant was considerably lower than in the uncoated components. Authors' own knee simulator tests according to standard test conditions ISO 142431 (2009) with uncoated CoCrMo and TiN-coated femoral components of a bicondylar knee endoprosthesis system showed a reduction of wear of the UHMWPE inserts combined with the TiN-coated femoral components after 2.5 million load cycles (Figure 15-6). Both tested surfaces showed scratches in flexion direction after the wear test; however, the coated surface was not worn through.

In general, most of the studies showed an increased surface roughness in the beginning of the wear tests compared to the uncoated references (Fisher *et al.*, 2004). Small pits and holes were found on the surface views under a microscope, which resulted from the polishing process after coating, where droplets and spikes left from the coating process were removed. This may lead to a higher initial surface roughness of the coated surfaces. However, a positive effect may

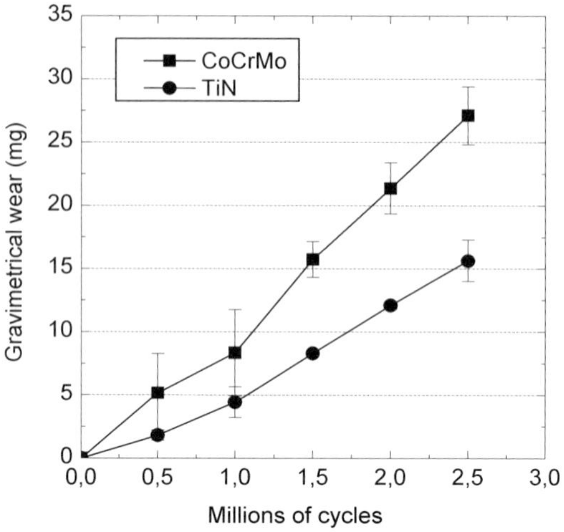

Figure 15-6. Gravimetrical wear of UHMWPE inserts (n = 3) combined with CoCrMo and TiN coated femoral components in a knee simulator test according to ISO 14243-1 conditions.

occur because of a possible increased lubrication due to pits or holes and could optimise the friction properties of such couplings (Falez *et al.*, 2000). Further investigations concerning surface roughness, surface properties and wear have to be performed to explain the partly inconsistent results of the wear tests with coatings of transition metal nitrides and carbides. The partly investigated ion concentration in the wear lubrication showed a reduced ion release for Cr, Co, and Mo by using TiN and CrN coatings (Fisher *et al.*, 2004).

5. Clinical Application

In recent decades, total joint replacements were successfully developed to meet the needs of long-term pain relief and mobility of the patients. The most important factors for satisfactory survival rates of the implants include a permanent implant osseous integration, a high joint stability as well as low amounts of wear debris from the articulating joint components. However, there are a lot of causes of implant failure reported in literature. In total knee and hip arthroplasty aseptic loosening, instability, and also implant-associated infections were

Table 15-2. Literature reports on wear simulation of different coated joint bearings.

Author	Coating	Against	Test conditions	Result (wear, surface analysis)	Further investigations
Fisher *et al.* (2004)	TiN, CrN, CrCN on CoCrMo, (reference CoCrMo)	TiN, CrN, CrCN, (reference CoCrMo)	Hip simulator; head size 28 mm; radial clearance 30 μm; bovine serum; 2×10^6 cycles	Wear of coated heads and inserts lower than CoCrMo, Damage of surface TiN > CrN = CrCN coatings were not worn through	At coated bearings Co, Cr, Mo ion concentration 20-fold lower
Williams *et al.* (2004)	CrN on CoCrMo, (reference CoCrMo)	CrN, (reference CoCrMo)	Hip simulator; head size 28 mm; diametrical clearance 30 μm; bovine serum; low, ISO, and microseparation swing phase load conditions, 5×10^6 cycles	Wear of CrN-CrN bearing lower than CoCrMo bearing wear at all test conditions (low, ISO, microseparation), Wear stripes were observed on the CoCr heads, partial little damage on CrN heads, coating was not worn through	CrN wear particles lower cytotoxic at macrophage and fibroblast cells
Leslie *et al.* (2009)	CrN on CoCrMo, (reference CoCrMo)	CrN, (reference CoCrMo)	Hip simulator; head size 39 mm and 55 mm; clearance 106–126 μm; bovine serum; 10×10^6 cycles	Wear of the CrN bearings was 88% and 71% lower than of the CoCrMo bearings for 39 mm and 55 mm, respectively	At coated bearings (39 mm and 55 mm) Co, Cr, Mo ion concentrations lower

(*Continued*)

Table 15-2. *(Continued)*

Author	Coating	Against	Test conditions	Result (wear, surface analysis)	Further investigations
Ortega-Saenz *et al.* (2013)	CrN, multilayer (TiN/CrN)×3 on CoCrMo, (reference CoCrMo)	CoCrMo (reference CoCrMo)	Hip simulator; head size 31.5 mm; bovine serum; 2×10^6 cycles	Wear of coated heads lower than CoCrMo, CoCrMo inserts against coated heads showed highest wear, Micropittings on CoCrMo bearings, coated heads undamaged	
Weisenberger *et al.* (2011)	TiN-coated femoral heads (reference uncoated heads)	TiN-coated acetabular liners (reference uncoated liners)	Hip simulator; head size 44 mm; bovine serum; ISO input waveforms; 5×10^6 cycles	Increased wear rates for the TiN-coated couples, A loss of coating on both the head and liner in the articulating region, The area where the coating wore away increased in size with test progression	
Galvin *et al.* (2008)	TiN, CrN on CoCr, (reference CoCr, alumina ceramic)	UHMWPE	Hip simulator; head size 28 mm; bovine serum; 5×10^6 cycles	Wear of UHMWPE was higher in combination with coated heads, Coatings undamaged	Highest contact angle at CrN
Gutmanas and Gotman (2004)	TiN on Ti6Al4V, (reference 316L SS)	UHMWPE	Hip simulator; head size 32 mm; Ringer's solution and distilled water; 4×10^6 cycles	Wear of UHMWPE with TiN-coated heads significant lower, No surface damage of TiN-coated heads	

(Continued)

Table 15-2. (*Continued*)

Author	Coating	Against	Test conditions	Result (wear, surface analysis)	Further investigations
Pappas *et al.* (1995)	TiN on Ti_6Al_4V	UHMWPE	Hip simulator; head size 47 mm; distilled water ; 48×10^6 cycles	Lower wear of UHMWPE with TiN-coated heads compared to 32 mm CoCr head (Pappas *et al.* 1990), Mostly no surface damage of TiN-coated heads	
Luo *et al.* (2009)	TiC on Ti_6Al_4V, (reference Ti_6Al_4V)	UHMWPE	Hip simulator; head size 28 mm; bovine serum; 1×10^6 cycles	Lower wear of UHMWPE with TiC-coated heads	
Peterson *et al.* (1988)	TiN on Ti_6Al_4V, (reference Ti_6Al_4V, CoCrMo)	UHMWPE (Poly Two)	Knee simulator; bovine serum; 100,000 steps of combined level walking and ascending/descending stairs activities	TiN-coated components showed no scratches and retained a polished surface, no correlation between wear mechanism and the femoral material, No wear measurement of UHMWPE	
Reich *et al.* (2010)	Multilayer CrN-CrCN+ZrN on CoCrMo, (reference CoCrMo)	UHMWPE	Knee simulator; bovine serum; 5×10^6 cycles; third body-wear	Lower wear of UHMWPE with multilayer coated femoral components, No surface damage of coated components even under third-body wear conditions	At coated bearings Co, Cr, Mo and Ni ion concentration lower

indicated as the main reasons for revision surgery (Suarez *et al.*, 2008). The most frequently used implant materials are SS, CoCr, or titanium and its alloys. Due to their less noble characteristics, the applied metals are prone to corrosion. An allergic reaction to one of the alloying elements of the substrate material (in particular nickel, chromium, and cobalt) may lead to an adverse response of the surrounding tissue, resulting in aseptic loosening (Bader *et al.*, 2008). A recent study of randomly chosen patients, representing the general population, indicated an average sensitivity to nickel of 13.1% (female 20.4%, male 5.8%). The prevalence of sensitivities to cobalt was 3% and to chromium was 1% (Schäfer *et al.*, 2001). Therefore, the sensitization of the patients to contact allergens such as nickel, chromium, or cobalt led to an increasing demand for alternative implant solutions. Coatings of transition nitrides and carbides on implant surfaces should help to reduce the release of metal ions.

Despite the widespread use of coatings on endoprostheses in clinical practice over several years, the number of clinical trails studies is relatively low. According to Gotman *et al.* (2011), this is due to the huge variety of coating compositions, coating processes, component types, techniques, and substrates. The few studies that have been found in the literature will be described more closely in the following section. Bergschmidt *et al.* (2011) compared the clinical outcome of TiNbN-coated CoCr femoral components with uncoated CoCr components. They performed a pre- and post-operative evaluation in two groups of patients. The first group was treated with a coated implant, whereas the second group, as a control group, was treated with uncoated implants with identical geometry. The evaluation was performed using scores such as HSS (Hospital for Special Surgery Score), WOMAC (Western Ontario and McMaster Universities Osteoarthritis Index), and SF-36 scores (SF = Short Form) regarding the clinical outcome and quality of life. Additional radiological evaluations were performed with standard anterior-posterior and lateral X-rays. The WOMAC and SF-36 score showed no significant pre- or post-operative differences between the two groups. HSS score was higher in the coated group (allergy patients) in the preoperative evaluation compared to the uncoated study group. In the post-operative evaluation, the HSS was also lower in the coated group compared to the control group. Müller (2006) investigated the subjective and clinical outcome of patients with hypersensitivity to metal. For this purpose, two patient groups were compared with each other. The first group included 67 patients with a hypersensitivity to metal, consecutively treated with TiN-coated total knee endoprostheses. The second group included 65 patients who had shown no hypersensitivity to metal in the past. These patients received uncoated CoCr femoral knee components. The evaluation was performed using KSS (Knee Society Score) and HSS score. According to the scores, patients with hypersensitivity to metal showed inferior results, despite the usage of a TiN-coated knee component in comparison to the other patient group (Müller, 2006). However, assessment of the results of both studies should be performed with caution as both publications were based on partly subjective scores. The HSS and KSS score gave results of 62% and 75%, respectively (Müller, 2006). Additionally, the authors of both studies mentioned that the scores found are in the range of several publications investigating total knee replacements. Thomsen *et al.* (2011) presented a case report of a patient who underwent a re-revision using a ZrN–(CrN–CrCN)–Cr multilayer coated femoral knee component. The preoperative problems of pain and eczematous reactions vanished after implantation. Additionally, the patient mobility was excellent with the multi-layered knee component. Lutzner *et al.* (2013) also reported good short-term follow-up results for patients who received a multilayer coated femoral component. Plasma metal ion concentrations did not change during the first year after implantation. However, longer-term follow-up results and additional clinical data will be needed.

In total hip arthroplasty, Raimondi and Pietrabissa (2000) as well as Harman *et al.* (1997) reported about delaminations of TiN-coated femoral heads, resulting partially in an increased surface roughness. It should be noted that such concerns were alleviated with coating technology progress in recent years. Buechel *et al.* (2004) showed an excellent clinical outcome after implantation of TiN-coated femoral heads. Patients were followed over a 2- to 12-year interval and demonstrated via Harris Hip Score excellent (82.3%), good (15.4%), fair

(2.3%), and poor (0%) results. In a clinical trail study by Hamelynck *et al.* (2011) 200 TiNbN-coated hip resurfacing prostheses were implanted. At intervals of 3, 6, 12, and 24 months post-operatively, blood samples were analysed according to chromium and cobalt ion concentrations. None of the patients showed a significant increase of chromium and cobalt ion levels in the blood post-operatively or ion levels above those of the normal population. Van Der Straeten *et al.* (2013) analysed the post-operative ion levels of patients with MoM TiN-coated hip resurfacing implants. In contrast, a sharp increase of the ion levels after two years was detected, which could be an indication of worn coatings.

Due to the lack of published clinical studies, it is somewhat difficult to conclusively evaluate the clinical performance of coatings. Therefore, in well-designed comparative clinical trials, the good preclinical results should be confirmed prior to clinical application.

6. Conclusions

Coatings for the articulating surfaces of total joint components have improved in recent years. Relevant delaminations of coatings, as found in the mid-1990s for TiN monolayers, belong to the past thanks to improved coating technologies. Intermediate basis layers provide reliable interfaces between substrates and the coatings. Furthermore, the number of coatings on the market is growing; therefore, the selection of the preferred layer can be made according to specific needs.

Coatings of transition metal nitrides and carbides are used for total joint arthroplasty in order to improve the wear properties of MoP and MoM bearings. Despite a slightly higher surface roughness, the experimental studies mainly showed decreased wear rates and undamaged surfaces for the monolayer-coated samples after tribometer and wear simulator tests imitating MoM or MoP bearings. Direct comparisons of wear results to other materials and coatings (e.g. ceramic, DLC, Oxinium®) are rare or difficult according to the different test conditions required. More attention should be paid to different performance results of the wear tests at different test parameters. Particularly in hip simulator tests, clearance is an important parameter for the wear behaviour but differs or is not specified in the cited studies. Excellent layer properties are useless if the clearance is inadequately dimensioned. Therefore, coated components should be carefully observed to avoid increased wear rates and consecutive clinical failures. A uniform tribometer test parameter set applied to all coatings could lead to the objective assessment of wear and friction properties of the different implant coatings before further experimental testing and clinical application. Subsequently, the coatings should be proven under realistic test conditions in joint simulators to ensure the adhesion of the coatings and to reproduce the *in vivo* situation.

For the new multilayer system of ZrN, a reduced wear rate could be detected (Reich *et al.*, 2010), whereby the decrease of wear debris cannot be clearly attributed to the multilayer structure of the coating. Furthermore, the favoured improved adhesion of multilayers cannot be clearly proven because a suitable standardised measurement method for the quantitative determination of adhesive strength is missing. This gap also affects monolayer coatings and has to be closed in the future.

Coated implant components for total hip and knee endoprostheses are primarily used for patients with a potential risk of metal allergy (Thull *et al.*, 1995). It has been proven by several studies that monolayer as well as multilayer coatings reduce the release of allergenic ions, in particular ions of Co, Cr, and Ni. Progresses in the coating technology can help to minimise process-related coating defects such as arc-related droplets. It should be noted that most of the tests regarding the ion release behaviour do not fully consider the chemical elements of the coating. Therefore, further investigations concerning the corrosion behaviour and the released elements of the coating material should also be performed.

In general, after more than twenty years of implant coating, two fundamental problems remain. First, there is a lack of clinical data regarding the assumed survivorship of coated endoprosthetic implants, as well as regarding the adverse reactions of patients postoperatively. Second, it is still difficult to compare nominally equal coatings of different manufacturers with each other. This is due to different test parameters, such as substrate material or layer thickness.

Furthermore, comprehensive test standards do not exist for the quantitative determination of layer properties such as adhesion or ion-release behaviour. Therefore, relevant procedures for surface testing and characterisation should be further developed, as should the coating technology itself.

References

Antunes, R.A., Rodas, A.C.D., Lima, N.B., Higa, O.Z. and Costa, I. (2010). Study of the corrosion resistance and *in vitro* biocompatibility of PVD TiCN-coated AISI 316 L austenitic stainless steel for orthopedic applications, *Surf Coating Tech*, **205**(7), 2074–2081.

Bader, R., Bergschmidt, P., Fritsche, A., Ansorge, S., Thomas, P. and Mittelmeier, W. (2008). Alternative werkstoffe und lösungen in der knieendoprothetik für patienten mit metallallergie, *Orthopade*, **37**(2), 136–142.

Balazsi, K., Lukacs, I.E., Gurban, S., Menyhard, M., Bacakova, L., Vandrovcova, M. *et al.* (2013). Structural, mechanical and biological comparison of TiC and TiCN nanocomposites films, *J Eur Ceram Soc*, **33**, 2217–2221.

Baumann, A. (2006). *Untersuchung zum Einfluss von PVD-Beschichtungen auf die Ionenabgabe von CoCrMo-Legierungen in SBF Puffer*, Prüfbericht DOT/Projekt Nr. 010-06.

Benarioua, Y., Lesage, J., Bemporad, E. and Chicot, D. (2006). Titanium carbide films obtained by conversion of sputtered titanium on high carbon steel, *Surf Coating Tech*, **200**(18–19), 5447–5454.

Bergschmidt, P., Bader, R., Finze, S., Schulze, C., Kundt, G. and Mittelmeier, W. (2011). Comparative study of clinical and radiological outcomes of unconstrained bicondylar total knee endoprostheses with anti-allergic coating, *Open Orthop*, **5**, 354–360.

Bobzin, K., Bagcivan, N., Immich, P., Pinero, C., Goebbels, N. and Kraemer, A. (2008). PVD–eine erfolgsgeschichte mit Zukunft, *Materialwiss Werkstofftech*, **39**(1), 5–12.

Bolton, J. and Hu, X. (2002). *In vitro* corrosion testing of PVD coatings applied to a surgical grade Co-Cr-Mo alloy, *J Mater Sci Mater Med*, **13**(6), 567–574.

Brama, M., Rhodes, N., Hunt, J., Ricci, A., Teghil, R., Migliaccio, S. *et al.* (2007). Effect of titanium carbide coating on the osseointegration response *in vitro* and *in vivo*, *Biomaterials*, **28**(4), 595–608.

Brunette, D.M., Tengvall, P., Textor, M. and Thomsen, P. (2001). *Titanium in Medicine: Material Science, Surface Science, Engineering, Biological Responses and Medical Applications*, Springer, Berlin.

Buechel, F.F., Helbig, T.E., D'Alessio, J. and Pappas, M.J. (2004). Two- to 12-year evaluation of cementless Buechel–Pappas total hip arthroplasty, *J Arthroplasty*, **19**(8), 1017–1027.

Buhl, R., Pulker, H.K. and Moll, E. (1981). TiN coatings on steel, *Thin Solid Films*, **80**, 265–270.

Chang, K.S., Kim, H.J., Park, J.C., Kim, B.O. and Han, K.Y. (1999). Surface characteristics and biocompatibility of bioinert nitrides ion plated titanium implant, *J Korean Acad Periodontol*, **29**(1), 209–231.

Cheng, Y. and Zheng, Y.F. (2007). Characterization of TiN, TiC and TiCN coatings on Ti-50.6 at.% Ni alloy deposited by PIII and deposition technique, *Surf Coating Tech*, **201**(9–11), 4909–4912.

Cho, S.M., Park, J.W., Han, H.S., Seok, H.K., Moon, M.W. and Kim, Y.C. (2013). Multifunctional composite coating as a wear-resistant layer for the bearing in total hip joint replacement, *ACS Appl Mater Interfaces*, **5**(2), 395–403.

Chou, W.J., Yu, G.P. and Huang, J.H. (2003). Corrosion resistance of ZrN films on AISI 304 stainless steel substrate, *Surf Coating Tech*, **167**(1), 59–67.

Clarke, I.C. and Willmann, G. (1994). Structural ceramics in orthopedics, in Cameron, H.U. (ed.), *Bone Implant Interface*, Mosby, Baltimore, 203–252.

Coll, B.F. and Jaquot, P. (1988). Surface modification of medical implants and surgical devices using TiN layers, *Surf Coating Tech*, **36**, 867–878.

Collins, G.J. and Shaw, D.M. (2000), Physical vapor deposition, in Collins, G.J. and Shaw, D.M. (eds.), *Plasma Processing for IC Manufacture*, Continuing Education Department of CSu, Colorado.

Davis, J.R. (1995). *Tool Materials,* ASM International.

Dobrzanski, L.A., Lukaszkowicz, K. and Labisz, K. (2009). Structure, texture and chemical composition of coatings deposited by PVD techniques, *AMSE*, **37**(1), 45–52.

Falez, F., La Cava, F. and Panegrossi, G. (2000). Femoral prosthetic heads and their significance in polyethylene wear, *Int Orthop*, **24**(3), 126–129.

Fisher, J., Hu, X.Q., Stewart, T.D., Williams, S., Tipper, J.L., Ingham, E. *et al.* (2004). Wear of surface engineered metal-on-metal hip prostheses, *J Mater Sci Mater Med*, **15**(3), 225–235.

Fisher, J., Hu, X.Q., Tipper, J.L., Stewart, T.D., Williams, S., Stone, M.H. *et al.* (2002). An *in vitro* study of the reduction in wear of metal-on-metal hip prostheses using surface-engineered femoral heads, *Proc Inst Mech Eng H*, **216**, 219–230.

Friedrich, S., Spies, H.J. and Ebersbach, U. (1999). Korrosionsverhalten von TiN-Hartstoffschichten auf einem niedriglegierten Stahl, *Materialwiss Werkst.*, **30**, 32–42.

Fuentes, G.G., de Cerio, M.J.D., Garcia, J.A., Martinez, R., Bueno, R., Rodriguez, R.J. *et al.* (2009). Gradient CrCN cathodic arc PVD coatings, *Thin Solid Films*, **517**(20), 5894–5899.

Galetz, M.C., Fleischmann, E.W., Konrad, C.H., Schuetz, A. and Glatzel, U. (2010). Abrasion resistance of oxidized zirconium in comparison with CoCrMo and titanium nitride coatings for artificial knee joints, *J Biomed Mater Res B Appl Biomater*, **93B**(1), 244–251.

Galvin, A., Brockett, C., Williams, S., Hatto, P., Burton, A., Isaac, G. *et al.* (2008). Comparison of wear of ultra-high molecular weight polyethylene acetabular cups against surface-engineered femoral heads, *Proc Inst Mech Eng H*, **222**, 1073–1080.

Gispert, M.P., Serro, A.P., Colaco, R., Pires, E. and Saramago, B. (2007). Wear of ceramic coated metal-on-metal bearings used for hip replacement, *Wear*, **263**, 1060–1065.

Gispert, M.P., Serro, A.P., Colaco, R., Pires, E. and Saramago, B. (2008). The effect of roughness on the tribological behavior of the prosthetic pair UHMWPE/TiN-coated stainless steel, *J Biomed Mater Res B Appl Biomater*, **84**(1), 98–107.

Gotman, I., Gutmanas, E.Y. and Hunter, G. (2011). Wear-resistant ceramic films and coatings, in Ducheyne, P. (ed.), *Comprehensive Biomaterials — Vol. 1 — Metallic, ceramic and polymeric biomaterials*, Elsevier, Amsterdam, 127–155.

Gutmanas, E.Y. and Gotman, I. (2004). PIRAC Ti nitride coated Ti-6AI-4V head against UHMWPE acetabular cup-hip wear simulator study, *J Mater Sci Mater Med*, **15**(4), 327–330.

Hamelynck, K., Woodnutt, D., Rice, R. and Bongaerts, G. (2011). Ceramic surface engineering of the articulating surfaces effectively minimizes wear and corrosion of metal-on-metal hip prostheses, *J Bone Joint Surg Br*, **93**(Suppl II), 222.

Harman, M.K., Banks, S.A. and Hodge, W.A. (1997). Wear analysis of a retrieved hip implant with titanium nitride coating, *J Arthroplasty*, **12**(8), 938–945.

Hendry, J.A. and Pilliar, R.M. (2001). The fretting corrosion resistance of PVD surface-modified orthopedic implant alloys, *J Biomed Mater Res*, **58**(2), 156–166.

Hsieh, J.H., Tan, A.L.K. and Zeng, X.T. (2006). Oxidation and wear behaviors of Ti-based thin films, *Surf Coating Tech*, **201**(7), 4094–4098.

Hubler, R., Cozza, A., Marcondes, T.L., Souza, R.B. and Fiori, F.F. (2001). Wear and corrosion protection of 316-L femoral implants by deposition of thin films, *Surf Coating Tech*, **142**, 1078–1083.

Isaac, G.H., Thompson, J., Williams, S. and Fisher, J. (2006). Metal-on-metal bearings surfaces: Materials, manufacture, design, optimization, and alternatives, *Proc Inst Mech Eng H*, **220**(2), 119–133.

ISO 10993-3. (2003). *Biological evaluation of medical devices — Part 3: Tests for genotoxicity, carcinogenicity and reproductive toxicity*, International Organization for Standardization.

ISO 10993-5. (2009). *Biological evaluation of medical devices — Part 5: Tests for in vitro cytotoxicity*, International Organization for Standardization.

ISO 14243-1. (2009). *Implants for Surgery — Wear of total knee-joint prostheses — Part 1: Loading and displacement parameters for wear-testing machines and corresponding environmental conditions for test*, International Organization for Standardization.

ISO 14577. (2012). *Instrumented indentation test for hardness and materials parameters*, International Organization for Standardization.

ISO 1519. (2003). *Paints and varnishes — Bend test (cylindrical mandrel)*, International Organization for Standardization.

Jabbari, Y., Fehrmann, J., Barnes, A.C., Zapf, A.M., Zinelis, S. and Berzins, D.W. (2012). Titanium nitride and nitrogen ion implanted coated dental materials, *Coatings*, **2**, 160–178.

Jagielski, J., Piatkowska, A., Aubert, P., Thome, L., Turos, A. and Kader, A.A. (2006). Ion implantation for surface modification of biomaterials, *Surf Coating Tech*, **200**(22–23), 6355–6361.

Jelinek, T.W. (1997). *Prüfung von funktionellen Schichten*, Leuze, Saulgau.

Kamali, A., Farrar, R., Hatto, P., Stone, M.H. and Fisher, J. (2005). Wear of ultrahigh-molecular-weight polyethylene against titanium-nitride-coated counterfaces, *Proc Inst Mech Eng H*, **219**, 41–47.

Kertzman, Z., Marchaj, J., Suarez, M., Staia, M.H., Filip, P., Kohli, P. *et al.* (2008). Mechanical, tribological, and biocompatibility properties of ZrN-Ag nanocomposite films, *J Biomed Mater Res A*, **84**(4), 1061–1067.

Kienel, G. and Röll, K. (1995). *Vakuumbeschichtung 2*, VDI, Düsseldorf.

Kim, H., Kim, C.Y., Kim, D.W., Lee, I.S., Lee, G.H., Park, J.C. *et al.* (2010). Wear performance of self-mating contact pairs of TiN and TiAlN coatings on orthopedic grade Ti-6Al-4V, *Biomed Mater*, **5**(4), 1–9.

Kim, N.H. and Chun, J.S. (1985). A study of the tool life of TiC and TiC plus AI203 chemical vapour deposited tungsten carbide tools, *J Mater Sci*, **20**, 1285–1290.

Knotek, O., Loffler, F. and Kramer, G. (1993). Process and advantage of multicomponent and multilayer PVD coatings, *Surf Coating Tech*, **59**(1–3), 14–20.

Leslie, I.J., Williams, S., Brown, C., Anderson, J., Isaac, G., Hatto, P. *et al.* (2009). Surface engineering: A low wearing solution for metal-on-metal hip surface replacements, *J Biomed Mater Res B Appl Biomater*, **90**(2), 558–565.

Luo, Y., Ge, S.R., Liu, H.T. and Jin, Z.M. (2009). Microstructure analysis and wear behavior of titanium cermet femoral head with hard TiC layer, *J Biomech*, **42**(16), 2708–2711.

Lutzner, J., Hartmann, A., Dinnebier, G., Spornraft-Ragaller, P., Hamann, C. and Kirschner, S. (2013). Metal hypersensitivity and metal ion levels in patients with coated or uncoated total knee arthroplasty: A randomised controlled study, *Int Orthop*, **37**(10), 1925–1931.

Mezger, P.R. and Creugers, N.H.J. (1992). Titanium nitride coatings in clinical dentistry, *J Dent*, **20**, 342–344.

Müller, G. (2006). *Titanium coated total knee prosthesis compared with Chrom-Cobalt-Molybdän prosthesis: Assessment of quality of life after total knee arthroplasty*, Doctoral Thesis, University of Giessen.

Neumann, H.G., Beck, U., Drawe, M. and Steinbach, J. (1998). Multilayer systems for corrosion protection of stainless steel implants, *Surf Coating Tech*, **98**(1–3), 1157–1161.

Nevelos, J. (2004). Surface engineering of prosthetic knee components, *Knee*, **11**(3), 163–167.

Odrey, N.G., Tongson, L., Biggers, J.V., Knox, B.E. and Ham, I. (1981). Cutting performance and chemical characterization of TiC-coated carbide cutting tools, *Thin Solid Films*, **79**, 83–89.

Oliver, W.C. and Pharr, G.M. (2004). Measurement of hardness and elastic modulus by instrumented indentation: Advances in understanding and refinements to methodology, *J Mater Res*, **19**(1), 3–20.

Onate, J.I., Comin, M., Braceras, I., Garcia, A., Viviente, J.L., Brizuela, M. *et al.* (2001). Wear reduction effect on ultra-high-molecular-weight polyethylene by application of hard coatings and ion implantation on cobalt chromium alloy, as measured in a knee wear simulation machine, *Surf Coating Tech*, **142**, 1056–1062.

Ortega-Saenz, J.A., Alvarez-Vera, M. and Hernandez-Rodriguez, M.A.L. (2013). Biotribological study of multilayer coated metal-on-metal hip prostheses in a hip joint simulator, *Wear*, **301**(1–2), 234–242.

Pappas, M.J., Makris, G. and Buechel, F.F. (1990). Comparison of wear of UHMWPE cups articulating with Co–Cr and Ti–N coated titanium femoral heads, *Trans Soc Biomater*, **13**, 36.

Pappas, M.J., Makris, G. and Buechel, F.F. (1995). titanium nitride ceramic film against polyethylene — A 48-million cycle wear test, *Clin Orthop Relat R*, **317**, 64–70.

Paschoal, A.L., Vanancio, E.C., Canale, L.D.F., da Silva, O.L., Huerta-Vilca, D. and Motheo, A.D. (2003). Metallic biomaterials TiN-coated: Corrosion analysis and biocompatibility, *Artif Organs*, **27**(5), 461–464.

Peterson, C.D., Hillberry, B.M. and Heck, D.A. (1988). Component wear of total knee prostheses using Ti-6A1-4V, titanium nitride coated Ti-6Al-4V, and cobalt-chromium-molybdenum femoral components, *J Biomed Mater Res*, **22**, 887–903.

Raimondi, M.T. and Pietrabissa, R. (2000). The *in vivo* wear performance of prosthetic femoral heads with titanium nitride coating, *Biomaterials*, **21**(9), 907–913.

Reich, J., Hovy, L., Lindenmaier, H.L., Zeller, R., Schwiesau, J., Thomas, P. *et al.* (2010). Präklinische Ergebnisse beschichteter Knieimplantate für Allergiker, *Orthopade*, **39**, 495–502.

Revell, P.A., Weightman, B., Freeman, M.A.R. and Vernon Roberts, B. (1978). The production and biology of polyethylene wear debris, *Arch Orthop Traum Surg*, **91**, 167–181.

Rieu, J. (1993). Ceramic formation on metallic surfaces (ceramization) for medical applications, *Clin Mater*, **12**, 227–235.

Schäfer, T., Böhler, E., Ruhdorfer, S., Weigl, L., Wessner, D., Filipiak, B. *et al.* (2001). Epidemiology of contact allergy in adults, *Allergy*, **56**(12), 1192–1196.

Serro, A.P., Completo, C., Colaco, R., dos Santos, F., da Silva, C.L., Cabral, J.M.S. *et al.* (2009). A comparative study of titanium nitrides, TiN, TiNbN and TiCN, as coatings for biomedical applications, *Surf Coating Tech*, **203**(24), 3701–3707.

Shah, H.N., Jayaganthan, R. and Pandey, A.C. (2011). Nanoindentation study of magnetron-sputtered CrN and CrSiN coatings, *Mater Des*, **32**(5), 2628–2634.

Suarez, J., Griffin, W., Springer, B., Fehring, T., Mason, J.B. and Odum, S. (2008). Why do revision knee arthroplasties fail?, *J Arthroplasty*, **23**(6), 99–103.

Thomsen, M., Rozak, M. and Thomas, P. (2011). Pain in a chromium-allergic patient with total knee replacement: Disappearance of symptoms after revision with a special surface-coated TKA — a case report, *Acta Orthop*, **82**(3), 386–388.

Thornley, R.H. and Upton, D.P. (1997). Effects of TiN coatings on tools, *Prod Eng*, **66**(5), 21–24.

Thull, R., Handke, K.D. and Karle, E.J. (1995). Examination of titanium coated with (Ti,Nb)ON and (Ti,Zr)O in an animal experiment, *Biomed Eng*, **40**, 289–295.

Tillmann, W., Herper, J. and Laemmerhirt, I.A. (2012). Development and tribological investigation of the coating system chromium carbonitride (CrCN) to different surface designs, *J Mater Sci Eng*, **2**(4), 223–229.

Van Der Straeten, C., De Roest, B. and De Smet, K. (2013). Randomized Controlled Trial comparing Nine Different Hip Resurfacing Designs, *Proc 59th Ann Meet Orthop Res Soc 2013*, San Antonio.

Vancoille, E., Celis, J.P. and Roos, J.R. (1993). Mechanical-properties of heat-treated and worn PVD Tin, (Ti, Al)N, (Ti, Nb)N and Ti(C, N) coatings as measured by nanoindentation, *Thin Solid Films*, **224**(2), 168–176.

Vanraay, J.J.A.M., Rozing, P.M., Vanblitterswijk, C.A., Vanhaastert, R.M. and Koerten, H.K. (1995). Biocompatibility of Wear-Resistant Coatings in Orthopedic-Surgery In-Vitro Testing with Human Fibroblast Cell-Cultures, *J Mater Sci Mater Med*, **6**(2), 80–84.

VDI Guideline 3198. (1992). Beschichten von Werkzeugen der Kaltmassivumformung, VDI.

VDI Guideline 3824. (2001). Quality assurance of PVD and CVD hard coating, VDI.

Warcholinski, B. and Gilewicz, A. (2003). Tribological properties of CrNx coatings, *JAMME*, **37**(2), 498–504.

Wei, C.H., Lin, J.F., Jiang, T.G. and Ai, C.F. (2001). Tribological characteristics of titanium nitride and titanium carbonitride multilayer films Part II. The effect of coating sequence on tribological properties, *Thin Solid Films*, **381**(1), 104–118.

Weisenberger, J.N., Hovendick, S.M., Garvin, K.L., and Haider, H. (2011). How durable are titanium nitride coatings on total hip replacements?, *J Bone Joint Surg Br*, **93**(4), 474.

Williams, S., Tipper, J.L., Ingham, E., Stone, M.H. and Fisher, J. (2003). In vitro analysis of the wear, wear debris and biological activity of surface-engineered coatings for use in metal-on-metal total hip replacements, *Proc Inst Mech Eng H*, **217**(3), 155–163.

Williams, S., Isaac, G., Hatto, P., Stone, M.H., Ingham, E. and Fisher, J. (2004). Comparative wear under different conditions of surface-engineered metal-on-metal bearings for total hip arthroplasty, *J Arthroplasty*, **19**(8), 112–117.

Xin, Y.C., Liu, C.L., Huo, K.F., Tang, G.Y., Tian, X.B. and Chu, P.K. (2009). Corrosion behavior of ZrN/Zr coated biomedical AZ91 magnesium alloy. *Surf Coating Tech*, **203**(17–18), 2554–2557.

Zhang, S. and Zhu, W. (1993). TiN coating of tool steels: A review. *J Mater Process Tech*, **39**, 165–177.

Zywiel, M.G., Sayeed, S.A., Johnson, A.J., Schmalzried, T.P. and Mont, M.A. (2011). State of the art in hard-on-hard bearings: How did we get here and what have we achieved?, *Expet Rev Med Dev*, **8**(2), 187–207.

Index